Table of Contents

Part 1: The Context Surrounding Pharmaceutical Care

Part 2: Implementation of Pharmaceutical Care

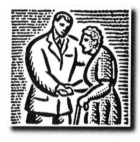

Foreword

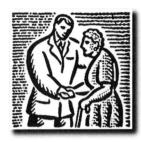

Foreword

David A. Knapp, Ph.D.

Now that the profession of pharmacy has successfully made it through the birth of a new century, it faces one of those pesky crossroads again. The difference today is that the pace has picked up. Those crossroads look more like interchanges on an Interstate than intersections on a main street. The traffic is thicker, speeds are higher, and the lanes are better marked because of information technology. But on this superhighway, slight changes of direction can quickly bring us either to our destination faster or to some place that we definitely did *not* wish to visit.

The most dominant feature of the health care landscape with which we must negotiate for the next quarter of a century will be the aging of the population. As the Rockies rise up on the horizon when we hurtle westward across the plains, so does the profile of the "baby boom" generation as it ages. We spot the Rockies from many miles away as we approach, but they lack reality until we get closer and then, all of a sudden, they are upon us, rising almost two miles straight up! We had better have the right vehicle and the right equipment to go forward. If we are driving, we can pull off the highway somewhere in the foothills and check our vehicle. We can put on the snow tires, tune up the engine, and top off the gas tank before we begin.

But pharmacists and other health professionals will not have the luxury to pull off and prepare as we approach the aging of the baby boomers. We will inexorably reach the foothills of the aging population by mid-decade, and the mountains will quickly follow. When people reach 60, their use of medications accelerates rapidly, reaching a rate that is three times or more that of younger adults. Aging patients also use more medications concurrently, increasing the risks of drug therapy. Since Medicare does not cover pharmaceutical care or prescription drugs, our Interstate to the future lacks the wide shoulders and guardrails it needs as we climb into the mountains.

Do we have the right mix of health professionals to take care of a patient population soon to be dominated by the elderly? Right now we do not. The number of geriatricians and other geriatric specialists is dismally low. The number of patients with cancer is expected to double within the next decade. Are we equipped to provide not only the diagnostic and therapeutic services needed but also the palliative and end-of-life care they will need?

What of the roles of pharmacists? At the individual patient care level, most pharmacists have the preparation, experience, and ability to provide pharmaceutical care as described in this book. But the system for facilitating the provision of this care is in disarray. We have not yet aligned marketplace incentives with professional abilities and desires. Our major delivery mechanism to patients in the community is entangled in the retail marketplace. The values of retailing and the values of health care are sometimes aligned but often not, creating for both patients and practitioners an often confusing, inefficient, and muddled setting for pharmaceutical care.

Even health care institutions, such as hospitals and nursing homes, have difficulty integrating pharmaceutical care and medication use across a system dominated by medical specialties. Drugs are ubiquitous, but most other medical care services are not. Organizing pharmaceutical care in health care systems requires a broad prospective that has often not been well communicated by pharmacists to health care administrators and management.

Do we have enough of the right kind of pharmacists to do the job in the twenty-first century? The last decade saw demand for pharmacists far outstrip supply (and that's before the aging of the baby boomers). But the demand for pharmacists is an overt phenomenon. It measures the jobs that society is now willing to pay pharmacists to do. Projecting workforce requirements for the future requires an additional element—the tasks that will need to be done to keep tomorrow's population healthy and to treat its ills. The shortage of pharmacists to meet potential patient care needs is even larger than that necessary to meet today's marketplace demands.

The profession has engaged some of the issues of workforce expansion head on. The supply of pharmacists is being augmented by the creation of a significant number of new schools and colleges of pharmacy. Most existing educational programs are expanding their enrollment. The paradigm of education changed dramatically in the 1990's and pharmacists are graduating from programs culminating in the doctor of pharmacy degree.

The concepts and philosophy of pharmaceutical care are being adopted across the health care system through professional associations and employers, albeit at a pace that is almost paralyzingly slow. Information systems are helping pharmacists to integrate data from the fragmented sources of care used by patients. The power of the computer can organize such data and display it in ways that make the pharmacist's job of managing medication easier. Other computerized information systems can organize and present data on the thousands of drugs now available, along with clinical information on their use and potential problems. Automated order fulfillment equipment is increasing the efficiency of the proper provision of drug products. Well over 100,000 certified pharmacy technicians are already at work within the profession.

The challenges that lie ahead are great. The workload to be borne will be enormous. Society has not yet learned from experience the impact of the baby boom generation as it proceeds through the life cycle. We are still unprepared for the surge in elderly patients that is coming. But the tools are there; the talented practitioners are there. What remains to be seen is whether or not individual pharmacists will perform not only what is demanded of them but what is needed from them by tomorrow's patients.

Pharmaceutical Care provides an outstanding travel guide to the superhighway of the future. It scans the countryside, reviewing where we've come from, where we are now, and where we're going.

The philosophy of practice and the nature of the problems we face are discussed in detail along with a framework for providing solutions.

An almost entirely new treatment of the implementation of pharmaceutical care provides the kind of information and analysis necessary for not only those who would study the road ahead but also those who must do the driving.

Calvin Knowlton and Richard Penna bring synergy to this project. Cal Knowlton is the driver. He has been a pioneer in providing pharmaceutical care services successfully in the marketplace. His firm, ExcelleRx, stands out as a superb example of harnessing information technology and modern communication to provide patient-centered pharmaceutical care services to hospice patients throughout the United States. He has also gained a national perspective on the delivery of pharmacy services through his leadership in the American Pharmaceutical Association. Along the way he has developed the skills of a scientist and has evaluated systematically the contributions of pharmacy.

Richard Penna is the navigator. He is intimately aware of the major highways and back roads of pharmacy and health care from a career as an association executive, first at the American Pharmaceutical Association and then at the American Association of Colleges of Pharmacy. He has long used his unique skills to steer the leaders of both organizations toward the coherent development of their ideas into practical plans. Adept at working both behind the scenes and in public forums, Dr. Penna's contributions were recognized by his recent selection to receive the Remington Honor Medal, pharmacy's highest award.

Knowlton and Penna have selected a terrific complement of authors to help untangle the complexities of pharmaceutical care and the search for better medication use in the coming years. The resulting book should find a place not only in the library of students, but also in the glove compartments of practitioners and leaders.

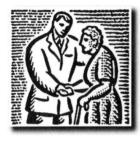 **Preface**

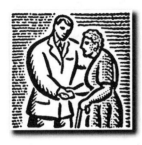

Preface

Calvin H. Knowlton, Ph.D.
Richard P. Penna, Pharm.D.

Why Was This Book Written?

Mrs. Smith: A Case Study

Mrs. Barbara Smith is a healthy 75-year-old woman who lives independently and maintains an active schedule, which includes volunteer work, reading, walking, and playing with her two young grandchildren. She drives her own car and depends very little on others for her day-to-day needs. The only medication she takes is digoxin, prescribed by her physician a number of years previously for a "heart irregularity." Constantly vigilant about her health, she visits her physician regularly and takes her digoxin religiously according to directions. Because of her extremely good health, she, her physician, and her family were astounded and surprised when Mrs. Smith developed a chest cold that rapidly progressed to pneumonia. Mrs. Smith required a week in the intensive care unit of her local hospital and two more weeks of hospitalization before she could return home. Even then, it was several months before she could return to her normal, vigorous schedule.

At first glance, one would attribute this episode to an unfortunate confluence of an unusually virulent bacteria and an elderly patient. But there's more to the story. Subsequent investigations determined that Mrs. Smith contracted pneumonia because she was malnourished. She became malnourished because she stopped eating. She stopped eating because she lost her appetite, and she lost her appetite because of a well-known side effect of digoxin. The dose of her digoxin was such that over time (perhaps years) small amounts began to accumulate in her blood until the drug began to exert one of its toxic effects (loss of appetite).

The point to this story is that no one—not Mrs. Smith's physician, not her nurse, not her pharmacist—thought to ask Mrs. Smith about her appetite even though the effect of digoxin on appetite is well known. These health professionals simply forgot! Routine greetings by physician, nurse, and pharmacist of "How are you?" were offered—and meant—strictly in their social contexts, not as health care questions.

This true story had a happy ending. Mrs. Smith recovered, and she is back to her

XIII

usual, active life style, but now her physician and pharmacist closely monitor her medication. Of course, there was a cost. Medicare paid a handsome sum of money to the hospital and physicians who cared for her during her stay. Her family (not to mention Mrs. Smith herself) paid a substantial emotional toll as a result of her battle with a life-threatening illness.

All this financial and emotional cost and suffering could have been avoided (1) if someone, some health professional, had looked upon Mrs. Smith as a person who was taking a needed, but very potent, drug and (2) if that someone had been concerned enough to worry about Mrs. Smith's therapeutic outcomes and ask a few simple questions periodically and especially whenever she renewed her prescription for digoxin.

The Response of One Profession

Pharmacy, like all health professions, is undergoing an enormous transformation as the changing nature of the U.S. health care system makes its influence felt. As the profession most concerned with drugs (raw drugs, purified drug entities, formulated drug products), pharmacy began examining its societal role as the profession that must be responsible for ensuring safe, effective, and (now) appropriate drug use. For the past thirty years, pharmacy has explored the drug-use process and has made some startling observations and conclusions, which this book will discuss. This book is about pharmaceutical care—a revolutionary philosophy of health care practice, a new way of dealing with the most popular therapeutic interventions used in health care. It is about the underlying trends in health care that make pharmaceutical care so critical to the successful treatment or diagnosis of illness. It is about what pharmaceutical care is and how it may be provided.

Our Health Care System Has a Drug Problem

The Extent of Drug-Related Illness

Several chapters in this book discuss in clear detail the disquieting statistics that demonstrate that drugs, for all their benefits, are associated with a major public health problem costing tens of billions of dollars annually. It's not the drugs themselves that are responsible for the morbidity and mortality associated with their use, it is how they are used—the drug-use process (or lack of a process)—that is at the root of the problem. The evidence is very clear that, when used within a systematic process focusing on the patient and the outcomes of therapy in the patient, the drug-use process becomes one of the most cost-effective health care interventions available. On the other hand, when used in the fragmented fashion so typical of today's drug-use process, the results are a costly array of therapeutic failures, drug interactions with diet and other drugs, and adverse reactions to the drugs themselves.

Who's at Fault?

No one person or group of persons (professions) can be blamed as causing our health care drug problem. Indeed, the evidence is quite clear that there is enough blame to go around for everyone: prescriber, nurse, pharmacist, patient, and system. Drug therapy goes wrong when

1. The prescriber (physician, dentist, podiatrist, optometrist, physician assistant, nurse practitioner, or patient) decides not to use a drug when one is indicated, prescribes the wrong drug or dose, or prescribes a drug when no drug is indicated.

2. The pharmacist does not get the drug to the patient when needed; the drug does not get to the patient's bedside in the hospital or nursing home; the pharmacist dispenses the wrong drug or the correct drug with wrong instructions; or the caregiver administers the wrong drug or dose to a patient.

3. The patient refuses to obtain the medication or fails to follow prescribed instructions.

4. No one monitors patients on medication for desired therapeutic endpoints or adverse reactions or to determine whether the patient is taking the medication as instructed.

What our health care system needs, therefore, is for someone—some group of health professionals—to step forward to take responsibility for ensuring that these causes of drug-related illnesses are substantially eliminated and controlled. The best way to ensure this result is for individual practitioners to assume responsibility for the outcomes of drug therapy in patients whom they serve—to care for the patients they serve.

Pharmaceutical Care, a New Health Care Discipline

Researchers and theorists within pharmacy have examined the nature and scope of the nation's health care drug problem along with its root causes. As a result of their findings, they propose that the public and the health care professions change their attitudes about the drug-use process. They suggest that the same degree of attention be given to the drug-use process as is given to the diagnostic process, rehabilitative process, and the nurturing process. They suggest that the best way that this can be achieved is for a profession to step forward and assume responsibility for the results (outcomes) of drug therapy in patients. This is the only way all the functions that comprise the drug-use process can be integrated into a safe, effective, and efficient systematic process that ensures that the outcomes of therapy are the ones desired and expected by the patient and those caring for the patient.

Researchers also propose that a new philosophy of practice be adopted to ensure that patients receive full benefit from pharmacotherapy. This philosophy of practice is called pharmaceutical care. It's a concept that in one sense is quite simple—a health professional must assume the responsibility of worrying about the therapeutic outcomes in patients under his or her care. At the same time pharmaceutical care is quite complex. It involves issues related to interprofessional collaboration, quality of life, identifying and quantifying outcomes, performing various functions and tasks, ethics, competence, and the concepts of responsibility and accountability.

For Whom Was This Book Written?

Is Pharmaceutical Care Just for Pharmacists?

The adjective *pharmaceutical* when used to describe *care*, indicates that the care is associated with pharmaceutical agents, not the individual who provides it. Consequently, this new philosophy is not reserved for any one profession or group of professionals. Although it is true that most of the underlying research and theory behind the concept were performed within the profession of pharmacy, it does not necessarily follow that pharmacists will step forward to provide pharmaceutical care. And "step forward" a profession must, if it is to be granted the right to be held accountable by society for the outcomes of drug therapy in patients.

This book is written with the expectation that the pharmacy profession will accept the challenge and step forward to accept the public's mandate to provide pharmaceutical care. However, because pharmaceutical care is, by definition, collaborative, and because other professionals are involved in the drug-use process, this book is intended for other health professionals and caregivers as well. Moreover, it is entirely possible (and probable) that pharmaceutical care will be provided by a variety of health professionals.

Pharmaceutical care is intended to provide information to practitioners (pharmacists, physicians, nurses) who are interested to learn more about improving the drug-use process and how they can assume greater responsibilities in caring for patients with pharmacotherapy.

Potential Audiences

This book is intended to be a resource for all who have an interest in the use of drugs as diagnostic or therapeutic interventions in health care. Although one would expect that a primary audience will be practitioners (pharmacists, physicians, and nurses), students are another major intended audience, especially pharmacy students. The editors recognize that, although pharmaceutical care is a part of every pharmacy school curriculum, there exists no organized resource on pharmaceutical care for students. Because the topic is alluded to in a typical pharmacy curriculum, the editors intend that this book will be used at several places in the curriculum.

Contributors

Daniel Albrant, Pharm.D.
President, Pharmacy Dynamics
1902 N. Nottingham Street
Arlington, VA 22205

Robert A. Buerki, Ph.D.
Professor
Ohio State University, College of Pharmacy
500 West 12th Street
Columbus, OH 43210-1291

Donna E. Dolinsky, Ph.D.
Professor and Director, Social & Administrative Sciences
Arnold & Marie Schwartz College of Pharmacy & Health Sciences,
Long Island University
75 DeKalb
Brooklyn, NY 11201

Bill G. Felkey, M.S.
Associate Professor
Pharmacy Care Systems-Auburn University
128 Miller Hall
Auburn, AL 36849

Brent I. Fox, Pharm.D.
Informatics Research Associate
Pharmacy Care Systems-Auburn University
128 Miller Hall
Auburn, AL 36849

Diane Giaquinta, Pharm.D.
Vice President
Worldwide Health Systems Management
Bristol-Myers Squibb
Princeton, NJ 08540

Charles D. Hepler, Ph.D.
Professor and Director, DuBow Family Center for Research in Pharmaceutical Care
University of Florida, College of Pharmacy
4140 NW 35th Street
Gainesville, FL 32605

Gregory J. Higby, Ph.D.
Director, American Institute of the History of Pharmacy
University of Wisconsin, School of Pharmacy
777 Highland Avenue
Madison, WI 53705-2222

Brian J. Isetts, Ph.D.
Associate Professor, Department of Pharmaceutical Care & Health Systems
University of Minnesota, College of Pharmacy
3510 Wild Turkey Lane
Red Wing, MN 55066

Calvin H. Knowlton, Ph.D.
Chief Executive Officer and Chairman
ExcelleRx, Inc.
530 Walnut Street, Suite 550
Philadelphia, PA 19106

Earle W. Lingle, Ph.D.
Associate Professor
University of South Carolina, College of Pharmacy
3735 Northshore Road
Columbia, SC 29206

John M. Lonie, M.A.
Instructor, Social & Administrative Sciences
Arnold & Marie Schwartz College of Pharmacy & Health Sciences,
Long Island University
75 DeKalb
Brooklyn, NY 11201

Lucinda L. Maine, Ph.D.
Executive Vice President
American Association of Colleges of Pharmacy
1426 Prince Street
Alexandria, VA 22314

Henri R. Manasse, Jr., Ph.D., Sc.D.
Executive Vice President and Chief Executive Officer
American Society of Health-System Pharmacists
7272 Wisconsin Avenue
Bethesda, MD 20814

Bernard J McKone, Dip Pharm, MPharm, FNZCP, FPS
President
Pharmaceutical Society of New Zealand
Owner of Quins Gore Pharmacy Ltd.
104 Main Street
Gore, New Zealand

Susan M. Meyer, Ph.D.
Senior Vice President
American Association of Colleges of Pharmacy
1426 Prince Street
Alexandria, VA 22314

Kavita V. Nair, Ph.D.
Assistant Professor
University of Colorado, School of Pharmacy
4200 East Ninth Avenue, Box C-238
Denver, CO 80262-0238

Peter M. Penna, Pharm.D.
Consultant
8912 52nd Street Court West
University Place
Tacoma, WA 98467

Richard P. Penna, Pharm.D.
Executive Vice President, Emeritus
American Association of Colleges of Pharmacy
1426 Prince Street
Alexandria, VA 22314

Michael T. Rupp, Ph.D.
Professor and Executive Director,
Center for the Advancement of Pharmacy Practice
Midwestern University¾College of Pharmacy, Glendale Campus
19555 North 59th Avenue
Glendale, AZ 85308

Marion Schaefer, Ph.D.
Professor
Institut fuer Pharmazie
Goethestrasse 54
D-13086 Berlin

Orsula Voltis Thomas, Pharm.D., M.B.A.
Vice President and Chief Marketing Officer
ExcelleRx, Inc.
530 Walnut Street, Suite 550
Philadelphia, PA 19106

Kasey K. Thompson, Pharm.D.
Director, Center on Patient Safety
American Society of Health-System Pharmacists
7272 Wisconsin Avenue
Bethesda, MD 20814

Robert J. Valuck, Ph.D.
Associate Professor, Department of Pharmacy Practice
University of Colorado, School of Pharmacy
4200 East Ninth Avenue, Box C-238
Denver, CO 80262-0238

Frank Verheyen, Ph.D.
Personal Counsellor of the Board of Management
Techniker Krankenkasse
Bramfelder Straße 140
22303 Hamburg

Louis D. Vottero, M.S.
Professor of Pharmacy Emeritus
Ohio Northern University
35 Plantation Drive
Vero Beach, FL 32966

Susan C. Winckler, J.D.
Group Director, Policy and Advocacy
American Pharmaceutical Association
2215 Constitution Avenue, NW
Washington, DC 20037

Stephanie A. Zarus, Pharm.D.
Chief Performance Officer
ExcelleRx, Inc.
530 Walnut Street, Suite 550
Philadelphia, PA 19106

William A. Zellmer, M.P.H.
Deputy Executive Vice President
American Society of Health-System Pharmacists
7272 Wisconsin Avenue
Bethesda, MD 20814

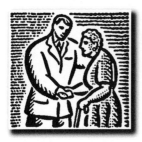

Part 1: The Context Surrounding Pharmaceutical Care

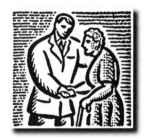

Chapter 1: The Profession of Pharmacy and Pharmaceutical Care

Robert A. Buerki, R.Ph., Ph.D.
Louis D. Vottero, R.Ph., M.S.

In a 1989 paper titled "Opportunities and Responsibilities in Pharmaceutical Care," Hepler and Strand[1] proposed a new philosophy of pharmacy practice that went far beyond the expectations of most pharmacy practitioners, even those dedicated to the patient-oriented practices embraced by the term "clinical pharmacy." They reviewed the alarming extent of drug-related morbidity and mortality in the American health care system and concluded that this problem could only be addressed by a fundamental change in the pharmacist's professional function. They referred to this concept as pharmaceutical care, which they defined as "the responsible provision of drug therapy for the purpose of achieving definite outcomes that improve a patient's quality of life." They stressed that the practice of pharmacy "must restore what has been missing for years: a clear emphasis on the patient's welfare, a patient advocacy role with a clear ethical mandate to protect the patient from the harmful effects of . . . 'drug misadventuring.'"

Rather than restrict the pharmacist's professional role to merely supplying and monitoring drug therapy, Hepler and Strand built upon concepts of clinical pharmacy to create "a process in which a pharmacist cooperates with a patient and other health professionals in designing, implementing, and monitoring a therapeutic plan that will produce specific therapeutic outcomes for the patient." Central to their shared vision is the establishment of a "mutually beneficial exchange in which the patient grants authority to the provider, and the provider gives competence and commitment to the patient." Leaders in pharmacy have embraced the concept of pharmaceutical care because they see within it an opportunity to respond to critical health care needs of society and to renew the sense of professional purpose in American pharmacy practice.

Pharmaceutical care involves professional care decisions beyond enhanced therapeutic outcomes. Practitioners who embrace the concept of pharmaceutical care will encounter increasingly complex moral and ethical situations which will require not only a deeper professional and personal commitment to patients as individuals but also a higher level of clinical knowledge as they deal with more complex patient care decisions. As a result, the status of the practice of pharmacy will be further enhanced as a socially necessary health care profession.

What Is a Profession?

Professions are found wherever humans live together in socialized groups. Professions emerged in the Middle Ages when specialized practitioners began to develop and provide an array of significant, unstandardized personal services that were central to human values. These services—such as health, education, religion, and welfare—were adapted to meet the needs of individuals and required knowledge and skills that the typical person did not possess. Pharmacy is among the oldest of the healing professions and its practitioners provide unique, personalized services that meet the fundamental needs of individuals, communities, and society.

One approach to understanding the purpose of professions in our society is to examine these unique, individual service needs and how an organized body of professionals meets those needs. We will begin by examining the nature of professions in general. We will then explain how professions differ from other service occupations and from strictly commercial enterprises. Finally, we will examine the unique power professionals possess, as well as their special prerogatives, duties, and obligations, and explain why pharmacy is properly considered to be a profession.

The word "profession" means "to testify on behalf of" or "to stand for" something. Members of a profession pledge or profess their fundamental commitment to serving society. People who are professionals stand for something and vow not only to provide their clients with knowledge but also to use a particular body of learning to solve a specific range of human problems.[2] In this context, pharmacists not only profess to be experts on drug therapy but also vow to help people make the best possible use of drugs.

Origins of Professions

In the medieval world, the term "professional" was not applied to lawyers, physicians, priests, or academics, who professed their commitment to apply their respective bodies of knowledge to the service of human need, but to monks, who professed their faith in God when they took up the contemplative life.[2] In the West, we trace our professional lineage more directly to late medieval cities in Europe, especially Italy. As Europe became more urbanized, artisans broke away from the manor estates and took up middle-class occupations. Pharmacy was one of a number of occupations that developed guild-like associations during this period.[3] At about the same time, occupations that had been confined to the learned world of the medieval clergy became secularized.

Toward the close of the twelfth century, the physicians and pharmacists of Florence, together with some others, formed a single guild. Supervision was rigid. During annual inspections of pharmacies, guild commissions confiscated drugs not meeting the guild requirements and excluded the culprits from professional practice for varying periods.[4] The separation of pharmacy/medicine practitioners and organization into different guilds was a prerequisite to professionalization; actual professionalization came more slowly. Historians date the legal recognition and regulation of pharmacy in the West, as an occupation separate from medicine, to the thirteenth century.[3]

The Work of Professionals

In their practice, professionals use a variety of observable techniques and tangible goods. They also use intangibles, such as skill, knowledge, and previous experience, that often go unrecognized by members of the public. The results of professional functions take the form of products, services, advice, opinion, and even a physical presence on behalf of another person or group.[5]

There is a uniquely public nature to the work of professionals. Professionals must use their knowledge not simply to display their virtuosity but also to serve human needs. Professionals serve not only the needs of friends but also those of strangers. Professionals must act altruistically. The seventeenth-century idea of "hanging out one's shingle" symbolized this readiness to "go public" and to serve the needs of strangers.[2]

Secondly, there is a special nature to the functions professionals perform. These functions are always more complex than the mechanical activities a client may observe. The seemingly simple chest tapping involved in auscultative percussion, for example, belies years of clinical experience. Furthermore, it is not unusual for professionals to practice in relative isolation from the routines of daily life and provide their services to society in abstract ways.[5]

Finally, there is an exclusive nature to the functions professionals perform. Professionals, through a representative body of peers sanctioned by the state, are given the unusual authority to determine who may be permitted to practice and under what conditions. For example, state boards of pharmacy define the kinds of activities pharmacists are allowed to perform, outline the social privileges and professional prerogatives they may claim, and establish controls to guarantee that these privileges and prerogatives are not abused.[5]

The Societal Need for Professions

Although many professions trace their origins to European medieval guilds, health professions in the United States emerged from other occupational groups. This emergence took place toward the end of the nineteenth century as a result of the expansion of urban society. These professions have since become integral parts of society. They have flourished because most people find modern life too complex to live without the benefit of expert consultation and specialized services.[5]

The services provided by professionals depend upon the application of formal knowledge, sometimes in highly modified form, to complex problems of immediate importance to clients. However, expertise in a profession extends beyond mere knowledge to include the skills, judgments, and experiences necessary to practice at a level of competency determined by academics, regulators, and the public.[5]

The complex, ever-changing needs of American society in the twenty-first century provide a special challenge to health professionals. In the murky world of managed competition, does a health professional still declare, promise, or vow anything that would make a requirement of integrity clear and compelling? Should a profession be understood as a value-free collection of knowledge and skills learned by training and accessible to consumers or as a value-driven form of human activity constituted as much by the ends it seeks as by the skills it requires?[6]

The Inherent Power of Professionals

Professionals exercise power over their clients and over other professionals through the services they provide and the environment in which they practice. Expertise is sometimes equated with the power to control and master the formal knowledge of the profession.[5]

Moreover, professionals often attempt to enhance their power of knowledge by transforming the formal knowledge base that is at the heart of their profession into a complex vocabulary of technical terms.[7]

Society grants varying amounts of discretionary power to each profession based on the value of the goods and services provided by the profession. These powers of position, once given, are very difficult to revoke. For example, pharmacists wield a certain power by controlling access to potent, often dangerous drugs. Physicians wield power by deciding which types of patients they will treat. Society often has difficulty controlling or limiting such discretionary power even when this power exceeds the best interests of society.[5]

Society also grants each profession certain functional powers that can have a profound impact on the professional–client relationship. In pharmacy, these powers go far beyond the traditional power to dispense to include developing and managing systems of drug distribution that provide access points to patients and ensure drug safety and compliance with legal and professional standards. These powers also extend to providing other cognitive services solidly based on professional knowledge and skills. Health professionals should employ these powers to effect a "good outcome" for their patients as determined by patients' individual life-plans, their understanding of their illness, and their concept of what constitutes appropriate treatment.[8] With this in mind, pharmaceutical care encourages pharmacists and physicians not only to agree upon a therapeutic plan but also to share their functional power with their patients by including the patients in both the formulation and the implementation of the plan.

Attributes of a Profession

Dictionary definitions for the term "profession" more or less agree that a profession involves specialized, intellectual learning that is used to render a particular service either by guiding or advising others or by practicing an art.[3] A. M. Carr-Saunders and P. A. Wilson[9] point out that there is no single test or touchstone for professionalism, characterizing it as "a complex of characteristics." Roy Lewis and Angus Maude[10] have written that "a moral code is the basis of professionalism." Beyond this common thread of morality, however, the promulgation of a satisfactory definition of the term has progressed little beyond the five criteria proposed by Abraham Flexner[11] in 1915 and elaborated upon by Isador Thorner[12] in 1942: 1) a relatively specific, socially necessary function upon the regular performance of which the practitioners depend for their livelihood and social status; 2) a special technique, competence in which is demanded, resting upon; 3) a body of knowledge embracing generalized principles the mastery of which requires theoretical study; 4) a traditional and generally accepted ethic subordinating its adherents' immediate private interest to the most effective performance of the function; and 5) a formal association fostering the ethic and improvement of performance.

Systematic Theory and Body of Knowledge

A profession relies upon a body of knowledge organized into an internally consistent system of abstract propositions that describe its focus of interest. Theoretical knowledge and understanding underpin the technique of every profession.[3] Moreover, as has been suggested above, patients use and benefit from this body of knowledge, even though they do not understand or use it directly.[5]

Professional Authority and Special Privileges

A profession serves society by doing for society what society cannot do for itself. In turn, society grants professionals special privileges when they demonstrate skill and knowledge. Professional discretion represents evidence of a social contract wherein society receives adequate professional services in return for granting professionals the privilege of internal control. Some authors claim that professionals have abused and distorted the social privileges granted them through internal control and discipline.[5]

Community Sanction and Social Utility

A profession serves a socially necessary function. It provides a service that has a high social utility. This function is typically sanctioned through a system of professional licensure. This system of licensure is viewed by some social critics as a monopoly that screens and protects the profession from censure rather than protecting society. Others argue that licensure serves as a positive influence for preserving professional commitment.[5]

Ethical Codes and Internal Control

A profession relies on formal and informal means of internal control and sanctions, traditionally codes of ethics and peer review mechanisms. A profession accepts responsibility to maintain a standard of conduct beyond compliance to law or demonstration of technical skill. Society expects a profession to generate its own statement of acceptable and unacceptable behavior, usually in the form of a formal code of ethics.[13]

Professional Culture and Organizations

Professions employ a wide array of values, attributes, norms, symbols, and specialized vocabulary that make up their culture. Professions also rely upon a network of organizations that foster the professional ethic and promote the improvement of performance. In addition to licensure, professional organizations often validate professional knowledge and competence through a collegially organized community of peers.[14] Starr[15] suggests that a professional's authority may be increased by membership in an organization that is generally recognized as being selective on the basis of consensually valid and professionally relevant competence criteria. For example, some professional associations have developed their own specialty certification programs.

The Process of Professionalization

Professionalism is a concept that develops around a given profession. Its basic characteristics include four aspects. The psychological aspect comprises an individual's personal sense of worth, ambition, self-esteem, and self-concept. The social aspect is how professionals evolve socially for a specific purpose. The sociological aspect centers on the profession's model, code of ethics, and theoretical knowledge base drawn from educational requirements. The legal–ethical aspect includes laws and moral issues related to the public good.[16] In contrast, professionalization is the dynamic process of becoming a professional.

Becoming a Professional

The process of becoming a professional begins with admission to a professional school where students are exposed to a variety of educational materials and problem-solving skills that will enable them to function within the current standards of the profession.[16] Students gradually develop a professional self-image in the course of their training. This professional development consists of learning and assimilating the traits they will need in order to play the role of the professional after graduation.[17] Renée C. Fox[18] has analyzed the professional development of medical students and Mary Jean Huntington has shown that with each succeeding year in school medical students were more likely to say that, on the occasion of their last contact with a patient, they thought of themselves more as a doctor than a student.[19]

Functioning as a Professional

Professionals behave in a manner that embodies both their technique and their commitment to provide individualized service. Professionals also subscribe to a traditional and generally accepted ethic which subordinates their immediate private interests to the most effective performance of their professional function.[12] It is not unusual, for example, for a pharmacist to be called in the middle of the night to fill an emergency prescription. In a broader sense, professionals also use their knowledge and skill to benefit mankind. Many health professionals volunteer to serve on lay health advisory boards or participate in community health screening programs.

Professional Responsibility

Professionals develop a public and moral sense of responsibility to others by internalizing a clear sense of purpose, a strong commitment to serve the public, and a deep understanding of the ethic of the profession. This responsibility is reflected in the way professionals behave toward their clients and toward each other. The true professional will understand and practice the virtues of his or her profession. Society expects its physicians to be competent, its lawyers to hold confidences, and its pharmacists to be trustworthy—virtues all these professions share, to be sure. Professionals also strive to maintain their professional competence—generally through self-study or organized continuing professional education activities—to improve their service to the public.

The Special Nature of Professional Practice

As we have indicated, professions have developed around the provision of services that have three general characteristics: requirement of knowledge and skills that the typical client does not have, provision of personal services that are central to human values, and adaptation of these services to the needs of individuals.[20] Professionals must balance the provision of these services with the countervailing forces of professional prerogatives, authority, and autonomy.

Professional Prerogatives: Rights and Choices

Professional prerogatives may be defined as those rights that belong to specific groups or classes of individuals, as sanctioned by society. Professional prerogatives address issues within the professional's discretion that are not specifically addressed by law. Within pharmacy, for example, many pharmacists draw attention to their "right" to decide whether or not to fill a prescription order and often speak of "exercising" or "not exercising" their professional prerogatives, demonstrating the voluntary nature of this activity.[21] The concept of professional autonomy is a basis for exercising professional prerogatives. That is, professionals practice in a manner that cannot accommodate external interference. In daily practice, the knowledge and skills needed are esoteric, the tasks performed are complex, and the professional judgments made are sophisticated; thus professionals could not practice effectively if they had to contend with such interference.[5]

Professional Discretion: Power and Societal Interest

Professionals not only exercise discretionary powers over their individual actions but also supervise the actions of their peers. For example, physicians' professional practices are regularly reviewed by peer-review committees composed of other physicians. Professionals also accept a social contract underlying their discretionary powers, balancing discretion and societal interest. Thus, pharmacists have the discretionary power to distribute certain dangerous or potentially habit-forming drugs within the community but typically exercise this power in a manner that is in the best interest of society.

Professional Autonomy: The Boundaries of Power

Society is reluctant to permit any profession to be completely autonomous. Full autonomy would provide professionals with a mechanism to define, control, and eventually monopolize the services of other interdependent professions to such an intolerable level that societal intervention would become inevitable. Thus, the virtual monopoly on prescribing medications enjoyed by generations of physicians is now shared by osteopaths, dentists, optometrists, nurse practitioners, and—in some states—by pharmacists. To avoid societal intervention, professionals typically seek to balance the relationship between their discretionary powers and the exercise of their professional autonomy.[5]

The Special Nature of Health Professionals

Health professions exist because there is illness. When they are ill, people are suffering an attack on their "wholeness," their humanity, and often their very identity. This vulnerability is unique in that a lack of health robs people of the ability to deal with their other vulnerabilities, such as the loss of personal freedom or privacy in a hospital setting. Moreover, because they do not have the knowledge or skills necessary to effect their own cure, ill people are forced to place themselves under the care of the health professionals who have these skills. Unfortunately, these health professionals may also inadvertently bring harm to their patients.[22] Health professionals should be alert to the sense of powerlessness that often accompanies illness and be prepared to respond to it.[8]

Pharmacy as a Health Profession

As health professionals, pharmacists make moral decisions that affect human purposes. Edward C. Elliott,[23] director of the deeply probing Pharmaceutical Survey (1946–49), made this point clear when he concluded that "the profession of pharmacy is fundamentally moral in nature." In his 1981 analysis of pharmacy's societal purpose, pharmacy educator Donald C. Brodie[24] stressed a pattern of professional behavior that demonstrates a "commitment to the common good." That same year, Pellegrino and Thomasma[25] elegantly encapsulated the moral dimension of the pharmacist–patient relationship when they declared that "any act which applies knowledge to persons involves values and consequently falls into the moral realm."

The Societal Need for the Profession of Pharmacy

For centuries, the profession of pharmacy has provided service of fundamental value to society. During the first half of the twentieth century, American pharmacy gradually lost three of the four professional functions that had characterized the work of pharmacists for nearly one thousand years—the procurement, storage, and compounding of drug products. At midcentury, pharmacists concentrated on the remaining professional function—dispensing drug products and managing the supply of medicines.[5] As drugs became more potent and federal and state legislation became more stringent, pharmacists took justifiable pride in being responsible and accountable for controlling drug distribution.

In the mid 1960's, pharmacists began to focus their professional attention upon assuring safe, effective, and cost-efficient therapeutic outcomes for their patients. By the late 1960's, the profession began to draw sharp criticism that it had become too commercialized.[26] By the mid 1970's, however, bolstered by challenging interprofessional practice settings and freer access to clinical data and other patient information, the profession opened a new clinical role for itself in the area of consultation. In recent decades, the societal need for both the distributive and the more highly specialized professional services provided by pharmacists has been well documented.[27] Today, American pharmacists face the challenge of providing pharmaceutical care, which requires accepting responsibility for providing drug therapy for the purpose of achieving definite outcomes that improve a patient's quality of life.[28]

The Evolving Societal Role of the Pharmacist

As we have suggested, at the turn of the century, American pharmacy began to move away from the path that had characterized its professional function since the earliest times, a function centered upon the knowledge and skills needed to compound drug products. The mechanized processes of industry and the emergence of new drugs placed the complexity of drug preparation far beyond the reach of the average pharmacist. Because drugs are inherently dangerous substances and the pharmacists' knowledge about their proper preparation, storage, and handling is greater than that of any other professional group, pharmacists began to develop a more technologically advanced role in quality assurance as it applied to drug distribution. This evolving professional function, as defined by society and the profession, ensured that the drugs provided to patients were safely and accurately dispensed.[5]

In recent years, pharmacy practice has experienced a gradual shift away from the technical paradigm, which emphasized drug products and their preparation, toward a more disease- and patient-oriented approach to pharmaceutical decision-making. This shift in favor of more active, direct involvement with patient care came about more naturally in institutional settings than it did in community practice settings. Pharmaceutical decision-making has been strengthened by the institutional pharmacist's access to clinical data and the underlying interprofessional support of changing practice patterns and functions of pharmacists.[5]

Values and Attitudes of the Pharmacist

In his analysis of the shift of moral values over time, Daniel Callihan[29] envisioned "a resurgence in social ethics of an emphasis on community, on the common good, on the hazards of an excessive dependence on the language of rights, and on an exultation of individual over community." Although human values are more commonly associated with such humanistic disciplines as philosophy and religion, health professionals are beginning to realize that the success of their medical interventions with their patients depends as much upon interpersonal, value-based relationships as it does upon technical competence. When the full range of personal and societal values associated with pharmacy practice is taken into consideration, even the seemingly benign activity of recommending a nonprescription medication takes on an added meaning. Rather than making a quick clinical judgment and recommending a product, pharmacists sensitive to their patients' individual needs may defer a "sale," recommend medical intervention, suggest a change in lifestyle, or just offer comfort and reassurance.

To what extent, for example, does the perceived socioeconomic status of the patient determine the extent and nature of the professional services pharmacists provide? To what extent does the pressure for cost-containment influence pharmacists' drug-product selection process? How does the acceptance of the concept of pharmaceutical care affect the value system of American pharmacists? Indeed, human values seem to be so completely integrated with modern health care practices that one might argue that the so-called "ideal" of a highly technical, purely clinical, and "value-free" practice of pharmacy is neither possible nor even desirable.

Values may be defined as beliefs or ideals to which an individual is devoted and which ultimately guide that individual's behavior. A closely held value system will be continually reflected through an individual's attitudes, personal qualities, and a consistent pattern of behavior. Unfortunately, value identification and acceptance are not included to any great extent in the curricula of our schools and colleges of pharmacy or in the programs of its professional pharmaceutical associations.[30] Indeed, becoming a professional is a socialization process, although often there is no formal process in place to make sure that professionalization actually occurs. Schools and colleges of pharmacy need to identify the attitudes and behaviors they expect, why they are necessary and important, and ensure that they are being taught.[31]

Table 1.1 depicts a set of essential values that might be acceptable to professional pharmacists. The table was adapted from a set of values and behaviors that were intended to guide educational programs for professional nursing. It is clear that the same set of values prevails for all of the health professions, although some professions may need to stress some areas in different ways.

In practice, professional pharmacists assign priorities to these values as they encounter their patients or when they engage in specific decision-making situations. Individual pharmacists, relying on and guided by these values, will demonstrate a behavior that is consistent with the strength of conviction that they hold for these values. It is often during these "testing" periods that individual novice pharmacists will grope for a suitable, satisfying response. Experience may provide some guidance, yet many pharmacists who are unable to act based upon a consistent, internalized value system, will attempt to deal with each new problem as it arises and may not approach similar problems in a consistent

Table 1.1. Values and Behaviors for Professional Pharmacists[a]

Values	Attitudes	Professional Behavior
Altruism	Commitment	Gives full attention to patients
(concern for the	Compassion	Assists other health care personnel
welfare of others)	Generosity	Sensitive to social issues
	Perseverance	
Equality	Fairness	Provides services based on needs
(having the same	Self-esteem	Relates to others without discriminating
rights, privileges,	Tolerance	Provides leadership in improving access to
or status)		health care
Esthetics	Appreciation	Creates supportive patient care environments
(qualities of objects,	Creativity	
events, and persons	Sensitivity	
that provide satisfaction)		
Freedom	Openness	Respects each individual's autonomy
(capacity to exercise	Self-direction	
choice)	Self-discipline	
Human Dignity	Empathy	Respects the right of privacy
(inherent worth and	Kindness	Maintains confidentiality
uniqueness of an	Trust	
individual)		
Justice	Integrity	Acts as a health care advocate
(upholding moral	Morality	Allocates resources fairly
and legal principles)		Reports incompetent, unethical, and
		illegal practices
Truth	Accountability	Documents actions accurately
(faithfulness to	Honesty	Protects the public from misinformation
fact or reality)		about pharmacy
	Rationality	

[a]Adapted from American Association of Colleges of Nursing. The Essentials of Baccalaureate Education for Professional Nursing Practice. Washington, DC: American Association of Colleges of Nursing; 1998.

manner. For this reason, professional pharmacists need to both identify the basic values that impinge upon their professional practice and use these values in a consistent, rational manner when they make professional judgments.

Professional versus Business Conflicts

The practice of pharmacy in the United States has always been associated with the merchandising of unrelated goods. The sale of general merchandise in drugstores was necessary to build an adequate cash volume to subsidize the pharmacists' professional functions. Moreover, having items besides drugs available in the pharmacy helped to establish the corner drugstore in the community. People could obtain in one place not only the prescriptions and other health goods needed in times of illness but also sundries and convenience items needed in times of health. The presence of departments beyond the prescription counter was not seen by pharmacists as deprofessionalizing when compounding was still an important part of their daily activities. Indeed, many pharmacists saw these departments as a natural extension of the prescription department.

In 1899, pharmacist George J. Seabury[32] noted, "Unlike the grocer, who is a . . . mere exchanger of articles that are daily requested of him, the pharmacist is expected, by his education and profession, to examine every article sold in his establishment and to be accountable for its quality." Over four decades later, sociologist Isador Thorner[33] agreed: "Distribution may be in the process of becoming scientific and is being taught in schools of business administration but it cannot become a profession until the seller's interest is institutionally subordinated to that of the user of drugs. The grocer has no moral obligation to his customers parallel to that of the physician, lawyer or pharmacist toward his client."

As the dispensing of prescriptions became a more centralized professional function of American pharmacists, however, many practitioners became torn over which of their functions—professional or mercantile—should assume primacy. Many sought to achieve an uneasy balance, a dilemma compounded by the commercial setting in which much of pharmacy is still practiced. The business and professional concerns of the pharmacist often conflict, and these conflicts can cause ambiguity in the way patients view pharmacists and their functions.

The Professional Image of the Pharmacist

Pharmacists have also had to contend with the pressures of competing public and professional expectations. Some indication of how the public views pharmacy is given by public opinion polls conducted during the last two decades. These polls show that the public accords pharmacists a high professional standing in terms of honesty and ethical standards. It is significant that the prime source of influence on the views of individuals was their personal experience with pharmacists and the quality of each individual patient–practitioner interaction. Pharmacists who demonstrate technical expertise and provide services consistent with their patients' views of professional services will be deemed professional. It is the collective judgment of the public that determines whether pharmacy is an occupation or a profession.[34,35]

Professional Practice in a Corporate Setting

Within the past 50 years, health care delivery in the United States has evolved from a cottage industry to one dominated by large corporations, managed care processes, and government regulation.[36] During this time, the practice of pharmacy has undergone dramatic changes as well: in the 1950's, most pharmacists either enjoyed the freedom of owning their own pharmacy or worked in small groups in the burgeoning institutional and drug chain settings, reporting directly to another pharmacist; professional decisions related to patient care reflected the personal values and ethics of one or, at most, a handful of pharmacists. In today's practice environment, whether they practice in community, institutional, mail-order, or Internet settings, a majority of American pharmacists are employed by corporations that are controlled by executives and administrators who make business decisions calculated to satisfy their stockholders. Many of these executives do not have a professional background in pharmacy, and their corporate policies tend to reflect a bottom-line mentality. Corporate employee pharmacists are often torn between exercising their personal value system and complying with a corporate ethic that may be far removed from the individual pharmacist–patient encounter.

For example, corporate pharmacists may be asked to dispense generic equivalent products routinely without regard for the wishes of their patients or downplay the offer to counsel patients guaranteed by federal law. This is not to say that corporate practice is ethically challenged by definition. Many corporations have pioneered systems which improve both the efficiency of drug distribution and the scope of patient-oriented health care services while respecting and supporting their employee pharmacists' personal value systems; still, many pharmacists are asked to carry out corporate policies that are in direct conflict with their own deeply held personal values—such as dispensing a "morning after" contraceptive medication—at the risk of being dismissed for not complying with a corporate policy. In all cases, pharmacists must decide whether they are advocates for their patients or merely agents of their employer.

The Covenantal Nature of Professional Relationships

The key ingredients of the notion of covenant are promise and fidelity to promise. A covenantal relationship is based upon the concepts of indebtedness and responsiveness.[37] The work of a health professional begins with a response to a patient's request for assistance or care. The patient thus provides the "gift" of a personal sanction to the health practitioner to initiate professional service. This "gift" creates a sense of indebtedness on the part of practitioners, providing them with an opportunity to perform their professional functions. Implicit in this covenant is the commitment not only to maintain a high quality of technical skill but also to safeguard patients from possible untoward effects related to drug therapy.

Trust is also inherent in the relationship between health care professionals and their patients. This condition is a reflection of the system of licensure that is imposed by society—a system that permits patients to place their most intimate thoughts, as well as their bodies, in the hands of professionals whose competency they cannot easily judge. In contrast to the practices of medicine and nursing, which are characterized by direct patient contact, the pharmacist often fills prescription orders in seclusion or partially shielded from the patient. Therefore, the patient must have even greater faith in the pharmacist's competence than he does in the physician's. As the practice of pharmacy expands to include more intense patient–pharmacist encounters, this trust will be increasingly challenged as patients have expanded opportunities to scrutinize and evaluate the professional services they receive.

Covenant or Contract?

In a contractual relationship, two parties agree upon some joint project in which both derive some benefit for the goods or services contributed by each party. Are the goods and services offered by pharmacists to their patients defined by such a relationship and reduced to simple transactional events? Doesn't the practice philosophy of pharmaceutical care imply a pharmacist–patient relationship that extends beyond a mere contractual arrangement?

Some of the aims of a contractual relationship might be desirable in the context of pharmacy practice: a clear expression of rights, clearly defined self-interests, the possibility of legal enforcement. Unfortunately, a contractual relationship suppresses the gift of trust that is essential in professional relationships. Furthermore, a contractual relationship may undermine pharmacists' attitudes toward professional behavior by encouraging a restrained response to patient care. Pharmacists could construe such a relationship to mean that they should do no more for their patients than what their contract calls for or to perform only specified services for certain fees, no more, no less.

Professional services in the health professions are directed to subjects who are by nature rather unpredictable as they deal with their own sickness or the ills of their loved ones. These services cannot be exhaustively specified in advance for each patient; pharmacists must be ready to deal with the contingent, the unexpected. Patients may require services that exceed those anticipated in the contract or incur additional costs beyond those originally agreed upon. Moreover, the services associated with pharmaceutical care are more likely to achieve the desired therapeutic results if they are delivered in the context of a fiduciary relationship in which patients have full trust in the pharmacists serving them.[38]

Caring as a Professional Responsibility

Care and medicine have become closely identified, if not synonymous, in the minds of many. For example, medicine, nursing, and other health-related activities are often referred to as "caring professions." Care often appears to be a more important regulative notion for determining the basis and direction of health-related activities than might be morally justified. Care, however, is a significant notion that reminds us that medicine serves as one of the ways we can help others maintain basic physical and psychological integrity. Moreover, care directs our attention to the concrete patient in need without subjecting him or her to manipulation for the good of others. However, it is important that the care given the patient be based on the respect due each of us, well or ill, for otherwise our attempts to care can lead to sentimental or paternalistic perversions.[39]

Summary and Conclusions

Accepting the mandate of pharmaceutical care will greatly increase the pharmacist's responsibility to patients; discharging that responsibility will require philosophical, organizational, and functional change in the practice of pharmacy.[1] Today, the profession of pharmacy faces daunting challenges to its traditional functional autonomy. The profession has responded to these pressures by increasingly relying upon paraprofessional help, robotics, and computer-assisted patient information systems to manage its interpersonal patient care functions. Just as pharmacy has learned it can no longer focus exclusively upon the safe distribution of drugs or even upon expanded clinical functions to justify its societal function, it may also learn it cannot solely rely upon the enhanced service mandate suggested by the concept of pharmaceutical care for its raison d'être.

References

1. Hepler CD, Strand LM. Opportunities and responsibilities in pharmaceutical care. *Am J Pharm Educ.* 1990; 53:7S–15S.

2. May WF. The beleaguered rulers: the public obligation of the professional. *Kennedy Inst Ethics J.* 1992; 2:25–41.

3. Sonnedecker G. To be or not to be—professional. *Am J Pharm.* 1961; 133:243–54.

4. Sonnedecker G. Kremers and Urdang's history of pharmacy. 4th ed. Philadelphia: J. B. Lippincott Company; 1976.

5. Mrtek RG, Catizone C. Pharmacy and the professions. In: Wertheimer AI, Smith MC, eds. Pharmacy practice: social and behavioral aspects. 3rd ed. Baltimore: Williams & Wilkins; 1989:23–57.

6. Lammers SE, Verhey A, eds. On moral medicine: theological perspectives in medical ethics. Grand Rapids: William B. Eerdmans; 1987.

7. Freidson E. Professional powers: a study of the institutionalization of formal knowledge. Chicago: Univ. of Chicago Press; 1986.

8. Brody H. The healer's power. New Haven: Yale Univ. Press; 1992.

9. Carr-Saunders AM, Wilson PA. The professions. Oxford: Clarendon Press; 1933.

10. Lewis R, Maude A. Professional people. London: Phoenix House; 1952.

11. Flexner A. Is social work a profession? *Sch & Soc.* 1915; 1:901–11.

12. Thorner I. Pharmacy: the functional significance of an institutional pattern. *Am J Pharm Educ.* 1942; 6:305–19.

13. Buerki RA, Vottero LD. Ethics. In: Wertheimer AI, Smith MC, eds. Pharmacy practice: social and behavioral aspects. 3rd ed. Baltimore: Williams & Wilkins; 1989:329–49.

14. Starr P. The social transformation of American medicine. New York: Basic Books; 1982.

15. Hepler CD. Pharmacy as a clinical profession. *Am J Hosp Pharm.* 1985; 42:1298–1306.

16. Sogol EM, Manasse HR Jr. The pharmacist. In: Wertheimer AI, Smith MC, eds. Pharmacy practice: social and behavioral aspects. 3rd ed. Baltimore: Williams & Wilkins; 1989:59–88.

17. Buerki RA. Pharmacist Smyth and druggist Smith—a study in professional aspirations. *Am J Pharm Educ.* 1977; 41:28–33.

18. Fox RC. Training for uncertainty. In: Merton RK, Reader GG, Kendall PL, eds. The student physician: introductory studies in the sociology of medical education. Cambridge: Harvard Univ. Press; 1957:207–41.

19. Huntington MJ. The development of a professional self-image. In: Merton RK, Reader GG, Kendall PL, eds. The student physician: introductory studies in the sociology of medical education. Cambridge: Harvard Univ. Press; 1957:179–87.

20. Larson MS. The rise of professionalism: a sociological analysis. Berkeley and Los Angeles: Univ. of California Press; 1977.

21. Buerki RA, Vottero LD. The changing face of pharmaceutical education: ethics and professional prerogatives. *Am J Pharm Educ.* 1991; 55:71–4.

22. Pellegrino ED. Toward a reconstruction of medical morality: the primacy of the act of profession and the fact of illness. *J Med Philos.* 1979; 4:32–56.

23. Elliott EC. The general report of the pharmaceutical survey, 1946–49. Washington, DC: American Council on Education; 1950.

24. Brodie DC. Pharmacy's societal purpose. *Am J Hosp Pharm.* 1981; 38:1893–6.

25. Pellegrino ED, Thomasma DC. A philosophical basis of medical practice: toward a philosophy and ethic of the healing professions. New York and Oxford: Oxford Univ. Press; 1981.

26. Francke DE. Let's separate pharmacies and drugstores. *Am J Pharm.* 1969; 141:161–9.

27. Trinca CE. Does pharmaceutical care respond to society's mandate for professional pharmacy services? Proc NABP/AACP Dist IV. 1991:[31–37].

28. Hepler CD, Strand LM. Opportunities and responsibilities in pharmaceutical care. *Am J Hosp Pharm.* 1990; 47:533–43.

29. Callihan D. Ethics and health care: the next twenty years. In: Bezold C, Halperin JA, Binkley HL, Ashbaugh RA, eds. Pharmacy in the 21st century: planning for an uncertain future. Bethesda, MD: Institute for Alternative Futures and Project HOPE; 1985:79–86.

30. Smith MC, Smith MD. Instruction in ethics in schools of pharmacy. *Am J Pharm Educ.* 1981; 45:14–7.

31. Berger B. Pharmacist–physician–patient relationships: caring, covenants, codes and commitment: Part 4—a profession changes. *US Pharm.* 2001; 26:80,82,85.

32. Seabury GJ. Shall pharmacists become tradesmen? 3rd ed. New York: George J. Seabury; 1899.

33. Thorner I. Comments on "Pharmacy, the functional significance of an institutional pattern." *Am J Pharm Educ.* 1942; 6:617–9.

34. Smith MC, Knapp DA. Pharmacy, drugs and medical care. 4th ed. Baltimore: Williams & Wilkins; 1987.

35. Hughes EC. The study of occupations. In: Merton RK, Broom L, Cottrell LS Jr, eds. Sociology today: problems and prospects. New York: Basic Books; 1959:442–58.

36. Schommer JC. Pharmacist workload and time management. *Drug Topics.* 2001; 145:45–54.

37. May WF. The physician's covenant. Philadelphia: Westminster Press; 1983.

38. May WF. Code, covenant, contract, or philanthropy. In: Haddad AM, Buerki RA, eds. Ethical dimensions of pharmaceutical care. New York and London: Pharmaceutical Products Press; 1996:49–72.

39. Hauerwas S. Care. In: Lammers SE, Verhey A, eds. On moral medicine: theological perspectives in medical ethics. Grand Rapids: William B. Eerdmans; 1987:262–6.

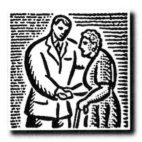

Chapter 2: From Compounding to Caring: An Abridged History of American Pharmacy

Gregory J. Higby, Ph.D.

Since the dawn of humanity, practitioners of the healing arts have prepared medicines from basic ingredients (drugs) for the treatment of disease. Archaeological digs from around the world have revealed evidence of various drugs and their dosage forms employed by prehistoric peoples. As civilizations developed in the great river valleys of the world, separate classes of workers specialized in healing. Most practiced a combination of empirical and supernatural medicine, although medicines were almost always in use. Plant drugs were especially popular, sometimes acting as the medium between this world and that of healing spirits.

Traditionally in the West, we tend to connect our medical heritage with the name of Hippocrates (circa 425 B.C.) and his school of medicine on the Greek island of Cos. Hippocratic physicians relied heavily on dietary regimens and environmental changes to produce good health and only used medicines occasionally. When they did use them, they left instructions with family members who prepared the simple medicines. For these doctors, the balance of four humors (blood, black bile, phlegm, and yellow bile) governed health.

An active approach to therapeutics came later with Galen, a Greek physician who practiced in Rome during the second century A.D. Galen believed that drugs should be given to patients in order to balance their bodily humors. For example, to treat a rash a Galenic physician might have applied cucumber, a drug with cool and wet characteristics. Galenists also used polypharmaceutical compounds, arguing that a patient's body pulled out the needed drug from what we call in modern times a "shotgun prescription." Although drug gatherers and sellers did exist in the Greco-Roman world, no distinct class of pharmaceutical practitioners developed.

Foundation in the West

If the roots of Western medicine can be traced back to Cos, those of pharmacy are more recent in origin. During the Middle Ages, the period between the fall of Rome (circa 400 A.D.) and the fall of Constantinople (1453), pharmacy as a specific occupation arose in the nations of Islam. Scholars such as Rhazes (860–932) and Avicenna (980–1063) built on the writings of Greek medical authorities and created a set of basic medical texts.

19

Traders in the expanding sphere of Arab influence brought new and exotic drugs from Asia into the materia medica as well. With demands for new drugs in elaborate dosage forms came specialists, first in ninth-century Baghdad and later throughout the sophisticated cities of Islam, the ancestors of today's pharmacists.

At those places where the expanding Islamic sphere collided with medieval European culture, the example of drug shops catering to the needs of physicians and the public was transferred. By the middle of the 1200's, pharmacy in southern Europe had separated from medicine to the extent that Frederick II, ruler of the Kingdom of the Two Sicilies, issued an edict to the effect. Apothecaries in European cities joined guilds and became established members of the emerging middle class of small merchants and protoprofessionals.

Renaissance and Early Modern Europe

Our modern world view began with that huge cultural shift we call the Renaissance. The mid-1400's were a time of great upheaval and promise: the fall of Constantinople to the Turks (1453) pushed the vestiges of Greek scholarship back into the West; Gutenberg printed his first run of Bibles (1453–1455); Christopher Columbus and Amerigo Vespucci were born (1451); and Leonardo da Vinci began his studies (1461). The end of the century brought new discoveries, both of land and of drugs. Vasco da Gama's successful sea voyage to India (the feat Columbus failed to accomplish) opened up the vast Asian drug and spice trade. New worlds, new diseases (notably syphilis), and new medicines encouraged the development of the pharmaceutical enterprise. After producing Bibles and hymnals, printers turned to medical and pharmaceutical books, especially herbals, which displayed beautiful woodcuts of medicinal plants. In contrast to herbals, which appealed to the public, books of formulas also appeared about this time. Some of these received the sanction of governments, becoming the first pharmacopeias.

For nearly 500 years, pharmacopeias have served the purpose of defining the characteristics of the drugs and preparations made by pharmacists. The appearance of pharmacopeias around 1500 is a milestone of the development of the pharmacy profession. Pharmaceutical sophistication had reached the level where physicians desired standards that would govern the preparation of their prescriptions.

Arrival in the New World

During the sixteenth and seventeenth centuries, apothecaries on the European continent solidified their position as middle-class professionals. In England, however, the ideology of laissez-faire capitalism blocked the full development of professional control. Instead, a haphazard system arose of university-educated physicians, apprentice-trained apothecaries (who practiced a combination of medicine and pharmacy), plus a group known as chemists and druggists who came to control the drug trade. A large variety of barber–surgeons, apothecary–surgeons, and other healers also contributed to the nearly chaotic character of health care in early modern England. It was during this period of turmoil that English settlers came to dominate the North American continent. Thus, the foundations of the American health care system lie in the disarray of the English system rather than the stability of the continental European system.

The Pre-Professional Period (1620 to 1820)

There was little to attract physicians and apothecaries to the colonies of the British New World. The populace knew little about medicine and was often illiterate. For that reason, other people of authority—political leaders, clergymen, and midwives—commonly provided medical care. With the aid of home medical guides, New World men and women practiced both medicine and pharmacy. They diagnosed illnesses and made up and administered simple medicines. When physicians did become common in the 1700's, pharmacists were still very rare. Physicians compounded their own prescriptions or had their apprentices do it for them.

Colonial Apothecary Shops

In colonial America, apothecary shops were only found in the largest cities. A major function of shops like Christopher Marshall's in Philadelphia (**Figure 2.1**) was to put together and service medicine chests for prosperous land owners or physicians. Early American apothecaries operated more as manufacturers and wholesalers of drugs and medicines than as retailers. Drugs and patent medicines could be bought from general stores, book sellers, and other merchants, who did not have the specialized skills necessary for operating a true apothecary shop.

Because most physicians dispensed their own drugs, prescriptions rarely found their way to shops like Marshall's. Most of the compounding he did was from old family recipes handed down over the generations. The close connection between medicine and pharmacy is well illustrated by Jonathan Roberts, the first hospital pharmacist in colonial America. In 1751, the Pennsylvania Hospital was established in Philadelphia. At first, physicians provided their own medicines, but after a large shipment of drugs arrived from London in 1752 it was decided to set up a pharmacy in the hospital. Roberts was hired to handle the "shop." His duties, like those of hospital apothecaries well into the next century, required him to go on rounds, practice some minor medicine, take care of the hospital's accounts and library, and perform odd chores along with managing his shop. When Roberts left the hospital in 1755, he was succeeded by John Morgan, one of the pivotal characters in the history of American medicine and pharmacy.

Morgan held the Pennsylvania Hospital apothecary job for only 13 months before going off to Europe to study medicine. In 1765, having returned from Europe, Morgan proposed the separation of the practices of medicine and pharmacy. Morgan

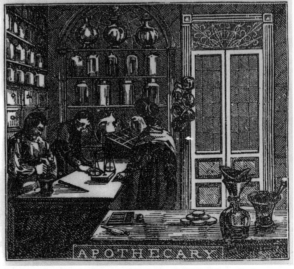

Figure 2.1. An Apothecary Shop in Colonial America.

argued that physicians should write out their prescriptions, which pharmacists would then compound and dispense as had been the practice in Europe for centuries. This would discourage over-drugging of patients, a common problem according to Morgan. Morgan did not merely suggest this division of labor, he brought his own pharmacist from Scotland.

Although Morgan attempted to follow this model of practice, he soon encountered problems. Patients were unhappy with the increased expense and inconvenience of receiving prescriptions from physicians that had to be filled by a pharmacist, and physicians relied heavily on the fees they received from the medicines they compounded and dispensed. By convention, American doctors diagnosed on credit, but dispensed medicines for cash or for goods. Later in life, Morgan found his practice shrinking. He was forced to open his own doctor's shop and practice medicine and pharmacy in one location. When he died in 1789, pharmacy and medicine were still not clearly distinct occupations in the United States.

Emergence of Independent Occupation

If Morgan failed to bring about the separation of medicine and pharmacy, when and how did it occur? From city directories and other documents, we know that apothecary shops and drugstores became more common in cities and towns after about 1810. Strangely enough, historians have not fully explained the emergence of the American drugstore. In their classic *History of Pharmacy*, Kremers and Urdang[1] point to four roots from which the American pharmacy developed. First they cite the so-called "doctor's shops" of physicians like John Morgan. Second, they describe the small number of shops operated by colonial apothecaries who specialized in selling drugs and related products, as much to physicians and landowners as to everyday customers. The third root was the general store, which sold opium to customers alongside flour without any legal restrictions. Finally, they cite the drug wholesalers, who repackaged the drugs and products imported from England for sale to physicians, apothecaries, general stores, and other outlets.

In the early nineteenth century, physician offices contained a wide range of pharmaceutical furnishings. Some stocked just a shelf or two of standard preparations, while fully equipped shops carried patent medicines and sundries. Some shop-doctors hired employee apothecaries, called "drug clerks." Graduates of medical schools had often missed out on the pharmaceutical training gained through a long apprenticeship and needed to hire someone with expertise to compound prescriptions. Even if they had sufficient expertise, successful shop doctors would often hire a drug clerk to keep shop while they practiced medicine inside and outside the shop. When they were successful enough to have a full, office-style practice, shop-doctors would often move and sell their pharmacy businesses to their clerks. This stimulated the growth of the retail drug trade. As a proprietor, a former drug clerk proudly took on the title of apothecary.

Wholesalers and the Establishment of Corner Drugstores

Many of the most prominent early American pharmacies arose from the "front ends" of wholesale businesses. This usually started by fixing up a public entrance to the warehouse for physicians and shopkeepers to enter for placing orders. Soon these front ends attracted walk-in customers interested in getting good buys or the freshest crude drugs. When new or exotic drugs came on the market, physicians would send patients to those wholesalers with the best trade contacts.

Nomenclature is another source of evidence that front-end wholesalers played an important role in the development of the American drugstore. Specialty retail establishments of the early to mid-nineteenth century were called shops. The term "store" was applied usually to businesses that carried a wide variety of goods, that is, a "storehouse." Apothecaries regarded store as a vulgar term, because it implied a lower class of retailing, such as the general store. Wholesalers—normally called druggists in the trade—referred to their establishments as drugstores. When many of them moved into retail, the name stuck.

Two additional factors not mentioned by Kremers and Urdang were critical to pharmacy's development as an independent occupation and the development of its special environment, the American drugstore. The first is so obvious that we tend to ignore its significance. The services of apothecaries, regarded generally as a luxury in America during the Colonial period, came to be considered essential in the early nineteenth century. The best evidence of this change in attitude is found in the records of early hospitals. The hospitals of the young republic usually employed medical apprentices as staff apothecaries. For example, the *Brief Account of the New-York Hospital*, published in 1804, states that

> A house Surgeon and Apothecary constantly reside in the Hospital. These offices are filled by the students of the Physicians and Surgeons belonging to the Hospital, which affords an excellent school for the young men appointed to those places.[2]

By 1811, however, the position of apothecary at the New-York Hospital had changed. The job was held by a full-time pharmaceutical practitioner, tested before hiring on his prowess as a compounder of medicines. Instead of being obligated to go on rounds, he was required to stay in his shop at all times.[3]

The by-laws of the hospital passed in 1819 not only required testimonials on the applicant's behalf, but also a $250 bond to ensure "faithful performance of the duties of his office, and that he will not cease to perform the duties of this office, without giving two months notice of his intention to leave his employment."[4] In a little more than a decade, pharmacy services moved out of the hands of the medical apprentice and into the hands of a trained individual with professional responsibilities.

Dispensaries—clinics established to treat the deserving poor and supported by public or private largess—followed the same pattern in the early nineteenth century. Full-time, responsible apothecaries replaced medical apprentices. By selecting mature apothecaries, the directors of hospitals and dispensaries obtained competent day-to-day management of their institutions. More importantly for the nascent occupation of pharmacy, full-time apothecaries provided reliable pharmaceutical services and probably encouraged prescription writing.

Beginning about 1815, study in medical schools began to replace the apprenticeship as the standard system for the training of doctors. Physicians who gained their clinical experience in hospitals and dispensaries instead of as apprentices learned to write prescriptions rather than compound them. After graduation these young physicians wrote out more prescriptions—in part to emulate their European-trained superiors and also out of habit.

The years following the War of 1812 were transitional for the country's pharmacies. Physicians continued to dispense but began to take advantage of the slowly growing number of retail apothecaries. For example, the fee bill approved by the New York County Medical Society in January 1816 contained a detailed section of "Pharmaceutical Charges," while in Boston, where there was a more developed cadre of apothecaries, the local medical association omitted pharmaceutical charges from its fee bill. The physicians there were writing out prescriptions. Advertisements and city directories of the time indicate that the number of doctors' shops was dropping off rapidly.

A small class of retail apothecaries presented no particular threat to urban physicians in the first decades of the nineteenth century, and provided several conveniences. New advances in chemistry and pharmacy added to the number of therapeutically active drugs available to physicians. It became difficult for physicians on rounds to carry all the drugs they needed to dispense. Well-educated physicians knew of the advances of pharmacy on the European continent and fostered pharmacy's progress in the United States.

About the same time, a change occurred in the American retail sector that would permanently affect the practice of American pharmacy. Specialized shops for all sorts of goods appeared as the major cities of the Atlantic Coast prospered. Rather than buying shoes in a general store, customers went to shops that sold only shoes. Apothecary shops fit into that trend. Early apothecary shops sold a great many more exotic items, such as tropical fruits and spices, than in later eras. Apothecaries dealt with wholesalers and importers of exotic goods because these merchants also handled drugs. In 1820, for example, one would usually go to an apothecary rather than a grocer to buy figs.

Summary of Pre-Professional Period

In the years following the War of 1812, a new, distinct occupation arose in American cities—the independent pharmacy practitioner. Before that time, pharmacy, that is, the making of medicines from drugs and other ingredients, was practiced primarily by physicians and their apprentices or by lay healers in the home. A complex set of economic, demographic, and other changes in the years following the war led to the emergence of American pharmacy practice and its unique location—the drugstore.

Period of Proto-Professionalism (1820 to 1850)

Two events occurred in 1820 and 1821 that make those years an excellent starting place for telling the story of American pharmacy's development as a profession. In January 1820, a group of about one dozen physicians met in Washington, DC, and founded the United States Pharmacopoeia. Their objective was to "prevent trouble or uncertainty in the intercourse of physicians and apothecaries."[5] Apothecaries, however, did not participate in the preparation of the new standard. Physicians believed it was their prerogative to found the standards for medicines in the United States and did not invite official collaboration with pharmacists until 1850.

Founding of the Philadelphia College of Pharmacy

In 1821, some prominent physicians in Philadelphia believed similarly that it was their privilege to designate which apothecaries in their city were "masters" of the pharmaceutical arts. When their scheme became known to the pharmaceutical community in Philadelphia, outrage led to direct action. The apothecaries and druggists of the city organized the Philadelphia College of Apothecaries, which was soon renamed the Philadelphia College of Pharmacy. The initial objective of this local association was to head off the certification program being developed by the elitist physicians. The grand scheme of the physicians never got off the ground. The College of Pharmacy, however, did and continues to the present as an active participant in the professional life of pharmacy in the United States.

In contrast to medical schools, pharmacy instruction of the early 1800's took place at night, so that the apprentices could work in shops, warehouses, and manufactories during the day. To obtain a diploma, students were required to attend the same set of lectures twice, write a thesis, and pass an examination. Since the emphasis was on the knowledge and not the diploma, only about 1 in 10 students in the early decades of the Philadelphia College of Pharmacy actually graduated. Their real education came through work and reading the texts of the day—the pharmacopoeias and the dispensatories. The Philadelphia College of Pharmacy was nevertheless an important institution, and it was no accident that the most important pharmaceutical book of the nineteenth century—the United States Dispensatory—was written by two of its professors, physicians George B. Wood and Franklin Bache.

Emergence of the "Pharmaceutist"

In the early 1830's, a growing number of pharmacists began calling themselves pharmaceutists—a term short for "pharmaceutical scientist." The rapid and profound advancements of French pharmacy had made American physicians aware of new potent drugs, such as morphine, strychnine, and quinine. In isolating these alkaloids, pharmacists had provided medical practitioners with potent plant drugs of reliable strength for the first time. Not only did this development attract the approbation of physicians, it increased the necessity for skilled pharmaceutical practitioners. In addition to discoveries such as the alkaloids, continental pharmacists also excelled in other areas of chemistry. In the larger East Coast cities, American pharmacists began participating in local scientific societies and discussion groups. Apothecary shops like that of Elias Durand in Philadelphia became gathering places for scientific investigators.

Relations with Physicians

The timing of the emergence of the American drugstore and the public recognition of the contributions of pharmacy was propitious. Physicians supported the appearance of pharmaceutists near their practices and welcomed them as subordinate colleagues. The pharmaceutists and apothecaries were small in number and did not compete directly with physicians for business. They also served a check against unscrupulous drug wholesalers and other importers and helped ensure drug quality.

The relationship between physicians and pharmacists varied over the next few decades. During the 1840's, medical schools increased their output of physicians, who flooded the markets in cities and towns. To survive, these physicians often reverted to setting up shop and selling drugs as well as advice. Pharmacists competed by doing the same—so that during the 1850's especially, the borders between pharmaceutical and medical practice in cities became fuzzy again. Pharmacists began "counter prescribing," that is, recommending favorite preparations "over the counter" for customers. They also solidified their position as the prime sellers of patent medicines, which enraged physicians, who saw nostrums as another competitor to their practices.

Nature of Antebellum Pharmacy Practice

Figure 2.2 is one of the oldest illustrations we have of an American pharmacy interior (circa 1836). Note that the work areas of the apothecary are right out front. This allows the apothecary to get the needed light from the windows and allowed customers to watch him in action. This was important since much of his sales were simply crude drugs sold in bulk for home use. The customers liked to see the powder being weighed and wrapped. In addition, the front counter position permitted the apothecary to exhibit his skill in compounding. In contrast, the pharmacist used a laboratory in the back, away from customer view, for the dirtier jobs of manufacturing.

In addition to medicines, apothecaries also sold the usual drugstore goods. In the 1830's, apothecaries started to phase out the sale of exotic food items, such as figs, raisins, and citrus fruits. In cities they stocked fewer general articles, such as glass, paint, and oils and concentrated on patent medicines, fancy soaps, toiletries, dyes, and flavorings. Books were a common drugstore merchandise in some parts of the country.

Pharmacy Practice at Midcentury

In some cases we have detailed records of the daily activities of midcentury pharmacists. For example, master pharmacist William Procter, Jr. filled six prescriptions on 27 February 1847, for a total charge of $1.20. The first was from a Dr. Mayer, who wanted fifteen grains of camphor dissolved in one-half ounce of ether, probably for his own use. The second prescription was for a tonic of ammonium hydrochloride and the syrups of ipecac, wild cherry, and balsam of Tolu, flavored with orange flower water. Procter asked 50 cents for this mixture, close to the maximum he charged for a single prescription. The third prescription Procter compounded called for a mixture of Dover's powder and potassium nitrate divided into six powder papers. Although this was an easy mixture to prepare,

Procter charged 19 cents for it because of its expensive ingredients—opium and ipecac. The fourth prescription Procter prepared that day called for one ounce of uva ursi or bearberry and was probably ordered for a urinary tract disorder. Procter charged four cents for this package. The fifth prescription was quite typical for the time, calling for the combination of two crude botanicals, American columbo and valerian, with two chemi-

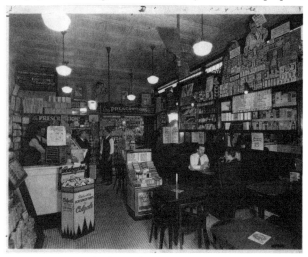

Figure 2.2. An Early Photo of an American Pharmacy Interior.

cals, an iron salt and bicarbonate of soda, and division of the mixture into powder papers. This was probably a stomach tonic. The last prescription called for zinc acetate to be added to a base of cerate of carrot. Procter charged 25 cents for this mildly astringent topical. The relatively high cost probably reflects the time required for preparation.

It is essential to remember that Procter, like most pharmacists of the day, spent more of his time manufacturing preparations than he did compounding or dispensing prescriptions. He made his own syrup of ipecac and syrup of wild cherry, as well as orange flower water and cerate of carrot. At that time, crude drugs, such as columbo and valerian would be bought in bulk and powdered and otherwise processed according to the pharmacopoeia, and pharmacists kept elaborate sets of apothecary jars and bottles filled with tinctures, syrups, extracts, and other preparations made on the premises. Pharmacists and their apprentices spent long hours powdering and sifting plant parts and percolating, macerating, filtering, and bottling preparations. Many preparations were produced in bulk for physicians to use in the office or from their bags. Much of the occupational identity of pharmacists was wrapped up in this special activity that separated them from other retailers. However, like the hat makers, tailors, and other shop owners nearby, pharmacists gained much of their recognition from the oven skills they had learned over years of practice.

While prescription business continued to grow, patent medicines kept most pharmacies in business. Extremely popular since Colonial days, these secret remedies usually contained alcohol and either laxative ingredients or opiates and were not the largely ineffectual nostrums of later years. In contrast with other goods, patent medicines were traditionally marked up at 100 percent, which made them very popular with shop owners.

Opiates and laxatives were also popular in compounded prescriptions. Among the most common drugs in prescriptions were mercury or its salts, opium or morphine, hyoscyamus, ipecacuanha, china rhubarb, iodine, antimony, quinine, lead, and squill. The most common dosage forms were solutions, mixtures, and powder papers, followed by pills, plasters, and ointments.

Almost all of the common drugs, even South American drugs like cinchona bark, were imported from Europe. Pharmacists purchased them in bulk from wholesale druggists and examined them carefully for adulteration. Adulteration was usually benign and common examples included bullets added to bulk opium and sawdust mixed into a sack of powdered root or bark. In the 1840's, a new problem grew in importance and led eventually to a significant professional development—the founding of the American Pharmaceutical Association.

Drug Law of 1848

In the 1830's, drug exporters in Europe came upon a new way to make a little extra profit. Crude drugs like cinchona bark were soaked in a solvent to draw out some of the active alkaloid, then carefully dried and packaged as sound crude drug. The solvent would then be processed and the alkaloid extracted, resulting in a double profit for the exporter.

In the 1840's, European authorities started to crack down on this practice, so drug exporters began shipping the spent crudes to the United States. Some of these packages were marked "good enough for America." It is important to realize that the medicines of the nineteenth century truly worked on the body—they tended to be strong laxatives, emetics, or diaphoretics. Although pure crystalline alkaloids were often available, conservative American physicians preferred the old botanical "purges, pukes, and sweats" of the old school of medical treatment. When the quality of botanical supplies began to fall, physicians soon noticed that their prescriptions were not working as well.

The decline in the quality of imported drugs led to the passage of the Drug Importation Act of 1848. This early federal law governing drug quality was initially a success and thousands of pounds of drugs were rejected at major ports. However, a change in administrations in 1849 brought in a group of political cronies as drug inspectors. The situation became worse than it had been before the passage of the law and so physicians and pharmacists called for more precise standards.

Most botanical drugs had no recognized standard of potency. For example, crude opium was generally expected to be at least 8% morphine, but this was only an informal standard. To facilitate the enforcement of drug purity laws, the College of Pharmacy of the City of New York called in 1851 for a national convention of pharmacists to draw up standards for the most popular imported drugs.

Summary of Pre-Professional Period

This call for a national convention of pharmaceutists marks the end of the proto-professional period. Pharmacy had at last achieved sufficient professional identity to allow for an assembly of apothecaries, pharmaceutists, and druggists to meet a national need. While a wide variety of social, economic, political, and scientific forces had molded the American drugstore during the proto-professional period, by the end of the 1840's it had developed the form and function that it would hold for the next century. When they met in New York in 1851, pharmacists stood on the verge of a new era.

First Period of Professionalization (1850 to 1910): The Drugstore Era

A key figure in the professionalization of American pharmacy was William Procter, Jr. Space does not permit a long discourse on his achievements, but no one has challenged his title as Father of American Pharmacy. This chapter will focus on a few of his accomplishments, which serve as important markers of pharmacy's progress.

In 1846, Procter became the first professor of practical pharmacy at the Philadelphia College of Pharmacy. The College had been teaching young pharmacists for a generation, but had never had a professor of pharmacy. Students had been taught the subjects of Materia Medica (natural history of drugs) and chemistry by two physician professors. Pharmacy was not deemed to be an academic subject and was relegated to the apprenticeship experience. Procter and a few of his young colleagues petitioned the college's board, which agreed with their arguments that pharmacy had progressed to the stature of a scientific discipline and appointed Procter to the professorship.

The professorship enabled Procter to enter the inner circle at the College. Most significantly, he joined the publishing committee of the College's periodical, the *American Journal of Pharmacy*. As the only journal of pharmacy in the United States, it exerted a great deal of influence over the young profession. Procter rose through the ranks, becoming editor in 1850. Procter's emergence as the first permanent pharmacist editor was indicative of the control pharmacists were taking over their occupation. They no longer needed physicians to run their schools and journals.

Founding of the American Pharmaceutical Association

When the New York College of Pharmacy called for its national convention in 1851, Procter and his Philadelphia friend and colleague Edward Parrish decided to go to New York to pursue a novel idea. They wanted the convention to achieve its original goal—the establishment of standards for imported drugs—but they also wanted the convention to go further and form a national pharmaceutical organization.

Procter and Parrish's call for a national organization was well received in New York, and a second national convention was called for Philadelphia in 1852. Using his position as editor of the *American Journal of Pharmacy*, Procter encouraged participation from all parts of the young nation. The time was ripe for such an organization. Rail and telegraph lines reached out across the countryside and on an intellectual and scientific level, if not a political one, the united states were becoming one nation.

The 1852 convention established a national organization, the American Pharmaceutical Association (APhA). For most of its history, APhA has counted only a small minority of pharmacists in its membership, but has exerted great influence on professional development. The founding of APhA came at an opportune time, when pharmacy needed a voice of leadership.

United States Census figures for druggists and apothecaries show that as the 1850's progressed, the growth of American pharmacy accelerated. From 1850 to 1860, the number of physicians per capita did not change significantly, rising from 1:572 to 1:576, while the number of druggists rose from 1:3778 to 1:2850—an increase of nearly 25%. This trend continued, at a slightly lower rate, through the rest of the nineteenth century.

A major cause of this trend was the entry of large-scale manufacturing into pharmacy in the late 1850's. With large firms doing much of the complicated work, less skilled men, who had recently been "mere shopkeepers," entered the ranks of pharmacists. Physicians, already disturbed by counter prescribing, saw pharmacy declining. As one physician put it in 1860, "It is an admitted and lamentable fact that many of those now practicing pharmacy are totally incompetent to fulfill the responsibilities of the true apothecary. They know nothing of the science of preparing medicines." The late 1850's also was a time of great economic strife, which increased the tension between physicians and pharmacists.

With the beginning of the Civil War, American pharmacy and medicine communities ceased their battles and called a truce. Business in the cities slowed to a crawl during the war and many pharmacists lost their stores. The war, of course, greatly helped the manufacturers of medicines, who sold huge quantities to the armed forces. Some of the far-sighted firms like Squibb reinvested their profits into new equipment and expansion during the post-war period.

The Classic Drugstore (and Soda Fountain)

The years following the Civil War were witness to the redesign of the American drugstore into its classic form. The work table, which had always been near the front of the shop to benefit from natural light through the front window and to attract customer attention, was moved to the rear of the store, where the laboratory had previously been, and was hidden behind a screen. The preparations necessary for compounding prescriptions were now made outside the pharmacy, so an extensive laboratory was no longer needed.

In part, these changes mirrored a trend followed by all retail specialty shops that had at one time featured in-shop manufacturing. Remote manufacturing—which took advantage of economies of scale and sweatshop labor—replaced the out-front style of the antebellum stores. The new arrangement was thought to be more elegant. In the case of pharmacy, it also added a bit of mystery to what the pharmacist did. However, the actual work of the pharmacist was becoming simpler as large manufacturers started to put out finished dosage forms in addition to ingredients for prescriptions.

Of course, moving the prescription department to the back of the store opened up the front for the sale of tobacco, fancy goods, and, best of all, soda fountain specialties. Nothing attracted more business to a pharmacy than a soda fountain. Soda water first entered American pharmacies early in the century, but became popular in the post-Civil War years. Pharmacists possessed the chemical knowledge necessary to handle the early carbonated water generators, which were cranky at best. They also had the knack for making fresh flavorings and mixing up complicated confections.

Another factor in the success of the soda fountain was the rise of the temperance and prohibition movements. Pharmacists were seen as solid members of the middle class and their promotion of carbonated beverages was viewed as a support for the major family values cause of that era. By 1929, almost 60% of American drugstores had a soda fountain. Along with the soda fountain, drugstores of the 1870's added tobacco, candy, and magazines to their offerings. The corner druggist, the man who could mix up a chocolate soda or a good cough syrup, was now established as part of American life.

Physician and Public Outcry

After the Civil War, relations between physicians and pharmacists were bumpy. The truce that existed during the war held briefly, but soon physicians discovered that pharmacists made excellent scapegoats for the failings of their therapeutics. This was particularly true in cases of poisoning. While many problems could be traced back to physicians, the low level of general competency among pharmacists had indeed led to cases of patients dying from poisonous prescriptions. Additionally, accidental poisonings, usually from rat bait, had been a problem in pharmacies for decades. To cope with these problems, journalists and some physician groups called for poison-control laws, which usually included some serious regulation of pharmacy practices.

A Professional Response

In response to the drive for regulation of pharmacy practice, APhA empowered a committee, headed by John Maisch, to draw up a model state pharmacy act. In acquiescence to the ambivalent attitude of many pharmacists toward legal regulation, the association published and distributed the model act to all state legislatures without endorsement. As small businessmen, most pharmacists did not want outside restriction of their trade.

During the 1870's, state legislatures began considering in earnest pharmacy bills sponsored by non-pharmacists. In response to this trend, pharmacists in many states organized statewide associations to coordinate support for their own bills, which were usually versions of the APhA model. Although not enthusiastic about regulation of their businesses, pharmacists wanted a voice in the process.

Most of the laws that were finally enacted called for the establishment of state boards of pharmacy, composed of leading pharmacists appointed by a state authority, to judge which pharmacists were competent to practice. These boards mailed elegant licenses to established practitioners and set up examinations to test newcomers. Laws usually called for three to four years of apprenticeship before licensure. No states required any formal pharmaceutical education.

The more ambitious state associations followed up their work for the passage of a state act and establishment of a board of pharmacy with efforts to get state support for a school of pharmacy. If a state university existed, legislatures would often set up a school simply by authorizing a professor of pharmacy. This one-man department would draw on other university faculty members to provide instruction in a full range of subjects—chemistry, botany, geology, and physics.

Paper Credentials and Models of Professionalism

Despite their humble beginnings, these state schools of pharmacy played an important role in the development of pharmacy as a recognized profession. Before the Civil War, perhaps only one in twenty American pharmacists had finished formal schooling in pharmacy, and that consisted of night courses to supplement apprenticeship training. However, by the 1870's professional credentialing was becoming quite popular in the United States and pharmacists saw clear advantages to basing their claims of status on diplomas and licenses. Even though state laws did not require a pharmacy school diploma for licensure until the early twentieth century, the prestige attached to the sheepskin and growing public expectations attracted students to the burgeoning number of schools much earlier.

This new model of professionalism called for the rejection of the old, individualistic model of personal achievement in favor of the modern idea of a "community of the competent" based on paper credentials. For professions like engineering and accounting, this new approach proved successful. Pharmacy, on the other hand, had problems adopting this model completely. Pharmacists were generally extremely conservative and supportive of free enterprise. This new approach was anti-market and so did not gain complete support. Instead, pharmacy adopted the new professionalism in a half-way fashion.

Disagreement over the new professionalism lead to the split that developed within the ranks of APhA. Near the end of the nineteenth century, APhA became dominated by academics, scientists, and the elite of practitioners. They welcomed the new professionalism as a route to greater status within American society. Some of the ordinary members of the association were concerned that the organization was ignoring the great commercial changes going on around them.

The 1890's were hard times for pharmacists, despite the gay nineties stereotype. Department stores were infringing on pharmacy's traditional turf and the first true chain drugstores were popping up. The Commercial Section of APhA grew restless and broke off to form the National Association of Retail Druggists (NARD) in 1898. Relations between the two groups were cordial at first but quickly deteriorated. The members of NARD had retained the old approach to professional advancement—individual achievement—and worked to resist the movement toward more education, more examinations, and more regulation of pharmacy practice. They opposed it for commercial reasons and out of a deeply held belief in the individual and his own drugstore.

This split within pharmacy and the subsequent contentiousness was indicative of the tension between these parallel paths to professional recognition. For most of the next century, this division hindered the profession's climb toward full professional status.

The Drugstore Era in Retrospect

Pharmacy's place in American culture is strongly tied to the vision of the pharmacist as the proprietor of a drugstore. The drugstore itself, that special combination of soda shop, prescription department, and general emporium is something of a cultural icon. The proprietors of drugstores were called druggists by the public, although they preferred the term pharmacist. Apothecary was still retained by a few pretentious shop owners or those who operated a prescription laboratory only.

By the turn of the century, the position of the pharmacist in the American health care system was firmly established. Physicians had agreed to dispense medicines only rarely and pharmacists reciprocated by limiting their diagnosing and prescribing to cases of minor ills and emergencies. The pharmacist was known to be the compounder of prescriptions, although this was not a common occurrence. During the drugstore era, pharmacists no longer needed their laboratories and moved the prescription departments to the back of the stores. There they compounded prescriptions when necessary, although compounding got simpler and less costly as the nineteenth century progressed. For most pharmacists, the prescription department provided only a small fraction of their income and served more as a device to separate them from other retailers.

Although pharmacists gave up their role as primary medical practitioners, they continued to act as secondary providers through the sale of over-the-counter remedies and first-aid items. As general stores and traveling salesmen declined in number, the pharmacist became identified with his role as medical provider.

The drugstore era saw the beginnings of modern professionalism in the passage of state pharmacy laws mandating examinations and licensing. Modern schools of pharmacy, starting with the University of Michigan in 1876, set the stage for scientific advancement and professional development. The path, however, was long, with road blocks set up both by the profession itself and by those within colleges and universities who opposed pharmacy schools.

At the end of the drugstore era, the seeds of great change were already sprouting. Department stores began adding pharmacies in the late 1800's—an experiment that had mixed success, but foreshadowed pharmacies in mass-merchandisers. The 1890's were actually difficult times, but when the new century brought on chain stores, deep price-cutting, and severe competition, the pleasant myth of the gay nineties drugstore, dressed up in all of its finery, became part of the mythos of American pharmacy.

Second Period of Professionalization (1910 to 1965): Educational Reform

During the next half century, pharmacists concentrated on educational reform as the vehicle for professional improvement. The pursuit of professional status charged forward with the pharmacy curriculum as its standard. Just as the old model of the drugstore has lingered on through tremendous changes in science and technology, the belief in increased education as the panacea for all the ills of the American pharmaceutical profession has persisted as well.

New York Law Brings Educational Requirements

In 1905, the state of New York started an important trend by passing a law stating that after 1910, all new registrants in that state would be required to possess a diploma from a recognized school of pharmacy. The minimum course was two years of study. By and large, pharmacists opposed the idea of mandatory formal education. The apprenticeship system, when checked by the state board examinations, seemed to guarantee basic competency. A wide variety of schools were available to those who wanted more education. For example, in 1905 there were over 50 schools offering B.Pharm., Ph.G., or Ph.C. degrees after two years of study; 20 schools offering M.Pharm. and D.Pharm. degrees after three years of study; about a dozen schools offering B.Sc. degrees after four years of study; and four schools offering M.Sc. degrees after five years of study.[6] But since most pharmacists in 1910 had no degree of any sort, this requirement seemed to be just one more example of too much government.

Pharmacy Leadership Seeks Extended Training

In 1915, two events took place which changed many pharmacists' minds about educational requirements and spurred their leaders into action. First, Abraham Flexner, the respected reformer of medical education, declared that pharmacy was not a profession. He argued that although pharmacists did contribute to society through their specialized skill, physicians bore the responsibility for the medicines ordered. Soon after Flexner's shocking assertion, the War Department decided that registered pharmacists, even those who had received bachelor's degrees, would not routinely receive commissions because their professional education was so minimal.[6] Perhaps the War Department had a good point. After the turn of the century, the compounding of prescriptions started its great slide and the work of a pharmacist required less specialized skill than it once did.

To help strengthen their position as professionals, pharmacists turned to the best schools and colleges of pharmacy. This is ironic because it was the efforts of the faculties of these schools that permitted mass manufacturers to take over the art and science of pharmacy. Since the 1850's, a handful of pharmaceutical investigators, such as William Procter, applied science to manufacturing problems. Procter, for instance, spent much of his time perfecting new techniques for extracting active constituents from crude drugs. He developed the process of percolation for the preparation of fluid extracts and similar products. His motivation? To popularize a technique whereby a pharmacist could manufacture his own fluid extracts and eliminate the need to purchase those made by large firms. What happened was just the opposite. Big firms copied Procter's technique on a large scale and eliminated almost any need for the pharmacist to continue doing his own percolating. This pattern would be duplicated again and again for the next 100 years.

The irony here is that as pharmacy professors developed new techniques they insisted that their students learn them. This pattern became even more apparent by the middle of this century. Pharmacy professors asked for more classroom hours to teach their students

about the science and technology manufacturers were using to take away the main rationale for the profession's being—the making of medicines.

Major changes occurred in pharmacy in the years around 1900 with the emergence
of effective synthetic drugs. Out of laboratories in Germany and France came drugs like
aspirin and Salvarsan. Aspirin and other antiinflammatories had an immense impact on
medicine, giving physicians safe drugs to use against fever, the dominant symptom of
acute infectious diseases. The advances in pharmacology had influenced therapeutics by
the turn of the century. Physicians stopped writing prescriptions containing many ingredients, hoping one would work. Instead, the new prescriptions usually called for simple
mixtures of one or two ingredients. Moreover, the new drugs were usually potent crystalline chemicals that were well suited for tabletting, a finished dosage form perfect for mass
production.[7]

Prohibition and Soda Fountains

Even if pharmacists in the 1920's spent less time compounding prescriptions, they had
plenty to do. In 1919, the eighteenth Amendment to the Constitution prohibited the sale
of alcoholic beverages in the United States. The corrupting influences of this failed social
experiment are well known, and they extended to pharmacy.

Since beverage alcohols, such as whiskey, were officially recognized as drugs in the
United States Pharmacopoeia, pharmacies could legally sell them on prescription. This
practice was abused and strict regulations using special prescription blanks were imposed.
However, even the most honest pharmacists were tainted by this business and pharmacists became the butt of numerous jokes and the subject of many tall tales about liquor.

With taverns closed, the soda fountain business boomed. Many drugstores became
little more than soda shops with some old dusty bottles in the back filled with tinctures
and fluid extracts. The popularity of druggists may have hit an all-time high during the
Prohibition years, but it is doubtful that they gained any respect.

During the fabulous growth of the 1920's, educators worked hard to repair the damage
inflicted on their profession by Flexner and the War Department. In meetings of the American Conference of Pharmaceutical Faculties, later called the American Association of Colleges of Pharmacy (AACP), educators decided to seek more stringent educational requirements for pharmacists. In 1923, a requirement of four years of high school study was imposed for admission to AACP member schools. In 1925, the two-year Ph.G. courses were
eliminated and a three-year minimum installed. Ohio State University required the four-
year bachelor's degree in 1925 and was followed by Minnesota and a few other brave institutions in 1927. In 1928, the association adopted the four-year bachelor of science degree as
the minimum course of study, although this requirement did not go into effect until 1932.

The objective of this effort was to convince the public (and physicians) that pharmacists were well educated, cultured, professional men. This change came at a fortunate
time. In contrast with the 1890's, the 1920's were years of unprecedented prosperity.
Times were good in pharmacy, which encouraged educational reform.

The Great Depression and Repeal

Those who rushed into pharmacy schools in the late 1920's to beat the B.Sc. requirement came out to find no jobs as the Great Depression deepened. For those who had

established stores, however, the Depression was less trying than it was for many other shopkeepers. People still got sick and needed medicines, the soda fountain attracted those with some money, and, no matter how bad things got, people still bought cigarettes.

In 1933, during the darkest days of the Depression, the twenty-first Amendment to the Constitution was passed and Prohibition was repealed. People headed to the bars and the soda fountain business started to decline. However, something made up for the loss of soda sales. When Prohibition ended, pharmacies had cases of liquor and the licenses to sell it. For better or worse, alcohol sales became a boon to drugstores in the 1930's as the public connected liquor with the place where it was dispensed legally during Prohibition. It is depressing indeed to report that many drugstores in the 1930's survived by selling booze, cigarettes, and chocolate sodas.

The 1930's also brought changes to the store itself. The gradual trend toward self service, which had begun in earnest in the 1920's, continued in the 1930's. By the late 1930's, when the economy had improved, drugstores carried more costly goods—expensive perfumes and, as mentioned, liquor. Store owners opened up the design of their shops so that they could see the entire floor easily from the prescription department in back. The basic store layout featured an elevated prescription department. From a step up, the pharmacist could look down with authority on the customer. In spite of this elevation, the special art of the pharmacist—compounding medicines—was rapidly disappearing as prefabricated dosage forms flooded the market.[6]

Status of Pharmacists in World War II

As the nation stood on the verge of World War II, the leaders among pharmacists were confident. For nearly ten years, the bachelor's degree requirement had been in effect, raising the standards of the profession. Internally, the profession was undergoing dynamic growth. New organizations—the American College of Apothecaries, the American Institute of the History of Pharmacy, and the American Society of Hospital Pharmacists—were founded during this time of optimism and high ideals.

Again, however, the United States government decided that pharmacists were not to be routinely given commissions in the military. The decision was especially galling since nurses were being commissioned as second lieutenants by the thousands, even though they had less training. Even freshman medical students were commissioned as ensigns in the Navy. However, the Division of Scientific and Technical Personnel of the War Emergency Advisory Committee had concluded that pharmacists were not generally recognized as professionals. The commercialism connected with pharmacy practice seemed to make their expanded training and education secondary.

Moreover, there was no reason to offer pharmacists a special incentive to join the military. All the pharmacists needed could be obtained through the draft because the nation had an overabundance of pharmacists. In 1940, the nation had a population of about 130 million and about 115,000 registered pharmacists working in some 58,000 stores. Today, about 170,000 pharmacists and about the same number of community pharmacies serve a population of 250 million, nearly double the population in 1940. Physicians and dentists, who were needed in much greater numbers in the war effort, continued to receive commissions.[6]

Pharmaceutical Survey and the Five-Year Program

Stimulated by the decision of the Advisory Committee and opinion surveys that indicated a low regard for pharmacists, the pharmacy profession decided that a major self-study was in order. On 15 April 1946, the Pharmaceutical Survey was inaugurated. This joint effort of all major pharmacy organizations and the American Council on Education was the most complete study of an occupation ever undertaken. Nearly every aspect of pharmacy was scrutinized, including education, legal controls, organizations, student recruitment, the content of prescriptions, state boards, licensing, and postgraduate education.

Looking back over the results of the survey in 1951, Director Edward C. Elliott commented on pharmacy's uncertain future:

Whether pharmacy is to be able to have and to hold a real professional status, or whether it is to become stabilized, in most of its practice, as one of the subordinate technological occupations of modern civilization, may be considered debatable questions. The developments of the past generation have tended to make pharmacy a dependent enterprise.

Mass manufacture of medicinals has caused the practicing pharmacist to serve more and more as a mere distributor. Furthermore, and for the most part, pharmacy endeavors to fulfill its traditional, as well as its ever-broadening, responsibilities amidst an expanding jungle of commerce. . . . Here are problems of fundamental importance. Unsolved, they are hazards to any future good fortune of the profession.[6]

The survey made recommendations for change in eleven different areas, but the most substantial and controversial changes were those suggested for the pharmacy curriculum. In the words of the General Report of 1949, "It is recommended that the American Association of Colleges of Pharmacy and the American Council on Pharmaceutical Education take the necessary initial steps for the development and establishment of a six-year program of education and training leading to the professional degree of Doctor of Pharmacy, this program to include two or more years of general education and basic science training."[8]

The General Report also encouraged improvements in the four-year program. In 1950, the University of Southern California started the first two-to-four Pharm.D. program, but outside of California this seemed too radical. With the four-year program appearing too conservative, the five-year compromise, already in place at Ohio State in 1948, seemed attractive. In 1954, the AACP recommended the general adoption of the five-year program, beginning with the entering class of 1960.

It is important to realize that when the Pharm.D. debate began in the 1950's, it occurred in the context of broadening the education of the future pharmacist. Much of the attraction of the professional doctorate was the added opportunity for more general or liberal education. Pharmacists who followed this new course of study would be well educated and thereby worthy of the respect of other professionals and of the public.

Economic Growth and the Changing Marketplace

While educators debated about the future of the profession, great changes were taking place among practicing pharmacists. The 1950's were boom times, with new, effective drugs on the market. New antibiotics such as tetracycline (1950) and erythromycin (1952) joined the penicillins. Other new drugs of note included warfarin (1954), brompheniramine

(1957), chlorpromazine (1954), methotrexate (1955), reserpine (1953), dextromethorphan (1954), tolbutamide (1957), hydrochlorothiazide (1959), hydrocortisone (1952), imipramine (1959), and griseofulvin (1959). Post-war pharmacists were dispensing tablets and capsules which actually cured diseases, rather than just ameliorating symptoms.

The number of prescriptions filled went up over 50%, during the 1950's, transforming the prescription department into the economic engine of the drugstore. A relatively stable number of pharmacists worked harder and faster. In the post-war era, suburbia boomed and so did the chains. By concentrating their stores in newer, growing areas of population, chains came to dominate community pharmacy in both urban and suburban areas.

This was the era of "count and pour" pharmacy. Pharmacists were restricted to machine-like tasks. The 1952 Durham–Humphrey amendment to the Food, Drug, and Cosmetic Act had removed much of the pharmacist's autonomy in practice and the APhA Code of Ethics made the pharmacist's limited role quite clear.

"The pharmacist does not discuss the therapeutic effects or composition of a prescription with a patient. When such questions are asked, he suggests that the qualified practitioner [that is, a physician or dentist] is the proper person with whom such matters should be discussed."[8]

Pharmacists gained respect from their connection with the new, effective drugs coming on the market, but their new reputation came at the cost of being considered over-educated for a diminished professional function. The pharmacy curriculum had continued to emphasize the physical sciences that underlie the making of medicines, even though compounding was disappearing from practice.[9] The prevalence of this conservative approach to pharmacy education is illustrated by the first sentence of Remington's *Practice of Pharmacy*—"Pharmacy is the science which treats of medicinal substances"—which had not changed in two-thirds of a century.[10] The description of the profession's scope in the 1956 edition indicated no significant expansion from the mid-1800's and did not mention the loss of some responsibilities.

Failure of Academic Reform Movement

In retrospect, it is clear that the period of academic reform solidified the place of pharmacy within academia without greatly elevating the position of the pharmacist within the health care system or society at large. The argument has been made that pharmacists of the 1950s were too concerned with products and not enough with patients. Instead, it may be more useful to view the supposed product orientation of the post-war era as a result of the overall calcification of the role of pharmacists. Professional leaders sought peace with physicians, and educators strived for recognition from their peers. Practitioners of pharmacy, a majority of whom were independent store owners, concentrated on the business side of their practice in the face of the chain store threat. The professional opportunities available to pharmacists were extremely limited by state and federal laws and by the customs of the physician–pharmacist–patient relationship that had evolved over the previous 100 years. Pharmacists concentrated on overall service to the customer because their other opportunities were so limited.

Attempts to use a more extensive pharmacy school curriculum to elevate the stature of pharmacy failed because in spite of the increased amount of time students spent in school, students were too busy studying advances in industry to get a well-rounded education. It was general education that was to transform pharmacists into "educated men." The irony is that pharmacy students of the 1950's and 1960's spent longer and longer hours learning the scientific basis of the techniques industry used to eliminate compounding, a large part of the traditional raison d'être of pharmacy practice.

The end result was that educational reform did not raise the stature of pharmacists within the structure of the health care system or within society at large. Pharmacists learned all the steps necessary for manufacturing medicines but found their practice reduced to counting and pouring. They came out of pharmacy schools tired, with their heads full of unusable information, and with no more general education than graduates of technical schools.

Third Period of Professionalization (1965 to 1990): Changing Practitioners

The decade of the 1960's was a period of turmoil for American society. The civil rights and anti-war movements shook the social order and new rules of thinking and behavior replaced the old. So it went for pharmacy as well. "Clinical pharmacy" was the rallying cry for pharmacy's revolutionaries, who were just as uncertain of what their revolution's results would be as the marchers in the streets.

Rather than a revolution, the clinical pharmacy era (1965–1990) is better seen as a transitional period in professional development. Pharmacists steeped in knowledge about drugs stepped out of the shackles of count-and-pour practice and asserted themselves as drug information experts. As much as any other 60's movement, clinical pharmacy grew out of the actions of the grass roots (i.e., practicing pharmacists).

The major clinical pharmacy concepts and innovations came from institutional pharmacists. From the nineteenth century up into the mid-twentieth century, hospital pharmacists had low status within pharmacy. In the 1800's, they were viewed as marginally competent individuals who did not have the strength of character to run a store. During the first decades of the twentieth century, they were still on the fringe of pharmacy.

The special nature of their practice, however, caused hospital pharmacists to band together in organizations from the 1920's on. They practiced manufacturing and compounding pharmacy long after it disappeared from drugstores. As their group identity solidified and organizational numbers reached a critical mass, these groups began to work together. In Denver in 1942 the American Society of Hospital Pharmacists was founded.

In the unique setting of the hospital, pharmacists in the 1940's and 1950's gained more control over the rising number of new drugs and products. Pharmacy and Therapeutics (P & T) committees and hospital formularies brought pharmacists into the therapeutic side of practice. By the mid-1960's, this involvement increased to the point where Donald Brodie could state:

> The ultimate goal of the services of pharmacy must be the safe use of drugs by the public. In this context, the mainstream function of pharmacy is clinical in nature, one that may be identified accurately as drug-use control.[11]

By "drug-use control" Brodie meant "the sum total of knowledge, understanding, judgements, procedures, skills, controls and ethics that assures optimal safety in the distribution and use of medication."[11]

This approach was adopted by programs like the famous ninth floor project of the University of California–San Francisco Medical Center. This project, initiated in 1966, utilized several of the basic components of later practice, including unit doses, pharmacy technicians, a drug information center, and patient drug profiles. As clinical pharmacy demonstrated its utility, hospitals added more staff pharmacists to facilitate greater drug-use control. During the 1970's and 1980's, the number of pharmacists in institutional practice more than doubled to about 40,000, or nearly one-quarter of all practitioners.[12]

In community pharmacy, the shift to clinical practice started about the same time, but the burdens of business and the distance from the clinical milieu made the transition slower and more difficult. In 1960, Eugene V. White of Berryville, Virginia, started using patient profile cards. Soon afterward he totally remodeled his store into an office-style practice. While few community pharmacists followed White's example completely, many did see a new avenue for professional growth.

A great and gradual paradigm shift had begun in community pharmacy. The person who stood across the counter from the pharmacist was undergoing a transformation from "the customer" into "the patient." After 150 years of caring about the wants of customers, pharmacists were caring about the needs of patients.

A few progressive schools of pharmacy quickly adapted to the new concept, adding a few courses in clinical therapeutics to their already full curricula. The 1970's was a difficult decade for pharmacy education as schools opened their doors to hundreds of part-time practitioner instructors who put more and more time demands on the tight five-year curriculum. Some schools opted for six-year Pharm.D. programs, while others cut back some on laboratory courses and all but eliminated general education to include clerkship experience in their five-year programs.

The rapid change at the leadership level of pharmacy is also demonstrated in the 1969 revision of the APhA Code of Ethics. The old 1952 code admonished pharmacists not to inform patients about their drugs. The new code began, "A pharmacist should hold the health and safety of patients to be of first consideration; he should render to each patient the full measure of his ability as an essential health practitioner."[13]

During the 1970's, graduates of pharmacy schools entered a health care environment relatively hostile to clinical pharmacy. Clinical pharmacy was dismissed as too expensive and time consuming, but the need for clinical skills was manifest. The huge therapeutic advances and the burgeoning drug industry of the 1960's forced pharmacists more and more into decision-making roles. As a profession, pharmacy moved slowly into providing drug information and counseling to patients.

Transition occurred in the 1970's and 1980's, in large part because pharmacy educators, who initially lagged behind practitioners as advocates of clinical practice, saw the prospects for the future. Clinical pharmacy restored meaning to their teaching. Rather than just supporting their own scientific disciplines, professors turned their teaching toward contemporary practice issues and the challenges of the future. In 1989, the American Council on Pharmaceutical Education (ACPE) shook the pharmacy establishment in the United States when it proposed that future standards would only accredit Pharm.D. programs. A paradigm shift within pharmacy was demonstrated by the statement of support for the entry-level Pharm.D. issued by the American Pharmaceutical Association, the American Society of Health-System Pharmacists, and the National Community Pharmacists Association (then NARD) in 1992.

Other Transitions

Other great transitional changes in pharmacy practice also occurred during the period from the mid-1960's to the 1990's. Health insurance developments in the 1950's and the passage of Medicare and Medicaid legislation in 1965 created a complicated, yet incomplete, system of third-party payment for pharmacy services. Attempts to reform the health care system in the 1990's, most notably by the Clinton administration, failed but did stimulate consolidation throughout the industry. Economic forces also led to the closure of thousands of independent pharmacies.

A most significant transition began in the 1960's as women entered the profession in large numbers. In 1950, only five percent of active pharmacists were women. Today the number is over one-third of all practitioners, and women may hold the majority of pharmacist positions by the year 2015.[14] This is the most rapid professional gender shift in American history. While it is too early to gauge the impact of this trend, some have argued that the feminization of pharmacy may contribute to a short-term workforce shortage.

Pharmacy embraced computerization well in advance of other health professions because of its utility in handling and processing insurance claims. Computers were quickly adapted, to provide a wide variety of information services necessary for the provision of patient care. Meeting the drug utilization review regulations of the Omnibus Budget Reconciliation Act of 1990 (OBRA '90) on a national basis would be impossible without the computerization of pharmacies across the country. In conjunction with computers, high technology applied to dispensing started to remove the last manipulative function from pharmacy practitioners.

At the beginning of the 1960's, pharmacy was truly a "profession in search of a role." Pharmacists had gained a monopoly over the dispensing of prescription drugs but lost much autonomy in their practices after the passage of the Durham–Humphrey Amendment and state anti-substitution laws. Because of the academic reform movement of the early to mid-twentieth century, pharmacy graduates received a long and rigorous training. They were prepared to take on the new challenges of the clinical pharmacy ideal.

The clinical pharmacy era is best characterized as a transitional period between the years of count-and-pour practice and the current era of pharmaceutical care. What changed during this time was not so much what pharmacists knew as how they applied their knowledge. Above all else, pharmacists shared their drug expertise with physicians and with patients. As a movement, clinical pharmacy has its primary roots in institutional practice, ironically the traditional backwater of the profession. In the community setting, customers became patients and pharmacists began to accept, albeit reluctantly, some responsibility for the proper use of drugs. In both settings, pharmacists had begun to care about their patients, even if they were not caring for them.

Fourth Period of Professionalization: Full Responsibility and Societal Recognition

If the futurists in American pharmacy are right, we are at the beginning of a new period in our history, the era of pharmaceutical care. The concept, which grew out of Donald Brodie's drug-use control, may complete the move away from count-and-pour practice in ways that clinical pharmacy could not. Pharmacy educators and leaders, who at first lagged behind practitioners, arrived at this concept after a decade or so of speculation on pharmacy's future.

Several general definitions of pharmaceutical care exist. Because this phase of professional development is young, these definitions tend to be a bit vague and idealistic. Still, when one reads that "pharmaceutical care is the responsible provision of drug therapy for the purpose of achieving definite outcomes that improve a patient's quality of life," the challenge is stimulating.[15]

For the historian, the most significant aspect of the pharmaceutical care movement is its voluntary assumption of responsibility without substantial compensation. Motivated by professional pride and the understanding of the problems associated with drug use, pharmacists are adopting the goals set out by the pharmaceutical care model. It may well be that by taking on the responsibility for the proper use of medicines, pharmacists will achieve the societal recognition as full professionals that they have sought for over 150 years. If so, society will confer this status on pharmacists because of what they accomplish in practice, not because of extended curricula or grandiose titles. The individual achievement approach to professional recognition, set aside for a century, may fulfill the dream that paper credentials could not accomplish alone.

In a sense, pharmacy is returning to a high level of professional responsibility after decades of settling for a secondary role. At the beginning of the 1800's, pharmacists became common in American cities and towns. Their major professional function was to provide drugs and medicines of reliable strength and purity. They used their specialized knowledge of botany, chemistry, and pharmacy in the selection and processing of crude drugs that became the ingredients of the medicines they compounded. In addition, these pharmacists invented the drugstore, that unique part of American culture where health care and retail intermingled. A century and a half later, American pharmacists invented clinical pharmacy. This new approach to practice has brought the profession to the threshold of a new era and, after a century, pharmacists' search for a role has come to the beginning of its end.

References

1. Kremers E, Urdang J. History of pharmacy, 4th ed. Philadelphia, PA: Lippincott; 1976.
2. Society of the New-York Hospital. A brief account of the New-York Hospital. New York: Isaac Collins and Son; 1804.
3. Society of the New-York Hospital. An account of the New-York Hospital. New York: Collins & Co.; 1811.
4. Society of the New-York Hospital. By-laws and regulations ordained and established by the governors of the New-York Hospital. New York: Mahlon Day; 1820.
5. Pharmacopoeia of the United States of America. 2nd ed. Boston: Publisher; 1928.
6. Mrtek RG. Pharmaceutical education in these United States—an interpretive historical essay of the twentieth century. *Am J Pharm Ed.* 1976; 40:341.

7. Gathercoal EN. The prescription ingredient survey. Washington, DC: American Pharmaceutical Association; 1933.

8. Elliott EC. The general report of the pharmaceutical survey: 1946-49. Washington: American Council on Education; 1950.

9. Higby GJ. Evolution of pharmacy. In: Genaro AR, ed. Remington's pharmaceutical sciences. Easton, PA: Mack; 1990.

10. Martin E, Cook EF, eds. Remington's practice of pharmacy. Easton, PA: Mack Publishing; 1956.

11. Brodie DC, Benson RA. The evolution of the clinical pharmacy concept. *Drug Intell Clin Pharm.* 1976; 10:507.

12. Pharmacy Manpower Project. Ann Arbor, MI: Vector Research; 1993.

13. Buerki RA, Vottero LV. Ethical responsibility in pharmacy practice. Madison, WI: American Institute of the History of Pharmacy; 1994.

14. Seventh report to the President and Congress on the status of health personnel in the United States. Washington, DC: U.S. Government Printing Office; 1990.

15. Hepler CD, Strand LM. Opportunities and responsibilities in pharmaceutical care. *Am J Pharm Ed.* 1989; 53:12S.

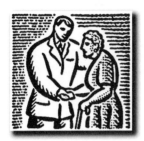

Chapter 3: Role of Pharmacy Organizations in Transforming the Profession: The Case of Pharmaceutical Care

William A. Zellmer, M.P.H.

Presented as part of a symposium on A Decade of Pharmaceutical Care, March 19, 2001, sponsored by the American Institute of the History of Pharmacy, at the annual meeting of the American Pharmaceutical Association, San Francisco, California.

This paper has also been published in Pharmacy in History, *#3, 2001, and the* American Journal of Health-System Pharmacy, *November 1, 2001.*

To what extent, and at what pace, can a professional organization influence change in the practice of pharmacy? In the framework of the "diffusion of innovations" model of Everett Rogers,[1] can a pharmacy association be an effective, forceful change agent? These are the underlying questions addressed in this chapter, using pharmaceutical care as a case study.

Research on the diffusion of innovations shows that (1) the time it takes for innovations to be adopted varies but the overall pattern of adoption is predictable, innovation to innovation; (2) the adoption process moves through distinct phases; and (3) different characteristics apply to categories of adopters based on how quickly they accept and implement an innovation.[1] Hence, we can expect that if, some years from now, the adoption of the pharmaceutical care practice model is plotted, it will resemble **Figure 3.1.**

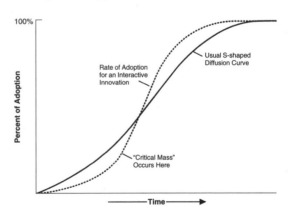

Figure 3.1. Typical Patterns of Adoption of Innovations. (Reprinted with permission of The Free Press, a Division of Simon & Schuster, Inc., from Diffusion of Innovations, 4th ed. by Everett M. Rogers. Copyright © 1995 by Everett M. Rogers. Copyright © 1962, 1971, 1983 by The Free Press.)

Change agents have an important role in fostering the adoption of innovations. Rogers[2] has said that the typical sequence of the change agent's role looks like this:

1. Develop the need for change.

2. Establish an information exchange relationship with the client.

3. Diagnose the problems of the client.

4. Create intent to change in the client.

5. Translate intent into action.

6. Stabilize adoption and prevent discontinuances.

7. Move toward a terminal relationship (client self-sufficiency).

This list describes reasonably well what several national pharmacy organizations have been trying to do with respect to fostering the adoption of pharmaceutical care. Simply stated, the goal of these groups is to shift the focus of the pharmacist in frontline practice from one practice model to another. The old model is "dispensing a drug product accurately to a patient." The new model is "helping a patient make the best use of medicines."

In exploring how well pharmacy organizations are doing in fostering this transformation, we must keep in mind the tremendous complexity of the situation. Both the *status* of pharmacy practice at any point in time, and the *direction of change* over time, are the result of the interplay of many forces within a very complex system. In the United States, few if any of these forces are under the direct control of pharmacy organizations. Many of the forces can certainly be influenced by pharmacy groups, but often only indirectly or weakly. Moreover, the most important factors affecting the practice focus of the pharmacist are not necessarily the same factors over which pharmacy organizations have the greatest influence (**Figure 3.2**).

This chapter looks primarily at the work of only four entities, namely, the Joint Commission of Pharmacy Practitioners (JCPP), the American Association of Colleges of Pharmacy (AACP),[a] the American Pharmaceutical Association (APhA),[b] and the American Society of Health-System Pharmacists (ASHP). Also included are collaborative ef-

Rank Order, Power (Importance) of Factors on Pharmacist Practice Focus	Rank Order, Factors by Susceptibility to Influence by Pharmacy Organizations
1. Desire of practitioners	1. Pharmacy education
2. Health care financing	2. Laws
3. Consumer expectations	3. Desire of practitioners
4. Pharmacy education	4. Consumer expectations
5. Physician expectations	5. Physician expectations
6. Laws	6. Health care financing
7. Pharmaceutical marketing	7. Pharmaceutical marketing

(Based on observations and opinions of author.)

Figure 3.2. Factors that Affect the Practice Focus of the Pharmacist, Ranked by Power (Importance) of the Factor (left) and by the Factor's Susceptibility to Influence by Pharmacy Organizations (right). The most important factors affecting the practice focus of the pharmacist are not necessarily the same factors over which pharmacy organizations have the greatest influence.

forts by these groups, many of which involved other organizations. Many more pharmacy organizations, at both the national and state levels, have been doing excellent work on this issue, but it is impractical to mention all of them here.

1985 Hilton Head Conference

To most of the world of pharmacy, the October 1989 "Pharmacy in the 21st Century" conference was the seminal event in the pharmaceutical care movement. It was there that C. Douglas Hepler presented the paper he co-authored with Linda Strand entitled, "Opportunities and Responsibilities in Pharmaceutical Care." However, pharmacists who have been members of ASHP for 15 years or more tend to go back a bit farther, to the 1985 ASHP Hilton Head Conference, which convened in Hilton Head, South Carolina, to assess the progress of the clinical pharmacy movement and to make plans for continuing to advance clinical practice.[3] Something far more significant than that came out of Hilton Head, namely, a recognition that pharmacy as a whole is inherently a clinical profession, and that it does not serve patients well to operationalize clinical pharmacy as an appendage to the profession as opposed to the basic thrust of the profession.

Dr. Hepler was one of the keynote lecturers at Hilton Head, speaking on "Pharmacy as a Clinical Profession." He addressed the nature of professions and the covenantal character of professional service. The following excerpt from Dr. Hepler's Hilton Head address demonstrates the linkage of what he said there with what followed in 1989:

> I believe it is essential that the pharmacy profession have goals that focus upon outcomes [that result from] serving the drug-related needs of society. If pharmacy is to serve as the primary force in society for the safe and appropriate use of drugs, then we must commit ourselves to that goal.[4]

ASHP leaders spoke and wrote extensively about the ideas from the Hilton Head conference, and the Society's Foundation funded a number of parallel state and regional programs. This stimulated widespread reexamination by hospital pharmacists of their professional mission and the creation of overt plans to transform their departments into a clinical enterprise.[5]

Joint Commission of Pharmacy Practitioners

The Hilton Head conference set the stage for inviting Dr. Hepler to address the 1989 Pharmacy in the 21st Century conference sponsored by JCPP. This was the second in a series of invitational "P21" pharmacy strategic planning conferences.[6] The first convened five years earlier through the leadership of Jerome Halperin, who at the time was an official with the Food and Drug Administration.[7] The first conference was funded by professional and trade organizations in pharmacy and the pharmaceutical industry and included participation by representatives of all the national pharmacy-related organizations. JCPP subsequently assumed responsibility for planning and funding another conference in the spirit of the 1984 program. A conference of this nature has been conducted every five years since under JCPP's leadership.

JCPP, created in 1977, is a federation of national pharmacist organizations[c] with liaison membership by other pharmacy groups such as AACP. On a quarterly schedule, the chief executive officers and the elected presidents of these organizations meet in the Washington, DC, area to examine current issues facing the profession and explore if they wish to collaborate on any issues. When it comes to taking on a project such as planning and conducting the P21 conferences, typically staff members of the constituent organizations form a committee to get the job done.

This is an important detail because when it came time to ask, "How should we keep alive the ideas presented and the areas of consensus developed at the 1989 P21 program?" a mechanism existed for that to occur through the staff committee that had planned the conference. This staff committee continued to meet after the conference to discuss the implications of pharmaceutical care and what could be done collectively through JCPP or by individual organizations to foster implementation of the concept.

Stimulated by the great enthusiasm at the conference for the pharmaceutical care philosophy, JCPP drafted a "provisional draft mission statement for pharmacy practice" that was published in a number of pharmacy periodicals in the summer of 1991 with an invitation to comment.[8,9] Supported by one page of background information, the mission statement itself was only one sentence long; it said: "The mission of pharmacy practice is to help people make the best use of medications." JCPP's review of the several comments that were generated from practitioners did not result in any significant changes. It then fell to individual organizations to carry the mission statement forward.

It is worth emphasizing again the key role of the staff planning committee for the 1989 P21 conference.[d] These individuals were pharmacists responsible for the practice development programs of the national pharmacist organizations. They labored over putting together an influential program and exceeded their expectations. They worked together well and were able to focus on advancement of the profession while transcending the sometimes narrow-minded self-interests of individual organizations that have been known to spoil similar attempts at collaborative work. They served as vectors, carrying the infectious enthusiasm from the P21 program into their separate organizations. It is because of their efforts that the outer reaches of pharmacy in the United States began to hear about pharmaceutical care shortly after October 1989, and those conversations are still going on today.

When it came time to plan the 1994 P21 conference—the third in the series—it was natural to focus on how to actualize the pharmaceutical care philosophy, or, as the program stated, to conduct "a conference dedicated to understanding and overcoming the obstacles to delivering pharmaceutical care." This conference analyzed the barriers to implementing pharmaceutical care in four areas of practice—ambulatory care and community pharmacy; acute care and institutional practice; long-term care and chronic care; and managed care. Strategies were identified for overcoming the barriers in each sector of practice at three levels of responsibility—individual practitioners, businesses or organizations that employ pharmacists, and pharmacy associations.[10]

The 1994 P21 conference deepened the profession's understanding of what is required to make pharmaceutical care reality. Although JCPP systematically examined the collective recommendations of the 131 participants, it was left up to the individual member organizations of JCPP and others to put the ideas into play. Although this conference in itself was not a turning point, it performed an important role in getting a large number of opinion leaders from all sectors of the profession to examine the pharmaceutical care philosophy in the face of the complexities of making change in practice. Likewise, it identified some concrete and feasible changes in practice that would move the field closer to a transformation, and it undoubtedly stimulated many practitioners to begin making those changes.

Official Organizational Support for Pharmaceutical Care

When assessing the role of individual pharmacy organizations in fostering pharmaceutical care, one important indicator is the official policies of the organizations. There is a remarkable story here. Recall that the P21 conference was held in October 1989. In 1990, AACP's House of Delegates endorsed a paper that declared "that the mission of pharmacy practice is to render pharmaceutical care."[11] Reflecting the pharmaceutical care philosophy, APhA adopted a policy in 1991 affirming "that the mission of pharmacy is to serve society as the profession responsible for the appropriate use of medications, devices, and services to achieve optimal therapeutic outcomes."[12] Also in 1991, the ASHP House of Delegates voted unanimously to endorse the concept of pharmaceutical care.[13] Clearly, these national pharmacy organizations were captivated by the promise of the pharmaceutical care concept, and they acted quickly to note as much in their policies.

Multiorganizational Initiatives

Many significant joint organizational efforts over the past decade have advanced the pharmaceutical care philosophy. Seven of them are discussed briefly here.

The *Scope of Pharmacy Practice Project,* 1992–1994, sponsored by AACP, APhA, ASHP, and the National Association of Boards of Pharmacy (NABP), conducted a national task analysis of practicing pharmacists and pharmacy technicians. The pharmaceutical care philosophy, and the functions and tasks of pharmacists in this practice model, served as the framework for the study. The results of the task analysis of pharmacists were used by NABP to revise the national board examination for licensure. APhA and ASHP used the technician results as the basis for beginning to plan for a national certification examination for technicians.

The creation of the *Pharmacy Technician Certification Board* (PTCB) in 1995 is relevant because it was recognized early in the pharmaceutical care movement that expanded use of pharmacy technicians would be necessary to free up pharmacist time for direct patient care activities. In order for pharmacists to feel comfortable in delegating more work to technicians, pharmacists must have confidence in the knowledge, skills, and abilities of these coworkers. Certification of technicians is one important way to build this confidence. PTCB was created jointly by ASHP, APhA, and two state organizations—the Michigan Pharmacists Association and the Illinois Council of Health-System Pharmacists, which previously conducted their own technician certification programs.

During President Bill Clinton's first administration, health care reform was one of the top issues on the national scene, and coverage of prescription drugs and pharmacist services was a priority for pharmacy organizations. On the heels of the 1989 P21 conference, it was natural for pharmacy groups to frame their advocacy in a way that would advance the concept of pharmaceutical care by including in health benefit plans coverage of pharmacists' patient care services. Emerging from this line of thinking was the *Consumer Coalition for Access to Pharmaceutical Care* (CCAPC), consisting of AACP, ACCP, AMCP, APhA, ASCP, ASHP, National Pharmaceutical Association, and National Consumers League. This coalition crafted a strong case for giving pharmacists financial incentives to help patients make the best use of medicines.

After health reform fizzled, the coalition continued for a while to consider, among other issues, how to expand the research base supporting a pharmaceutical care role for the pharmacist. This line of thinking led the coalition to support the work of *Johnson and Bootman* and resulted in their famous paper in 1995 in the *Archives of Internal Medicine*[14] that estimated that for every dollar spent on prescription medications in ambulatory care, another dollar was spent on the direct cost of dealing with adverse drug events (ADEs). Pharmacy organizations then advocated that to the extent to which ADEs are preventable by pharmacists, the health care system has an immense incentive to compensate pharmacists for preventing those problems.

In recent years, 11 national pharmacy organizations, calling themselves the *Alliance for Pharmaceutical Care*,[e] have exhibited at the National Conference of State Legislatures, featuring practicing pharmacists who demonstrate concretely what pharmaceutical care is all about; the exhibit further makes the case for compensating pharmacists for their role in managing drug therapy.

Thirty-eight states have now explicitly sanctioned a role for pharmacists in *collaborative drug therapy management*, either through amendment of the pharmacy practice act or board of pharmacy regulations. This has occurred through advocacy by state pharmacist organizations with support from their national counterparts. The unifying theme of pharmaceutical care made possible this concerted effort, which, long-term, may prove to be the basis for wide-scale compensation of pharmacists as providers of a health care service, not only purveyors of a product.

There are currently several important experiments being conducted around the country for compensating pharmacists for drug therapy management services, notably the Medicaid programs in Mississippi, Wisconsin, and Iowa. In this regard, it must be mentioned that there is a national program to credential pharmacists in disease-specific therapy management, namely, the *National Institute for Standards in Pharmacist Credentialing*, which involves NABP, NACDS, NCPA, and APhA.

American Association of Colleges of Pharmacy

In April 1989, six months before the P21 conference, AACP appointed its Commission to Implement Change in Pharmaceutical Education[11] (Dr. Hepler was a member of the commission). The original purpose of the commission was to examine the future of health care and make recommendations relative to the pharmacy curriculum needed to prepare practitioners for that future. The commission released its first paper ("What is the Mission of Pharmaceutical Education?") the following year.

The commission met for three years. During that time, the profession was engaging in widespread discussion of the pharmaceutical care philosophy. Sensing that pharmaceutical care was being adopted as the new mission of pharmacy practice, the commission set about the task of determining the nature and scope of the curriculum needed to prepare a practitioner to deliver it. The commission concluded that an entirely new practitioner would be required to deliver pharmaceutical care. It outlined the educational outcomes that such a practitioner should have and that a curriculum should achieve.

This set the stage for the big questions, "How long should the curriculum be, and what should the degree be?" According to Dr. Penna, the answers became rather simple when the issues were approached in the logical sequence used by the commission. Discussion related to the entry-level degree did not occur until late in the commission's work.

The commission recognized that a comprehensive curricular revision was required to prepare pharmacists for providing pharmaceutical care. Little expertise was available on how to accomplish this type of reform, and there was still considerable resistance in academe toward any change of this nature. AACP recognized that change agents needed to be identified and that those change agents required training and empowerment to work for reform on their campuses. Hence, AACP organized its summer institutes for this purpose—the AACP Institute on Curricular and Pedagogical Change.

Five-member teams from 25 colleges of pharmacy were accepted for each institute. The focus of the early programs was on how to change curricula and on how to use educational outcomes as the skeleton around which to build a teaching and learning strategy. Each team was expected to build a curricular change plan for implementation back home.

According to Dr. Penna, the results of these institutes were astonishing. Institute participants left the program with new skills and a deep commitment to curricular change. As a result of this process, when the American Council on Pharmaceutical Education announced its new standards for pharmacy education, the colleges of pharmacy were ready.

American Pharmaceutical Association

Already mentioned have been a number of APhA's collaborative efforts and its quick policy endorsement of pharmaceutical care. Further on the policy front, APhA issued a white paper in March 1992 on "The Role of the Pharmacist in Comprehensive Medication Use Management."[15] The paper, which was guided by a task force chaired by Calvin Knowlton, boldly articulated 20 principles that called for the profession to assume leadership in medication use management. This important paper commented on the needs to reprofessionalize pharmacy, to integrate pharmacy practice into the broader health system, to integrate practice within the profession, to empower pharmacists to practice appropriately, and to develop new payment systems for pharmaceutical care.

APhA formulated "Principles of Practice for Pharmaceutical Care" in 1994.[16] Developed by a working group of pharmaceutical care leaders, this document differentiated pharmaceutical care from traditional practice activities.

In the period 1995–1997, APhA and the National Wholesale Druggists' Association cooperated in the Concept Pharmacy Project, which researched the elements of innovative care delivery and distilled the findings into multimedia education and advocacy products. The project included an instrument that measured an individual's or group's readiness to implement pharmaceutical care activities. Concept Pharmacy was a precursor to the Alliance for Pharmaceutical Care exhibit at the National Conference of State Legislatures.

In 1996, APhA conducted a National Pharmacy Consumer Survey, which benchmarked traditional service and patronage issues as well as examined consumers' receptivity to the concept of pharmaceutical care and their willingness to pay for it. Of the consumers polled, 69% found the services described highly attractive (i.e., they would be interested in receiving such services from a pharmacist); 15% said their pharmacist currently delivered those services. Only a small percentage expressed willingness to pay out-of-pocket for those services, and what they would pay was equivalent to the coinsurance or copayment associated with a covered insurance benefit.[17]

These findings led APhA to formalize its work on reforming payment systems to support pharmacists' patient care activities. A committee that met from 1995 to 1997 focused largely on state Medicaid programs and private employers, and it assisted the Wisconsin and Mississippi Medicaid programs in designing their innovative programs. Another committee appointed in 1999 has helped analyze service payment issues associated with a potential Medicare outpatient prescription drug benefit. APhA and St. Anthony Press published a manual on coding and reimbursement for pharmacists.

In recognition of the need for more research-based evidence on the value of pharmacists' services and for explicit measures of quality of practice and medication use, APhA increased the capacity of its foundation during the 1990's. This led to the birth of Project ImPACT (Improving Persistence and Compliance with Therapy). Project ImPACT-Hyperlipidemia, a 29-site demonstration project of pharmaceutical care services delivered to nearly 400 patients with hyperlipidemia over a two-year period, was the first such project. It showed extraordinary increases in patient compliance with therapy and achievement of therapeutic goals. A pilot project is underway in asthma care, and plans are being made to conduct similar projects in osteoporosis and anticoagulation services. The APhA Foundation also provides incentive grants to stimulate practice innovation and offers training programs (e.g., Advance Practice Institute) in which emerging practice leaders receive intensive multi-day skill building in pharmaceutical care.

On the education front, APhA created the American Center for Pharmaceutical Care, based on the work of the Iowa Pharmacists Association, which offered, in partnership with state organizations, a certificate training program to assist community pharmacists in redesigning their physical practice environment, work flow, and personnel expectations to facilitate delivery of pharmaceutical care. The association has also offered certificate training programs in several disease-specific areas, including asthma, dyslipidemia, diabetes, and immunization administration. The APhA publishes an ongoing educational piece, "Dynamics of Pharmaceutical Care." These programs are initially delivered live and then disseminated as printed monographs.

In 1995, APhA convened the Task Force on Certification for Pharmaceutical Care to examine the need for and best approach to use in credentialing pharmaceutical care practitioners. The task force recommended that a generalist credential should be developed collaboratively with other partners. This recommendation has not been implemented, and the profession has moved in a number of other directions on the credentialing issue.

American Society of Health-System Pharmacists

One of ASHP's core strengths is the development of standards for hospital and health-system pharmacy practice, and shortly after its 1991 endorsement of the pharmaceutical care philosophy, ASHP began incorporating this practice model into new and revised practice standards. This is important because ASHP's standards are used widely by accrediting bodies, such as the Joint Commission on Accreditation of Healthcare Organizations, in developing their own requirements and by federal and state agencies in establishing practice regulations. The ASHP standards are also used on a voluntary basis by pharmacy department directors who are looking for authoritative advice on upgrading services, and the standards are applied in assessing pharmacy departments that conduct accredited residency training programs.

With respect to residency accreditation, a significant milestone occurred in 1991 when ASHP merged two previous standards—one for training in hospital pharmacy practice and a second for training in clinical pharmacy practice—into one document, which was called the "Accreditation Standard for Residency in Pharmacy Practice (with an Emphasis on Pharmaceutical Care)."[18] Those requirements for postgraduate training in pharmaceutical care remained in force for 10 years and have been updated recently.

In 1993, ASHP adopted its Statement on Pharmaceutical Care,[19] which was designed to assist pharmacists in understanding the concept. The statement included the following viewpoint, which expresses how this practice model may be applied in the hospital setting:

ASHP believes that, in organized health care settings, pharmaceutical care can be most successfully provided when it is part of the pharmacy department's central mission and when management activity is focused on facilitating the provision of pharmaceutical care by individual pharmacists. This approach, in which empowered frontline staff provide direct care to individual patients and are supported by managers, other pharmacists, and support systems, is new for many pharmacists and managers.

In 1996, ASHP adopted the document Guidelines on a Standardized Method for Pharmaceutical Care,[20] which identified ten functions in the provision of pharmaceutical care and gave details on implementing each of those functions in practice. Earlier, ASHP had identified these functions as the basis for its Clinical Skills series of publications and as the framework for its Residency Learning System, which outlines a process for residency instruction.

One of ASHP's most significant efforts to foster the pharmaceutical care model of practice in the institutional environment was its March 1993 San Antonio conference on implementing pharmaceutical care.[21] With the support of the ASHP Research and Education Foundation, this program brought together some 200 pharmacists to explore the full implications of assuming responsibility for the outcome of drug therapy, which is inherent in the concept of pharmaceutical care. The conference produced a road map for practitioner action. ASHP and the ASHP Foundation fostered a number of state and regional programs based on the San Antonio effort, and ASHP conducted follow-up programming at its major educational conferences over the next few years.

In ASHP's analysis of what it must do to help members implement pharmaceutical care, it determined that many of its existing publications and educational programs were applicable or could be made so with modification. Also, many services on the drawing boards were applicable. It created the designation "Project Catalyst" to tie together all of the services relevant to pharmaceutical care.

A major conclusion by ASHP was that its members would need the most help in the area of staff development—in preparing frontline distribution-oriented pharmacists to make a transition to direct patient care responsibilities. This decision led to an array of services, most of which are still viable, including:

- The Clinical Skills Program, which is a multi-module self-study clinical educational tool for frontline pharmacists; separate tracks focus on patient care responsibilities in acute care, drug information, and ambulatory care.

- The Competitive Edge, a certificate program in outcomes research and outcomes management.

- Certificate program training through the ASHP Research and Education Foundation in several areas of therapy management, including anticoagulation, asthma, and stem cell transplantation. Other programs are being developed in diabetes, oncology, and pain management.

- A series of articles and educational programs on practice change, led by ASHP staff member Dr. Christine Nimmo in collaboration with Dr. Ross Holland of Australia.[22-26]

- A book on staff development, designed to be of special assistance to those pharmacy departments that have made a commitment to preparing their staffs for direct patient care.[27]

Comment

It is easy, of course, to measure activity, and, indeed, there has been a great deal of activity by pharmacy organizations over the past decade focused on fostering the implementation of pharmaceutical care. However, what has actually changed in practice?

We each have our impressions about the general state of pharmacy practice in community pharmacy, but there are no good national data on this point. The availability of information is somewhat better in hospital pharmacy because ASHP has regularly surveyed practice since the early 1970's. **Tables 3.1** and **3.2** show representative data from surveys in 1999 and 2000. The findings in Table 3.1, which show that pharmacists indeed are "out and about" in hospitals, are important because pharmaceutical care cannot be provided from the central pharmacy. As shown in Table 3.2, in more than half of the hospitals surveyed, pharmacists are monitoring the drug therapy of at least 25% of the patients.

Table 3.1. Percentage of Hospitals with Pharmacists Deployed on Patient Care Units (Selected Data)[28]

Hospital Size	% of Hospitals
< 50 beds	13
≥ 400 beds	82
all hospitals	29 (with 59% of time on clinical activities)

Table 3.2. Percentage of Hospital Patients Whose Drug Therapy Is Monitored by Pharmacists[29]

% Patients Monitored	% Hospitals
< 25	43
25–50	19
51–75	17
> 75	20

Regardless of practice site, it is not yet the norm for pharmacists to be engaged in direct patient care; however, this does not mean that progress is not being made. There are many indicators that suggest pharmacy is on track with respect to implementing pharmaceutical care, including the following:

- There is widespread acceptance among pharmacy thought leaders that prescription dispensing will not continue to sustain the profession financially.

- There is a growing body of research evidence that supports a direct patient care role for the pharmacist.

- Pharmacists in ambulatory care are increasingly being compensated by third-party payers for providing drug therapy management services.

- There is beginning to be recognition in Congress of the need to compensate pharmacists for managing patient drug therapy, as reflected in the Medicare Pharmacists Services Coverage Act of 2001 (S.974), introduced by Senator Tim Johnson (D-SD).

- Three forths of the states have sanctioned pharmacist involvement in collaborative drug therapy management.

- Employment of pharmacists to provide direct patient care services has a firm footing in hospitals where the payment system for inpatient care provides a strong incentive for doing so.

- The cooperative spirit among national pharmacist organizations that was manifested so well following the 1989 P21 conference continues.

- The education of the pharmacist is now based on pharmaceutical care.

- There is widespread acceptance among practicing pharmacists that the occupation of pharmacy technicians needs to be enhanced, in part to free the pharmacist for direct patient care functions.

- Patient safety (including medication-use safety) is recognized as a major public health problem.

- A number of important drug products have been removed from the market in recent years because their well-known risks were not well managed, and public policy makers and the pharmaceutical industry are beginning to show interest in a role for pharmacists in the use of such high-risk products.

There are also worrisome indicators. One relates to the current pharmacist shortage and attempts to curtail health care spending, which results in highly stressful work situations in all sectors of practice. In this environment, it can be difficult to move beyond the status quo. And it is difficult to glean lessons from history. As pharmacy historian Higby observed, ". . . reform in pharmacy has never occurred in the midst of a crisis. Pharmacy has a tendency to become conservative in hard times."[30] At times there seems to be an overwhelming bias among practitioners to accept, not to challenge, the status quo. All of health care is becoming more financially driven and increasingly the professional imperative is given short shrift to the business imperative. Many of pharmacy's most innovative practice leaders have left to pursue other opportunities outside of practice. And, finally, the leaders in organized medicine and the pharmaceutical industry, by and large, remain to be persuaded of the wisdom of a role for pharmacists in drug therapy management.

One of the lessons this author has learned in 30 years of association work is that fundamental change in pharmacy comes slowly. This can be difficult to accept because we like to measure progress against the yardstick of our own lifetimes. Realism about the pace of change can be especially troubling to a pharmacist elected to leadership of an organization for a one-year term, who wants to change the profession during the months he or she wields the gavel. This is where the American Institute of the History of Pharmacy could be helpful to the profession by continuing to remind us of how things used to be and by documenting how changes of the past have occurred.

There are many reasons to be optimistic that the philosophy of pharmaceutical care will continue to be a beacon for pharmacy. Its light has already penetrated the hearts and minds of pharmacists, the place where real change begins. The hard work of making the ideal a reality is occurring all around us.

Conclusion

When the final chapter of this saga is written many years from now, it will show that in the early years of pharmaceutical care, the profession's organizations played a critical role in diffusing this idea deeply into the profession. Further, history will record that pharmacy organizations were effective change agents and influenced in a positive way several critical factors that affected the focus of the practicing pharmacist.

References

1. Rogers EM. Diffusion of innovations. 4th ed. New York: The Free Press; 1995.
2. Ibid., p 337.
3. Directions for clinical practice in pharmacy—proceedings of an invitational conference conducted by the ASHP Research and Education Foundation and the American Society of Hospital Pharmacists, February 10–13, 1985, Hilton Head Island, South Carolina. *Am J Hosp Pharm.* 1985; 42:1287–342.
4. Hepler CD. Pharmacy as a clinical profession. *Am J Hosp Pharm.* 1985: 42:1298–306.
5. Zellmer WA. Perspectives on Hilton Head. *Am J Hosp Pharm.* 1986: 43:1439–43.
6. Conference on pharmacy in the 21st century, October 11–14, 1989, Williamsburg, Virginia. *Am J Pharm Educ.* 1989; 53 (Winter Supplement).

7. Bezold C, Halperin JA, Binkley HL et al., eds. Pharmacy in the 21st century—planning for an uncertain future. Virginia: Institute for Alternative Futures and Project HOPE; 1985.

8. Anon. JCPP calls for pharmacists to comment on provisional draft mission statement for pharmacy practice. *Am J Hosp Pharm.* 1991; 48:1847–8.

9. Zellmer WA. Expressing the mission of pharmacy practice. *Am J Hosp Pharm.* 1991; 48:1195. Editorial.

10. The third strategic planning conference for pharmacy practice—a conference [1994] dedicated to understanding and overcoming the obstacles to delivering pharmaceutical care (undated supplement to *Am Pharm*).

11. Penna RP, ed. The papers of the Commission to Implement Change in Pharmaceutical Education. Alexandria, VA: American Association of Colleges of Pharmacy; 1994.

12. Anon. New policies adopted by the 1991 APhA House of Delegates. *Am Pharm.* 1991; NS31(6):29.

13. Oddis JA. Report of the house of delegates. *Am J Hosp Pharm.* 1991; 48:1739–48.

14. Johnson JA, Bootman, JL. Drug-related morbidity and mortality—a cost-of-illness model. *Arch Intern Med.* 1995; 155:1949–56.

15. The role of the pharmacist in comprehensive medication use management: the delivery of pharmaceutical care—a background position paper issued by the Board of Trustees, American Pharmaceutical Association, March 1992.

16. American Pharmaceutical Association. Principles of practice for pharmaceutical care. Washington, DC: American Pharmaceutical Association; 1996. www.aphanet.org (accessed 2001 May 15).

17. Metge CJ, Hendricksen C, Maine L. Consumer attitudes, behaviors, and perceptions about pharmacies, pharmacists, and pharmaceutical care. *J Am Pharm Assoc.* 1998; 38:37–47.

18. ASHP accreditation standard for residency in pharmacy practice (with emphasis on pharmaceutical care). *Am J Hosp Pharm.* 1992; 49:146–53.

19. ASHP statement on pharmaceutical care. *Am J Hosp Pharm.* 1993; 50:1720–3.

20. ASHP guidelines on a standardized method for pharmaceutical care. *Am J Health-Syst Pharm.* 1996; 53:1713–6.

21. Implementing pharmaceutical care—proceedings of an invitational conference conduced by the American Society of Hospital Pharmacists and the ASHP Research and Education Foundation. *Am J Hosp Pharm.* 1993; 50:1585–656.

22. Holland RW, Nimmo CM. Transitions, part 1: beyond pharmaceutical care. *Am J Health-Syst Pharm.* 1999; 56:1758–64.

23. Nimmo CM, Holland RW. Transitions in pharmacy practice, part 2: who does what and why. *Am J Health-Syst Pharm.* 1999; 56:19; 81–7.

24. Holland RW, Nimmo CM. Transitions in pharmacy practice, part 3: effecting change—the three-ring circus. *Am J Health-Syst Pharm.* 1999; 56:2235–41.

25. Nimmo CM, Holland RW. Transitions in pharmacy practice, part 4: can a leopard change its spots? *Am J Health-Syst Pharm.* 1999; 56:2458–62.

26. Nimmo CM, Holland RW. Transitions in pharmacy practice, part 5: walking the tightrope of change. *Am J Health-Syst Pharm.* 2000; 57:64–72.

27. Nimmo CM. Staff development for pharmacy practice. Bethesda, MD: American Society of Health-System Pharmacists; 2000.

28. Ringold DJ, Santell JP, Schneider PJ. ASHP national survey of pharmacy practice in acute care settings: dispensing and administration—1999. *Am J Health-Syst Pharm.* 2000; 57:1759–75.

29. Pedersen CA, Schneider PJ, Santell JP et al. ASHP national survey of pharmacy practice in acute care settings: monitoring, patient education, and wellness—2000. *Am J Health-Syst Pharm.* 2000; 57:2171–87.

30. Higby G. In: The third strategic planning conference for pharmacy practice—a conference [1994] dedicated to understanding and overcoming the obstacles to delivering pharmaceutical care. Undated supplement to *Am Pharm.*

Footnotes

[a]Appreciation is expressed to Richard Penna, Pharm.D., for the information in this paper from AACP.

[b]Appreciation is expressed to Lucinda Maine, Ph.D., for the information in this paper from APhA.

[c]JCPP member organizations: Academy of Managed Care Pharmacy (AMCP), American College of Apothecaries (ACA), American College of Clinical Pharmacy (ACCP), APhA, American Society of Consultant Pharmacists (ASCP), ASHP, and National Community Pharmacists Association (NCPA); liaison members: AACP, National Association of Boards of Pharmacy (NABP), and National Council of State Pharmacy Association Executives (NCSPAE).

[d]Members of the planning committee: William N. Tindall (NARD), chairman; Maude A. Babington (ASCP); Marsha K. Millonig (NACDS); Richard P. Penna (AACP); Dorothy A. Wade (National Pharmaceutical Council); C. Edwin Webb (APhA); and William A. Zellmer (ASHP).

[e]Members of the Alliance for Pharmaceutical Care: AACP, ACCP, AMCP, APhA, ASCP, ASHP, Healthcare Distribution Management Association (HDMA) (formerly National Wholesale Druggists' Association), National Association of Chain Drug Stores (NACDS), NCPA, NCSPAE, and United States Pharmacopeia (USP).

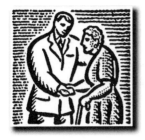

Chapter 4: Health Care in the United States

Earle W. Lingle, R.Ph., Ph.D.

Pharmaceutical care is not practiced in a vacuum. Various factors, such as the organization of health care delivery systems, reimbursement methods, laws regulating the practice of pharmacy and medicine, and many others, influence pharmaceutical care. This chapter will discuss the U.S. health care system. By reviewing its structure, financing, problems, and potential for reform, we can better understand how pharmaceutical care can best meet the needs of our growing, aging, and heterogeneous population.

Structure of the U.S. Health Care System

The term "health care system" is actually a misnomer, and what we currently have is a sickness care system that lacks an emphasis on maintaining health. Another argument might be made that it is actually a non-system because of the lack of coordination between the different actors. It may also be maintained that it consists of a group of sub-systems, each with different objectives, members, providers, and services.

One method of defining the structure of the health care system is according to *who* is paying health care providers for services: a patient or a third-party payer. If a patient pays the provider directly, the payment is referred to as an out-of-pocket expense. A third-party payer is defined as an entity that provides payment to a health care practitioner for services provided to a patient with whom the third party is affiliated. A third party may either be privately owned or publicly administered. Because of their influence in today's health care system, third-party organizations need to be more closely examined.

Private Health Insurance

Evolution

In the early 1900's health insurance policies were similar to accident and disability insurance in that they were loss-of-income policies, providing cash payments during certain specific illnesses, such as typhoid, smallpox, and diphtheria. They did not provide payment for health care services but were meant to replace lost income resulting from the disease episode.[1]

The Great Depression influenced the establishment of private health insurance to pay health care providers. In 1929, a group of teachers began paying fifty cents per month to Baylor Hospital in Dallas to provide each teacher with up to 21 days of care annually. This was the beginning of what became known as Blue Cross plans. These plans were followed by Blue Shield insurance programs that paid physicians instead of hospitals. Premiums were usually determined by averaging the costs for each community.[2]

During World War II, because workers were scarce and the government had imposed controls on wages, employers offered health insurance as a fringe benefit to attract employees. As more businesses sought health insurance packages, the number of insurance companies offering them rapidly increased. Insurance companies determined premium payments by experience rating—pricing premiums on the basis of an individual's or a group's medical claims history.

A recent development in private health insurance has been the decision by major employers to self-insure. Instead of paying premiums to an insurance company, these businesses predict the expense for their employees and assume the risks for these costs. The advantages for businesses are such that the number of employers that are self-insuring has rapidly grown. However, some self-insured businesses have either reduced or dropped their employees' coverage of cancer, AIDS, and other diseases that may prove costly.[3]

Types

Private health insurance companies offer a multitude of policies in an attempt to carve out niches in different markets. In addition, they may combine coverage to meet the needs of individual employers or employee groups. The following are the major categories of private health insurance.[1]

- *Hospital/Medical Insurance.* Provides coverage for specific benefits related to hospital room, board, services, and supplies during a hospital stay. It may also be combined with payment for doctors' hospital visits and surgical services.
- *Major Medical Expense Insurance.* Usually covers a wide range of medical charges and provides protection for large medical expenses.
- *Medicare Supplemental Policy.* Insurance policy often referred to as "Medigap" providing additional coverage for persons covered by Medicare, the government-sponsored health insurance program for the elderly.
- *Disability Income Protection.* Provides income for a worker who has become disabled. The benefit is usually related to a percentage of the beneficiary's earnings.

Coverage

In 2000, approximately 72% of the U.S. population was covered by some form of private health insurance.[4] Insurance provided by employers covered 64% of the population.[5] However, workers in smaller companies and those who are in retail trade, service industries, or self-employed were less likely to have employer-sponsored health insurance.

Employer-provided health insurance has been stimulated by tax policy. Health insurance benefits can be considered a substitute for wages. Employers can deduct their share of the premium payments as operating expenses. In addition, the benefits are not subject to employees' personal incomes or Social Security taxes.[6]

In 1999, health insurance companies collected $401.2 billion in premiums and paid out $355.3 billion in benefits. The difference, $45.9 billion, was used for administration of the plans, taxes, and company profits.[7]

A survey of small and large employers found that monthly premiums for employer-sponsored health insurance had increased at a greater rate (11%) than the growth of inflation (3.3%) or the growth of wages for non-supervisory workers (4.4%) from 2000 to 2001.[8] This was the largest increase since 1992. Employers cited that a primary factor behind rising premiums was an increase in health care expenditures, specifically for prescription drugs. They were pessimistic in their assessment that prescription drug costs could be controlled.

Public Insurance Programs

Federal, state, and local governments have become involved in health care for one or more of three purposes: 1) to either provide services or mandate the provision of services for the public good, 2) to purchase services for the public good, or 3) to redistribute income. Some health care services cannot be provided in a normal market setting because of little desire by the public to purchase them or small profit incentives for companies to provide them. The government may either provide these services directly or pass regulations to mandate their purchase or provision, for example, the regulation of pharmaceuticals by the Food and Drug Administration.

The government may purchase goods and services for the public good by providing medical research grants through the National Institutes of Health or purchasing health care services from health professions for certain segments of society.

The government affects income distribution by taxing citizens with higher incomes to pay for health care for persons who are considered poor. This is the basis for the Medicaid program. It is not possible to survey government's involvement in all aspects of health care in this chapter. However, because of the current interest in health insurance coverage, it is important to examine the evolution of public health insurance and government's two largest programs, Medicaid and Medicare.

Evolution

The industrialization of the U.S. and some social reform began in the early 1900's. With the Great Depression of 1929 through 1932 serving as a motivating factor, along with the resulting high unemployment, society began to change its view of government's role in helping citizens. In 1932, the Committee on Costs of Medical Care reported that a form of national health insurance was needed for this country. However, the politically powerful interest group of organized medicine vehemently opposed. The American Medical Association (AMA) reacted in an editorial in its journal: "The alignment is clear—on the one side the forces representing the great foundations, public health officialdom, social theory—even socialism and communism—inciting to revolution; on the other side, the organized medical profession urging principles of sound practice of medicine."[9] For the next 30 years, the mention of increased involvement in health care brought about concerns of socialism and communism expressed by AMA and their supporters.

President Franklin D. Roosevelt believed there was a need for publicly financed health care but he knew the odds were against such a program and instead supported Social Security. The Social Security Act of 1935 was important because it was the basis for future public health insurance. In addition to providing a payroll deduction plan for retirement, Social Security assists people in paying for essentials such as food, shelter, and medical care. Persons are eligible if they are poor and meet the criteria for one of four categories:

blind, disabled, elderly, or single-parent families with dependent children. People eligible for one of these categories are sometimes referred to as the categorically needy.

Over the next 25 years various proposals for public health insurance were put forward, yet no other major legislation was passed until 1960. The passage of the Kerr–Mills Medical Assistance for the Aged Act provided medical assistance for the elderly. The act was steered through Congress by Representative Wilbur Mills and Senator Robert Kerr. The reasoning behind the act was that since medical expenses consumed such a large part of many elderly persons' incomes, public assistance should be provided to those who were not poor enough to be eligible for the welfare payments discussed above.

Buoyed by the support of then-Senator John F. Kennedy and Representative Lyndon B. Johnson, comprehensive public health insurance for the elderly gained momentum. In 1965, after the assassination of President Kennedy and after President Johnson's election, Congress enacted legislation with primarily three sections: 1) a federally-administered hospital insurance program for the elderly (age 65 and older), disabled, and persons with end-stage renal disease (Medicare Part A); 2) a federally-administered supplemental health insurance program that the elderly, disabled, and persons with end-stage renal disease could purchase (Medicare Part B); and 3) a state-administered health insurance program for the categorically needy and some other poor persons.

Since 1965 there have been various efforts to reform the health care system. Probably the most extensive proposal was the Health Security Act proposed by President Bill Clinton in 1993. After intense debate, one of the major reasons for its defeat was the concern that the federal government would have too much control over the nation's health care system. However, some incremental changes have occurred in government programs. For example, the State Children's Health Insurance Program (CHIP) was adopted by Congress in 1997 to provide health insurance coverage to children of working parents or other low-income families who do not have employer-sponsored health insurance or do not qualify for Medicaid. In December 2000, 2.7 million children were enrolled in state CHIP benefit plans.[10]

Medicare

Medicare is the single largest health insurer in the U.S., covering approximately 39 million persons—34 million elderly persons and 5 million people who are under 65 and who have disabilities or renal disease.[11] This represents approximately 13% of the U.S. population. It is administered by the federal government with a uniform package of medical care benefits for eligible persons regardless of income. Medicare does not pay all medical expenses for its beneficiaries as it does not cover all services and there are certain cost-sharing responsibilities for each person. It is funded by a combination of payroll taxes, general tax revenue, and premiums. In general, Medicare does not cover medical care not reasonable and not necessary for the treatment of a specific illness or injury. Part A of Medicare, also known as the Hospital Insurance plan, pays for part of the costs of inpatient hospital care and related care provided by skilled nursing facilities, home health agencies, and hospices. Medicare Part B, Supplementary Medical Insurance, covers services and supplies provided by physicians and outpatient hospital facilities. In addition, some home health care, vision care, physical therapy, and mental health services are covered. Pharmaceutical benefits are limited to inpatient hospital coverage, hospice care, and some specific medications for outpatients. A more comprehensive outpatient drug benefit has been considered by Congress and continues to be debated. Persons entitled to Part

A coverage can enroll in Part B by paying a monthly premium. In 2001, this premium equaled $50 per month.

Medicare beneficiaries also have the option to enroll in private health maintenance organizations (HMOs) instead of the traditional fee-for-service Medicare program. In 1997, Congress expanded the types of plans from which beneficiaries could choose to include a variety of managed care plans and medical savings accounts. This part of the Medicare program is called Medicare+Choice. By December 2000, 5.6 million (14%) Medicare beneficiaries were enrolled in a Medicare+Choice plan and they accounted for an estimated 18% of Medicare payments.[12] However, the number of managed care plans participating in Medicare+Choice decreased from 346 in 1998 to only 178 in 2001, producing concerns about the future of this segment of Medicare.

A major concern with Medicare is that expenditures are increasing faster than revenue. Because of the aging population and smaller families, there are fewer workers per Medicare beneficiary to fund the program. The number of beneficiaries in 2030 will be more than 90% greater than in 2000, but the number of workers paying into Medicare will be only about 15% greater. Although there were five workers per beneficiary in 1960, this has now decreased to four workers per beneficiary in the year 2000 and it will reach only 2.3 workers per beneficiary in 2030.[11] Part A is currently financed with a 2.9% payroll tax and estimates are that Part A costs will equal 3.76% of payroll in the year 2000 and 8.62% in 2030. It is projected that Part A expenses will exceed its revenues beginning in 2016, and by 2030 revenues will cover only 66% of its expenses. The Part B program is growing more rapidly than Part A. Part B expenditures have shown increases from $10 billion in 1980 to almost $100 billion in 2000 and are estimated to reach $150 billion (using current dollars) by the year 2030.[13]

A deficiency in the Medicare program benefit structure is that it covers physician visits, but provides only limited coverage for outpatient prescription drugs. Poisal and Murray[14] estimated that 73% of Medicare beneficiaries had some type of drug coverage in 1998. They also found that beneficiaries without drug coverage spent an average of $546 out of pocket in 1998 compared with $325 paid by beneficiaries with coverage. Outpatient drug coverage already occurs under Medicare's hospice benefit and in Medicare HMO programs, although the coverage is limited in scope. Some Medicare beneficiaries also have drug coverage through private insurance either purchased by themselves or provided as part of their past employer's retiree benefits package. Others receive drug benefits by being eligible for Medicaid. Not considered in the above estimates were the benefits paid by 24 states that have developed assistance programs for mostly low-income Medicare beneficiaries.

Even though the number of elderly who do not have drug coverage is a minority, pressure continues to mount on Congress to add a drug benefit to Medicare. The cost of such a benefit would depend on the comprehensiveness of the benefit and its administration. The Congressional Budget Office estimated that spending by Medicare beneficiaries on prescription drugs will total $104 billion in 2004, more than the expenditures for Medicare Part B and 47% of the total Medicare expenditures of $222 billion in 2000.[15] The addition of a Medicare drug benefit is needed by many elderly persons; however, it would significantly increase Medicare's costs when there is already concern about the program's solvency.

Medicaid

When Medicare and Medicaid were established in 1965, the major debate was over Medicare. With relatively little consideration, Medicaid was included as a political compromise and opponents were assured that expenditures would remain relatively small. During the 1998–99 fiscal year, Medicaid covered 44 million persons, approximately 14% of the U.S. population, and expenditures had reached $176 billion, an increase from $74 billion in 1990.[16]

Medicaid is administered jointly by state and federal governments. Although a state can choose whether or not to participate in the program, all 50 states plus the District of Columbia participate in Medicaid. Once a state decides to provide services under Medicaid, federal regulations require that certain services be offered, identify the population groups eligible for benefits, and specify reimbursement. The federal government also contributes funds, the amount of which varies by state and is based on a state's per capita income as compared with the national average. The federal share may range from 50 to 83% but the average federal contribution is 57%.

Recipients must meet certain criteria to qualify for Medicaid benefits. Each state sets income and asset limits for qualification; therefore, there are large state variations in coverage. A beneficiary must meet the criteria for being categorically needy—low-income children, pregnant women, blind, elderly, disabled, or parents meeting specific income requirements. In addition, some states also include persons who are considered medically needy—blind, elderly, disabled, or low-income families whose income is above the Medicaid limit but whose medical expenses are so high that their income is reduced to below the eligibility limit. It is estimated that because of the eligibility categories and differing state income limits, approximately 75% of the nonelderly population with incomes below 200% of the federal poverty level are not eligible for Medicaid.[17]

Federal regulations require states to provide a basic set of services if they are medically necessary, including inpatient and outpatient hospital services, physician services, laboratory and x-ray services, nursing home care, home health care, and others. States may also elect to provide optional services including outpatient prescription drugs, dental care services, vision care, and services provided by intermediate-care facilities. All states and the District of Columbia offer outpatient prescription drugs although the programs vary. Prescription drug coverage is the most utilized Medicaid service.

One particular problem with the Medicaid program is the expenditure for long-term care, including nursing home care. Medicaid is the only public health insurance program that pays for such care. To become eligible for Medicaid and have reimbursement for long-term care, some elderly transfer their assets to their children and spend any remaining income and assets on their health care. Although only about four percent of Medicaid beneficiaries used long-term care in 1998, long-term care was responsible for approximately 25% of total Medicaid expenditures, and as the population increases in age, higher costs can be expected.[18] Medicare coverage of nursing home care continues to be debated, but the expense makes it politically difficult to enact.

Some persons who are elderly, blind, or disabled may be eligible for both Medicare and Medicaid. These persons are said to be dually eligible. In some cases, Medicare provides the primary coverage for hospital insurance (Part A), and states may pay the premiums for supplemental medical insurance (Part B) so that Medicare will also cover those services. In addition, state Medicaid programs may pay the patient cost-sharing and may provide the services Medicare does not, such as outpatient prescription drugs and long-term nursing home care.

Summary

Medicare and Medicaid play a major role in the delivery of health care in this country. Public insurance programs cover approximately 1 in 4 persons in the United States. Medicare and Medicaid paid approximately one-third percent of all national health expenditures in 1998.[7] If these programs go unchanged and the present trends continue, they will place significant pressures on state and federal budgets.

Managed Care Programs

As health care expenditures increased in the 1970's and 1980's, new health care delivery systems were being developed to change the incentives for providing care. These systems are based on three principles: managing the care of patients, using a select group of health care providers, and placing the providers at financial risk.[19] Because of the management of the patient's care, these organizations became known as managed care. The traditional fee-for-service system encourages the use of more services even though the services may not be the most appropriate or produce the preferred outcome. Theoretically, managed care systems would provide incentives to produce a more efficient use of medical services.

Types of Managed Care

Different types of managed care programs have evolved. The two major categories are HMOs and preferred provider organizations (PPOs). There are also different models within these categories.

HMOs are health care organizations that provide a comprehensive set of medical care services to an enrolled group of patients. The enrollee pays a fixed amount per month regardless of the amount of services used. This places the HMO at financial risk if total costs are greater than aggregate premiums, but it has a financial gain if the costs are lower than the premium revenue. As a result, incentives are provided to patients and health care providers to minimize use and therefore costs.

There are several different models of managed care that are considered HMOs. The staff model employs salaried physicians and owns the clinical facilities in which they practice. In a group model the HMO contracts with one or more physician groups to provide care and usually reimburses them on a capitated basis. Capitation is a type of reimbursement system in which the medical group or individual practitioner provides services for a fixed payment per patient over a defined time period regardless of the patient's use. Similar to the group plan is the network model in which physician providers contract with the HMO to provide services for their enrollees. The principal difference between the two is that HMO enrollees usually compose a small part of a network physician's practice. The fourth model is known as an individual practice association (IPA). In this situation the IPA contracts with various individual physicians or associations of independent physicians to provide services for their enrollees. These doctors may be paid on a capitated or fee-for-service basis.

PPOs are the second main type of managed care programs. These organizations contract with a network of doctors, hospitals, and other practitioners to provide services for a discounted reimbursement. Enrollees in PPOs usually have lower cost-sharing if they go to a health care provider in the network; however, they have the option to go to a physician or other health care provider outside of the network and pay a greater share of the costs. In an exclusive provider organization (EPO), if the enrollee goes to a non-network provider the patient must pay that provider's fee out of pocket.

A more recent development in HMOs is the point-of-service (POS) plan. This may be thought of as a combination HMO/PPO model because it integrates characteristics of both. The POS plan contracts with a network of providers and each enrollee has a primary care physician who acts as a gatekeeper to control the use of specialists. Physicians are paid via fee-for-service or capitation, and enrollees who use health care providers not contracting with the POS share a greater amount of the costs.

Managed care can be practiced in settings other than those described above. Managed care techniques are being increasingly adopted by insurers and include a variety of decisions before services are provided. These cost-control methods include prior authorization for hospital admissions, second opinions for surgical procedures, provider utilization review, patient caseworkers, and others.

The differences between these types and models of managed care organizations are becoming less distinct as each borrows options from others in an attempt to make their plans more attractive for potential enrollees. Even now, it is difficult to determine in which of these categories many managed care plans fall.

Trends

The number of HMOs has fluctuated since the early 1980's. In 1989, it was estimated that there were 623 HMOs in the United States. By 1992, the number had decreased to 562. This decrease may have been due to the consolidation of different HMOs and the disappearance of smaller ones. However, the number of HMOs had increased to 820 by 1999. Most of the HMOs are IPA plans (68%); there were only 28 staff model plans operating in 1999 (**Table 4.1**). Enrollment in HMOs was 104.6 million people in 1999, a three-fold increase since 1989. This growth is expected to continue with the offering of POS options. IPA plans had the most enrollees, approximately 58 million in 1999 (Table 4.1). Although PPOs did not become popular until the early 1980's, the number of enrollees has risen dramatically. Estimates vary because of differing definitions, but it is estimated that in 1999 more than 106 million people were enrolled in one of the 1079 operating PPOs. This is an increase from 38.1 million and 824 PPOs in 1990.[20] Staff model HMOs is the only type of HMO that has suffered a decrease in number and enrollment since 1989.[20,21]

Table 4.1. Numbers of HMOs and Enrollment by Type of Plan[20,21]

	1989 Plans	1989 Enrollment (x 1000)	1992 Plans	1992 Enrollment (x 1000)	1996 Plans	1996 Enrollment (x 1000)	1999 Plans	1999 Enrollment (x 1000)
Group	85	9,845	71	11,320	96	19,508	89	21,397
IPA	386	15,428	363	20,819	502	45,281	554	57,537
Network	86	5,432	72	6,859	105	8,362	149	23,753
Staff	66	4,327	56	4,744	46	4,189	28	1,882
TOTAL	623	35,032	562	43,742	749	77,340	820	104,569

A large majority of HMOs and PPOs use pharmacy benefit managers (PBMs) to administer their drug benefit. Managed care organizations may contract with PBMs to perform various functions, such as monitoring drug therapy compliance of enrollees, adjudicating claims, negotiating prices with manufacturers and reimbursement with pharmacies, developing a network of pharmacy providers, providing dispensing services through their own mail-order pharmacy, and developing cost-containment programs.

Effects of Managed Care

There is some disagreement on the current effectiveness and future promise of managed care to decrease health care costs. An earlier study estimated there would be an approximate 10% reduction in national health care spending if all services were delivered through staff or group model HMOs. However, this would only be a one-time drop and would have no effect on the rate of increase.[22] One might reason that managed care would produce cost savings because of adverse selection—serving a younger, healthier population. However, enrollment in staff and group HMOs—the most effective managed care plans in reducing costs—has been stagnant, suggesting that managed care has had little impact on health care spending.

Enrollment in managed care plans grew because managed care costs less than fee-for-service care. Managing care meant the use of practices to control use, such as restricted formularies and prior authorization of hospital stays. It appears that patients have chosen managed care plans primarily on the basis of cost and not quality of care.[23] In addition, patients are confused about their own care. In 2000, 66% of managed care enrollees reported that they had never been enrolled in a managed care plan and only 14% of a national sample reported they were extremely or very familiar with managed care.[24]

The future of managed care appears uncertain. Some patients have lost trust in the system because of concerns about cost controls that may be viewed as rationing and restricting access to providers. Some managed groups have taken action to eliminate administrative practices that restrict patients' choices by implementing programs that increase coordination of care.[25] Whether or not such actions will allow managed care to control costs while maintaining or improving quality of care remains to be seen.

Financing Health Care

National health expenditures were approximately $1.2 trillion in 1999. In other words, health care costs equaled $3.3 billion per day or $2.3 million per minute. It is estimated that if our current laws and medical practice remain unchanged, medical care costs will more than double to $2.6 trillion by the year 2010 (**Figure 4.1**).[7]

Another important way of examining health care costs is by looking at the percentage of the U.S. gross domestic product (GDP) that is spent on medical care (Figure 4.1). GDP is the value of all goods and services produced in this country; therefore, the more we spend on health care the less there is available to purchase other goods and services, such as education and housing. Health care expenditures equaled 8.8% of GDP in 1980, grew to 13% in 1999, and are estimated to increase to 15.9% in the year 2010.[7]

Use of Funds

National health expenditures are usually divided into two categories: (1) research and construction and (2) health services and supplies. Research and construction reached $39.8 billion in 1999, only three percent of the total spent on health care. Health services and supplies can be divided into personal health care, administration of public programs, and the net cost of health insurance, as well as government public health programs. Because personal health care is responsible for approximately 87% of national health expenditures, it is important to concentrate the discussion on personal health care expenditures.

Personal health care (PHC) includes those services provided and associated with individual health care. In 1999, the per capita PHC costs were $3808.[26] Hospital care, inpatient and outpatient, was responsible for 37% of PHC expenditures (**Figure 4.2**), compared with 47% of the costs in 1980. Hospital costs also include expenditures for pharmaceuticals used in this setting and physician fees/salaries paid by hospitals. Some of this decrease is due to the implementation of capitated payments and the expansion of alternative care settings, such as home health care. Expenditures for physician services were approximately $26.9 billion in 1999. This amounts to 25% of PHC costs, compared with 22% in 1980. Nursing home expenditures have remained stable with about 8% of total PHC in 1980 and 8.5% in 1999.[27]

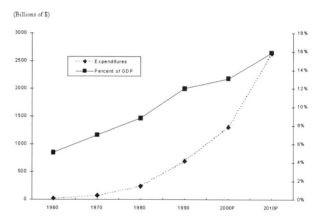

Figure 4.1. U.S. Health Care Expenditures, 1960–2010 (projected).[7]

The costs of prescription pharmaceuticals have increased from 5.6% in 1980 to 9.4% in 1999 (Figure 4.2). Although total pharmaceutical expenditures are relatively small, they are rapidly growing. It is estimated that prescription drugs will be responsible for 16% of PHC by 2010. The development of new and more expensive drug products, an aging population, and the effect of direct-to-consumer advertising have all had an influence on increasing prescription drug use and expenditures.[7]

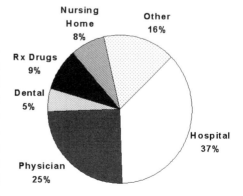

Figure 4.2. Percent of U.S. Personal Health Care Expenditures by Type of Service, 1999.[27]

Source of Funds

Payment for PHC usually originates from one of four sources: (1) private insurance companies, (2) federal government, (3) state and local governments, or (4) direct out-of-pocket payment from the patient to the provider. The first three listed are called third parties because they become the third player in the patient-health care provider relationship to pay all or a portion of the provider's fee. The source of PHC payments vary by the service provided.

Overall, third parties were responsible for paying approximately 82% of all PHC expenditures in 1999 (**Figure 4.3**).[27] The tremendous growth in third parties is evident from the fact that only 45% of PHC costs in 1960 and 60% in 1970 were paid by third parties. Most of the early increase was due to the implementation of Medicare and Medicaid in 1965. More recently, employer-provided insurance has contributed to the increase. In 1999, the federal government paid 33% of

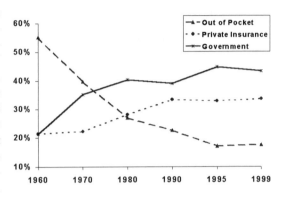

Figure 4.3. Percent of U.S. Personal Health Care Expenditures by Source of Payment.[27]

PHC while state and local governments paid 10.5%. Therefore, governments are already paying for about 43% of its citizens' personal health care. Private health insurance paid another 34%. Since 1980, out-of-pocket payments have decreased from 27% to only 18% in 1999.

Private insurance and government programs vary in terms of the extent to which they cover different health care services. Out-of-pocket payments concern most consumers because they are direct payments to the provider. Only three percent of hospital expenses and 11% of physician services are paid out-of-pocket, whereas 35% of prescription drugs are paid directly by patients (**Figure 4.4**).[26] Even though patients pay a relatively greater amount out-of-pocket for prescription drugs than other services, this amount has been steadily decreasing. In 1980, 69% of prescription drug expenditures were paid directly by patients. As recently as 1990, 59% of prescription drugs were paid out-of-pocket.

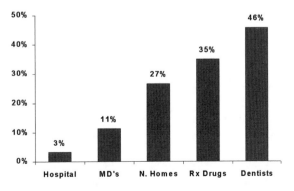

Finally, it must be understood that even though we say

Figure 4.4. Percent of U.S. Personal Health Care Expenditures Paid Out-of-Pocket by Type of Service.[27]

governments or insurance companies pay for medical care, these payments are derived from individuals. By paying health insurance premiums; federal, state, and local taxes; and increased prices for goods and services to help pay that business's health insurance for employees and by an employee receiving a lower salary to help pay for their own employer-sponsored health insurance, the individual ultimately shoulders the responsibility of paying for health care.

Problems of the U.S. Health Care System

The problems facing our health care system are interrelated and actions that affect one influence the others. However, these problems may be divided into three categories: (1) costs, (2) access to care, and (3) health status of the population.

Health Care Costs

The previous discussion on health care financing indicates the current and potential problems with increasing health care costs. Such a problem not only has ramifications for health care delivery but also is a foreboding sign for the soundness of the economy. To formulate successful strategies to contain rising costs, it is important to understand the causes underlying the problem.

One of the largest factors causing an increase in health care expenditures is economy-wide inflation. General inflation has been estimated to account for almost 25 to 50% of the annual growth.[27,28] Because this is affected by various factors, such as Federal Reserve Board policies or OPEC's price for oil, economy-wide inflation is difficult to control as a factor of increasing costs.

Another cause of rising health care costs is the increase in the elderly population. Almost 13% of the U.S. population (35 million persons) is 65 years of age or older. The population is expected to increase to 20% (approximately 70 million persons) by the year 2030.[29] The elderly use more services, on average, than the nonelderly and the intensity of their care is often much greater and, therefore, more expensive. For example, in 1995 per capita health care expenditures were $1946 for the population under age 65; however, for those persons age 65 or over the per capita health care expenditure was $8953.[30]

Another major factor has been the cost of technological advancements. This includes new equipment, products, and procedures. Newhouse[31] found that technological change in medicine represents a large proportion of the increases in expenditures we have seen. Although some technological advancements, such as pharmaceuticals that substitute for surgery, may result in lower initial expenditures, on balance, new products and procedures result in higher expenditures because they are more expensive and they increase the size of the market.

Consider, for example, the development of non-ionic contrast material as a radiological dye. The former dye had a mortality rate of 1 in every 30,000 uses; however, the new non-ionic contrast material mortality rate is only 1 in every 250,000 uses. The problem is that the new dye is ten times more expensive and it could add $1 billion to the cost of health care. These costs are passed along not only to the users but also to other patients. We are also confronted with the prospect of new developments from biotechnology laboratories that have tremendous promise for many of mankind's ills—but we must also face the costs of developing such products. What has occurred in the area of technological advancements over the past 20 years will probably only be surpassed by what will be developed in the future 20 years. However, someone has to pay for these advancements. Any attempt to control the use of these technologies has already been met and will continue to be met with the ethical concerns of rationing health care.

Another reason for increasing health care costs is what could be known as the health insurance effect. Health insurance has the influence of insulating consumers from their health care costs and diminishes the role that price of product/service plays in determining the quantity used. Research has shown that 34% of adults with health insurance did not know the amount of their family's most recent hospital bill.[32] Seventy-eight percent of the respondents did not know what contribution their employer makes for their insurance. Therefore, there is little incentive for patients to question the ordering of tests or procedures on the basis of financial considerations. In addition, prices increase because there is little incentive for suppliers or providers to lower them to gain market share.

As the number of lawsuits and liability awards increase, so do the liability insurance premiums for health care providers. These increased costs are then passed along to patients or insurers. The threat of such lawsuits encourages practitioners to practice defensive medicine—health care practitioners' actions primarily undertaken to reduce their exposure to malpractice liability.[33] Although difficult to measure, the practice of defensive medicine has been estimated to represent five to nine percent of health care expenditures.[34] This would equal approximately $60 to $108 billion in 1999 alone.

Of course there are many other reasons for increased health care costs. Some of these include the lack of information available to patients in order to make educated decisions regarding their medical care, administration costs of private health insurance, the duplication of services, competition for patients in many locations, fraud, and unnecessary care. Attempts to contain costs should take into account the factors above if they are to be adequately controlled.

Access to Care

Access to medical care is a critical issue for many persons in the United States. Lack of access to care may result in deterioration of a person's health and the eventual use of intensive and expensive medical care that may have been prevented. Because of the high costs, access to care in the United States may be measured in terms of the number of Americans who are uninsured. Estimates vary according to the number of persons uninsured for an entire year versus the number uninsured at any point during a year. Also, because most persons 65 years of age or older are covered by Medicare, the percentage uninsured also may represent the percentage of the nonelderly population. For example, the U.S. Census Bureau estimated that approximately 38.7 million persons, 14% of the U.S. population, were uninsured for the entire year in 2000.[7] Another estimate projected that 42 million nonelderly Americans, or 17.5%, were uninsured in 1999.[33] Add to these estimates many more Americans who are under insured and have little insurance protection against catastrophic medical expenses.

It is often assumed that the uninsured are persons who are unemployed and ineligible for public funds. However, often this is not the case (**Figure 4.5**). Only about 18% of the uninsured are in a family where no one is employed and 71% of the uninsured are in a family where at least one person is employed full time.[35] Persons who have the greatest risk of being uninsured include younger adults, particularly men; low-income families; racial and ethnic minorities; families with only part-time workers or no workers at all; and workers employed in low-paying jobs or small businesses.

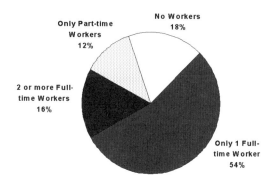

Figure 4.5. Nonelderly Uninsured by Family Work Status, 1999.[35]

One ramification of these findings is that a combination of programs, one providing incentives for employers to provide benefits and the other providing insurance for the unemployed and their families, could provide access to health insurance in our current system. However, using our present health care system, which has greatly contributed to the current crisis of increased health care costs, is controversial.

A final point regarding access is that the question should be, Access to what? Because a person has access to insurance does not necessarily mean they have access to medical care. As an example, consider pregnant Medicaid recipients. Even though they have publicly financed insurance, there is still a problem with low birth-weight babies in this population. There may not be transportation available for some to be able to travel to a health care provider in order to receive proper prenatal care. There may be others who do not seek it. In the situation where a person does have access to insurance, what can or should be done to ensure that care is given? Whose role is it to ensure this care?

Quality/Effectiveness of Care

There is little doubt that, overall, the present quality of health care in the United States is probably the highest it has ever been. But it is also apparent that this high quality of care is not available to all. Aggregate measures of the population's health status, such as infant mortality rates and life expectancy, are no better in this country than in other countries that spend less per capita on health care.

One of the problems with ensuring quality is that it has different meanings to different persons. To consumers quality may represent the opportunity to choose a provider or insurer, to an insurer it may suggest the appropriateness of care, and to a clinician it may mean the effectiveness of therapy. However, implicit in the concept of quality medical care is that services should be cost-efficient and cost-effective because unnecessary, excessive, or inappropriate services do not help the patient and may be harmful, or waste the patient's resources.[36]

In general, the main concerns over the quality of medical care in the United States have developed from an excessive or inappropriate use of services. These include the variable rates of hospitalization across the country, the overuse or underuse of various diagnostic tests, excessive or inappropriate surgery (such as tonsillectomies and caesarean sections), early discharge from hospitals because of diagnosis-related groups, variable results of surgeries, and the excessive or inappropriate use of prescription drugs.

The occurrences of medical errors have also received considerable media attention. An Institute of Medicine (IOM) study estimated that 44,000 to 98,000 people die in hospitals each year as the result of medical errors. If accurate, the lower estimate would make it the eighth leading cause of death in the United States ahead of motor vehicle accidents, breast cancer, and AIDS. The IOM report also estimates that medical errors cost the United States approximately $37.6 billion per year, of which an estimated $17 billion are associated with preventable errors.[37] It is also estimated that adverse drug events injure or kill 770,000 people each year in hospitals. Depending on the institution's size, annual hospital costs are estimated to be as much as $5.6 million per hospital.[38]

There is little doubt that quality and effectiveness of medical care are inseparable from access to care and the funds available to pay for the care. To consider the three separately during discussions of improving our health care system not only would be imprudent but also counter-productive. An example of this policy problem is the provision of pharmaceuticals. Most policy makers understand the importance of access to drug benefits in order to complete the provision of medical care, yet they are concerned about the costs, direct and indirect, and how such a benefit could be financed. In addition, the quality of the benefit must be ensured. Pharmaceutical care may be useful in ensuring quality but bring about additional questions regarding the provision and documentation of services, as well as reimbursement.

Representatives of insurers, corporations, the government, and consumers have generally come to the agreement that some changes must occur to affect the access, costs, and quality of the current U.S. health care system. Without such reform we will continue to spend an increasing amount of our resources on health care instead of other pressing social needs, and it will be increasingly difficult to ensure access to effective health care for all Americans.

Reforming a Disjointed Health Care System

Proposals to address the problems regarding access, costs, and quality of medical care vary widely. They represent the diversity of political, economic, and social philosophies found in U.S. society.

Basic Questions for Reform Proposals

In general, when considering different methods by which to change the incentives within our health care system several questions need to be asked to better understand the proposal:

1) What are the objectives of the plan? Does it attempt to affect costs, access, and/or quality?

2) Should all beneficiaries receive the same benefits or will there be a set of basic benefits which all receive?

3) If there is a set of basic benefits, what services are included and who decides what these will be?

4) How much are we, as a society, willing to spend for health care? How will this be measured—aggregate expenditures, per capita expenditures, percent of GDP?

5) How will these expenditures be financed?

6) Who will administer the program—private insurers, federal government, state governments, or a combination?
7) How will quality of care be measured, monitored, and ensured?
8) How much autonomy will patients be allowed regarding their choice of insurance plans, providers, and specific medical decisions?

Probably, the most difficult issues to address are those related to the financing of the plan and the cost controls used. In determining the financing, policy makers must assess the fairness in funding the plan. These different funding mechanisms may produce economic disincentives that must be considered, and lawmakers will certainly measure the political ramifications. Second, decisions must be made regarding the proper cost controls. Some degree of freedom may be taken from the beneficiary in the choice of a health care provider. This already has been found to be a political no-win decision. Also, policies limiting reimbursement for health care providers have to be defined. This again may bring about political fallout and unwelcome disincentives regarding access to care for beneficiaries.

Views on Health Care Reform

Proposals to reform our health care system lie on an ideological spectrum. On one end of the range are proposals that are egalitarian in nature and consider health care to be a social good available to all at the same level. An example of this would be to extend comprehensive medical care benefits to the entire population with payments for such services made by the federal government as the single payer. At the other end are those that maintain health care is a basic good that should be regulated and distributed through a free market. These proposals would remove restrictions that supporters maintain do not allow the free market to work. Most proposals are somewhere between these two and provide a basic set of benefits to all or a needy portion of the population.

According to this country's modern history, it appears that the more likely scenario would be a series of incremental changes. Social policy in the United States tends to evolve slowly, taking calculated steps but not giant leaps. Most of the U.S. population is satisfied with their health care although they believe some changes are needed; but they are also concerned about extending the welfare state. In addition, the complexity of both our health care system's problems and the proposed solutions make it difficult to develop a public consensus around any proposal. The perceived effects of reform on an individual's own personal health care and the increased funding needed to implement a reformed system result in a citizenry supportive of more prolonged and methodical change.

This incremental change might result in health insurance reform whereby small businesses and individuals share their risks through health share purchasing cooperatives, regulations prohibiting "preexisting condition" clauses in policies to prevent health insurance companies from refusing to insure persons with health problems, and insurance premiums based on a community rating of all persons in a geographical area and not based on experience rating of an individual's or a business' past medical care experience. Also, tax system reform may be proposed in order to help individuals or groups purchase health insurance. Another change in the tax system may attempt to lessen the health insurance effect by providing incentives for employers to offer and employees to accept less comprehensive health insurance plans. Finally, malpractice reform could seek to reduce malpractice premiums for health care providers and decrease the practice of defensive medicine.

Pharmaceutical Care and its Place in the U.S. Health Care System

The need for a reduction in health care costs, better access to medical care, and a commitment to improved quality and more effective health care bode well for the concept of pharmaceutical care and for practitioners. The pharmacist is in a unique position to positively affect each of the challenges the health care system faces.

The practice of pharmaceutical care has the ability to affect not only the well-being of patients but also their cost of care. For example, a study on medical errors found that the participation of a pharmacist in patient rounds resulted in a reduction in adverse drug events from 33 to 11.6 per 1000 patient days and a reduction in hospital costs of $270,000 per year.[39] By focusing on a patient's health outcomes, the pharmacist may not only ensure the proper therapeutic use of drug therapy but also decrease the occurrence of deleterious outcomes. This results in more cost-effective patient care and a control of costs precipitated by care and concern for patients. Other chapters will provide more support for this statement.

Pharmaceutical care also assists with concerns regarding the problem of access to care. Because of pharmacists' accessibility and reputation in the community, they have a unique opportunity to improve access to care for patients. Pharmacist availability in the community facilitates the provision of primary care and the coordination and continuity of care.

Quality of medical care is also positively influenced by pharmaceutical care. As we have seen, adverse drug effects have had significant harmful effects on the quality of medical care. Inappropriate drug therapy regimens result in treatment failures. Pharmaceutical care can assist in achieving optimal patient outcomes.

As health care organizations become more integrated, pharmacists will have better access to clinical information needed to perform their responsibilities. This will be enhanced by the development of new information systems. These systems should also provide a more effective method for determining patient outcomes. In addition, more persons will have health insurance benefits and be less affected by financial barriers to care.

Yet there are also challenges for pharmaceutical care providers. Managed care networks may omit some providers from participating unless they can document the effectiveness of the services they provide. Decreases in product reimbursement will decrease the margins on ingredient costs and will necessitate better management skills and the need for reimbursement for services provided. Again, documentation of effectiveness will be required. Payers also may attempt to share their risks with pharmaceutical care providers through capitated payments instead of a fee-for-service reimbursement. The calculation of the appropriate reimbursement levels will be critical for both the payer and the provider of care.

Summary

The U.S. health care system provides the best medical care in the world for those who have access to it. But it is also beset with problems of high costs, impeded access, and concerns regarding quality—dilemmas that are interrelated and difficult to unravel. The resolution of these problems will not be easy, quick, or perfect.

Pharmacists, as well as other health professionals, are at a crossroads where some will be winners and others will be losers. Only through the provision of care that recognizes the patient as the paramount concern will the profession progress. There are many challenges the health care system offers pharmacy, but there are also many opportunities.

References

1. Health Insurance Association of America. Source book of health insurance data 1991. Washington, DC: HIAA; 1992.
2. Jonas S. Health care delivery in the United States. New York: Springer Publishing; 1986.
3. Mariner WK. Problems with employer-provided health insurance—The Employee Retirement Income Security Act and health care reform. *N Engl J Med.* 1992; 327:1682–5.
4. Hoffman C, Schlobohm A. Uninsured in America, a chart book. Washington, DC: Kaiser Commission on Medicaid and the Uninsured; May 2000.
5. U.S. Census Bureau. Health insurance coverage: 2000. Current population reports. Washington, DC: U.S. Department of Commerce, Series P60-215; September 2001.
6. Schroeder S. Prospects for expanding health insurance coverage. *N Engl J Med.* 2001; 344:847–52.
7. Heffler S, Levit K, Smith S et al. Health spending growth up in 1999; faster growth expected in the future. *Health Aff.* 2001; 20:193–203.
8. Kaiser Family Foundation and Health Research and Educational Trust. Employer health benefits, 2001 summary of findings. Washington, DC: Kaiser Family Foundation; 2001. http://www.kff.org/content/2001/20010906a/EHB2001_sof.pdf (accessed 2001 Oct 11).
9. The Committee on the Costs of Medical Care. *JAMA.* 1932; 99:1950–2. Editorial.
10. Kaiser Commission on Medicaid and the Uninsured. CHIP program enrollment: December 2000. Washington, DC: Kaiser Family Foundation; September 2001. http://www.kff.org/content/2001/4005/4005.pdf (accessed 2001 Oct 12).
11. Board of Trustees, Federal Hospital Insurance Trust Fund. 2001 annual report of the board of trustees of the Federal Hospital Insurance Trust Fund. Baltimore, MD: Health Care Financing Administration; 2001.
12. Kaiser Family Foundation. Medicare at a glance. Washington, DC: Kaiser Family Foundation; June 2001. http://www.kff.org/content/archive/1066/Medicare%201066.pdf (accessed 2001 Oct 11).

13. Board of Trustees, Federal Supplementary Medical Insurance Trust Fund. 2001 annual report of the board of trustees of the Federal Supplementary Medical Insurance Trust Fund. Baltimore, MD: Health Care Financing Administration; 2001.

14. Poisal JA, Murray M. Growing differences between Medicare beneficiaries with and without drug coverage. *Health Aff.* 2001; 20:74–85.

15. Crippen DL. Medicare reform: providing prescription drug coverage for seniors. Congressional Budget Office testimony before the Subcommittee on Health, Committee on Energy and Commerce, U.S. House of Representatives. May 16, 2001.

16. Kaiser Commission on Medicaid and the Uninsured. Medicaid enrollment and spending trends. Washington, DC: Kaiser Family Foundation; February 2001. http://www.kff.org/content/2001/2113b/2113b.pdf (accessed 2001 Oct 11).

17. Kaiser Commission on Medicaid and the Uninsured. The Medicaid program at a glance. Washington, DC: Kaiser Family Foundation; January 2001. http://www.kff.org/content/2001/2004b/2004b.pdf (accessed 2001 Oct 11).

18. Health Care Financing Administration. A profile of Medicaid, chart book 2000. Baltimore, MD: Health Care Financing Administration; 2000.

19. Wallack, SS. Managed care: practice, pitfalls, and potential. *Health Care Fin Review.* 1992; 1991(Annual Supplement):27–34.

20. Aventis Pharmaceuticals. Managed care digest series 2000: HMO-PPO/Medicare-Medicaid digest. Bridgewater, NJ: Aventis Pharmaceuticals; 2001.

21. Marion Merrell Dow, Inc. Managed care digest, HMO edition. Kansas City, MO: Marion Merrell Dow, Inc.; 1993.

22. Staines VS. Potential impact of managed care on national health care spending. *Health Aff.* 1993; 12(Supplement):248–57.

23. Legnini MW, Rosenberg LE, Perry MJ et al. 2000. Where does performance measurement go from here? *Health Aff.* 2000; 19(3):173–7.

24. Employee Benefits Research Institute. 2001. 2001 Health Confidence Survey: Managed Care Confusion. Washington, DC: Employee Benefits Research Institute; 2001.

25. Dudley RA, Luft HS. Managed care in transition. *N Engl J Med.* 2001; 344:1087–92.

26. Center for Medicare and Medicaid Services. 2001. National health care projections: 2000–2010. 2001; www.hcfa.gov/stats/NHE-Proj/proj2000/tbles (accessed 2001 Oct 12).

27. Health Care Financing Administration. National health expenditures, 1999 highlights. 2000. www.hcfa.gov/stats/nhe-oact/hilites.htm (accessed 2001 Oct 12).

28. Levit KR, Lazenby HC, Cowan CA et al. National health expenditures, 1990. *Health Care Fin Review.* 1991; 13:29–54.

29. Administration on Aging. A profile of older Americans: 2000. Washington: U.S. Department of Health and Human Services; 2000.

30. Hodgson PA, Cohen HA. Medical care expenditures for major diseases, 1995. *Health Care Fin Review.* 1999; 21:119–64.

31. Newhouse JP. Medical care costs: how much welfare loss? *J Econ Persp.* 1992; 6:3–21.

32. Anderson K. Why health care costs are tough to cure. *USA Today.* March 11, 1991:3B.

33. Office of Technology Assessment, U.S. Congress. Defensive Medicine and Medical Malpractice. Washington, DC: U.S. Government Printing Office. July 1994; Publication OTA-H-602.

34. Kessler DP, McClellan M. Do doctors practice defensive medicine? *Qtr J Econ.* 1996; 111:353–90.

35. Hoffman C, Pohl M. Health insurance coverage in America. Washington, DC: Kaiser Commission on Medicaid and the Uninsured. December 2000.

36. Lohr KN, Yordy YD, Their SO. Current issues in quality of care. *Health Aff.* 1988; 7:5–18.

37. Agency for Healthcare Research and Quality. Medical errors: the scope of the problem. Washington, DC: U.S. Department of Health and Human Services. February 2000; Publication No. AHRQ 00-PO37. http://www.ahrq.gov/qual/errback.htm (accessed 2001 Oct 18).

38. Agency for Healthcare Research and Quality. Reducing and preventing adverse drug events to decrease hospital costs. Washington, DC: U.S. Department of Health and Human Services. March 2001. Publication No. AHRQ 01-0020. http://www.ahrq.gov/qual/aderia/aderia.htm (accessed 2001 Oct 18).

39. Leape LL, Cullen DJ, Clapp MD et al. Pharmacist participation on physician rounds and adverse drug events in the intensive care unit. *JAMA.* 1999; 281:267–70.

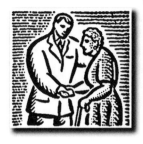

Chapter 5: Drug Use and the Health Care System

Robert J. Valuck, R.Ph., Ph.D.
Kavita V. Nair, Ph.D.

Traditionally, all of the health disciplines have been involved to some degree with drugs, but no particular discipline operating at the clinical level has exercised a broad responsibility for the total drug use process. Typically, the drug prescribing, dispensing, and administering functions have occurred independently, with no effective co-ordination. This situation has resulted in drug misuse, overuse, abuse, and serious untoward effects. The problems in drug therapy management, resulting from the isolation of these functions, led to the thinking that there was a need for one discipline to assume broad leadership and responsibility for the safe and appropriate use of drugs in society.[1]

Introduction

In 1969, President Johnson's Task Force on Prescription Drugs formally documented an array of problems with the use of prescription drugs in the United States health care system.[2] The Task Force proposed a series of system improvements, including enhanced physician education in clinical pharmacology and experimentation with various drug utilization review (DUR) methods, with the goal of achieving rational drug therapy for all patients.[3] In the course of the three decades between its final report and the present day, some of the solutions of the Task Force have been implemented. Most notably, formal retrospective and prospective DUR programs were required for Medicaid recipients by legislative provisions contained in the Omnibus Budget Reconciliation Act of 1990 (OBRA 1990).[4] However, many problems noted by the Task Force remain unresolved and in need of attention.

Henri Manasse, a longtime leader in the pharmacy profession, has suggested the label "drug misadventuring" as a broad term inclusive of any complication of drug therapy.[5,6] Manasse notes that the extensive use of pharmaceuticals in the United States has increased the risk of misadventuring. He cites estimates that drug misadventures contribute tens of billions of dollars annually to this country's spiraling health care costs. Ernst and Grizzle[7] have calculated that the cost of drug-related morbidity and mortality in the United States in the ambulatory setting alone may be as high as $177 billion annually as of the year

2000. Manasse advocates for the development of a comprehensive public policy dealing with this problem. Hepler[8] has suggested specific, system-level strategies to prevent drug-related morbidity by regulating practice to ensure optimal patient outcomes.

Indeed, some attention over the past 30 years has been centered on the identification, documentation, and, to some extent, the prevention of various forms of drug misadventuring. Strand et al.[9] proposed a useful descriptive typology for classifying, dealing with, and preventing drug-related problems (see **Table 5.1**) that has become a central part of the provision of pharmaceutical care. However, just as drug-related problems were the result of a lack of a coordinated system of drug use, efforts to address them have often been fragmented as well.

Table 5.1. Major Types of Drug-Related Problems

A patient is experiencing (or has the potential to experience) an undesirable event (medical problem, complaint, symptoms, diagnosis, or syndrome) that is of psychological, physiological, social, emotional, or economic origin, and is a function of the patient's

1. needing pharmacotherapy but not receiving it (a drug indication),
2. taking or receiving the wrong drug,
3. taking or receiving too little of the correct drug,
4. taking or receiving too much of the correct drug,
5. experiencing an adverse drug reaction,
6. experiencing a drug–drug, drug–food, or drug–laboratory interaction,
7. not taking or receiving the drug prescribed, or
8. taking or receiving a drug for which there is no valid medical indication.

Strand LM, Cipolle RJ, Morley PC. Pharmaceutical care: an introduction, p. 11. Kalamazoo, MI: The Upjohn Company; 1992.

This chapter is based on the premise that the drug-use *process* in the health care system is suboptimal and therefore is not conducive for the delivery of pharmaceutical care. In addition there are several forces, both internal and external to pharmacy, that create major obstacles to the delivery of pharmaceutical care. Therefore, the profession of pharmacy must endeavor to transform the existing process into a drug-use *system* designed to promote the rational prescribing, preparation, distribution, use, monitoring, and evaluation of drugs and drug therapy.

The Drug-Use Process in the U.S. Health Care System

In the mid 1960's, Brodie[10] was the first to advocate the notion of drug-use control as "the keystone to pharmaceutical service . . . the mainstream function of pharmacy." Brodie defined drug-use control as the system of knowledge, understanding, judgments, procedures, skills, controls, and ethics that ensures optimal safety in the distribution and use of medication. He further stated, "Drug-use control provides a purpose, it gives a direction, it recognizes need and fulfillment in the patient–pharmacist relationship, it is the basic ingredient which underlies the essentiality of pharmacy and its service." Brodie suggested that drug-use control encompasses the chain of events from the development of a drug to the completion of the drug's task in the patient's body. The term applies to community, institutional, and industrial pharmacy practice, as well as pharmacy education.

Evolution of the Drug-Use Process Concept

As the fundamental nature of pharmacy practice has evolved over the past 100 years, so has our conceptualization and understanding of the complexities of the drug-use process. Paralleling this professional role evolution has been an expansion and a revision of what has or should have constituted the drug-use process. In an era when pharmacists were primarily the compounders and the dispensers of medicines, the drug-use process might have been described as beginning with the discovery, extraction, or synthesis of raw drugs and ending with the sale of the finished, compounded prescription to the patient.[11] During the era of expansion of clinical pharmacy, the scope of practice grew to include the delivery of several pharmaceutical services (e.g., pharmacokinetic dosing, therapeutic monitoring, provision of drug information, nutritional support, and the compilation of medication histories). The notion of the drug-use process had shifted to place much less emphasis on compounding and considerably more emphasis on clinical service delivery.

Since the mid 1970's, many experts have argued that pharmacy should be defined as a *system* that renders a health service by concerning itself with knowledge about drugs and the application of this knowledge to man and animals.[12] More recently it has been advocated that this knowledge about drugs should constitute the theoretical base of pharmacy practice in the 1990's and well into the twenty-first century.[13] For this assertion to hold true, the drug-use process must be viewed in terms of the application of specialized knowledge to any and all aspects of drug use. Pharmacists' unique education and skills represent an enabling mechanism by which they may affect many aspects of drug use. Among the tools the modern pharmacist has available is consultation with physicians on therapies of choice—monitoring the ability of drugs to achieve therapeutic objectives and minimize adverse events in patients, and, ultimately, making recommendations accordingly.

Since the landmark description of the concept of pharmaceutical care by Hepler and Strand,[14] there have been numerous definitions of the concept[15] and suggestions and evaluations of models for implementing pharmaceutical care in practice. These include the Therapeutic Outcomes Monitoring (TOM) model of Grainger–Rousseau et al.[16] and the Pharmacists Implementation of Pharmaceutical Care (PIPC) model of Odedina et al.,[17] among others. Descriptions of actual implementation of pharmaceutical care concepts in practice are provided elsewhere in this text.

The Drug-Use Process Model

The concept of coordinated efforts to achieve the optimal use of drugs is encompassed in the multistage model referred to as the drug-use process.[18–20] This requires patients and all health professionals to play a role in the drug-use process and to consider that all actions related to drug therapy represent a continuum. The systems perspective espoused here (**Figure 5.1**) necessitates interrelated and coordinated decisions with a focus on patient problems and the means to achieve the desired therapeutic endpoints. As illustrated in the figure,

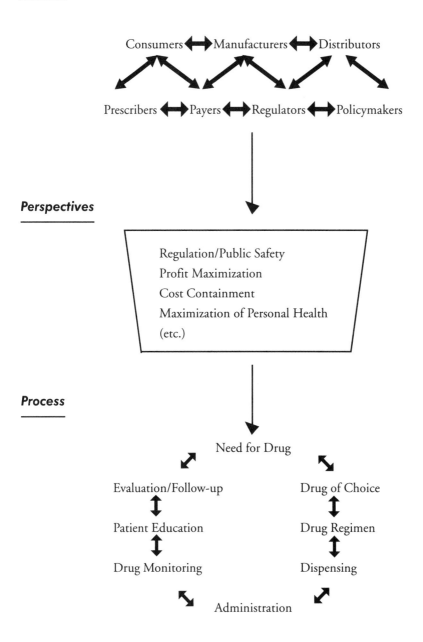

Figure 5.1. An Expanded View of the Drug-Use Process (modified from reference 21).

this perspective must also include an understanding of the fact that there are numerous players involved in the drug-use process, each with their own perspectives as to what constitutes appropriate or rational drug use. For example, consumers clearly have an interest in the drug-use process, and their interest is in maintaining their own personal health, safely and at reasonable cost. Regulators, on the other hand, are most interested in ensuring the safety of the general public. Pharmaceutical manufacturers are interested in developing new drug products and bringing them to market, with the goal of serving society and their stockholders. Payers (insurance companies, Medicaid agencies, etc.) are interested in providing comprehensive health coverage for their enrollees at reasonable cost.

Given these complex and diverse interests in the drug-use process, it is not surprising that it is disjointed and inefficient in manpower use and resource consumption. Physicians, pharmacists, and nurses spend significant amounts of time carrying out technical tasks in isolation, and many professional activities are poorly coordinated.[21] As a result, patients may be placed at risk.

The following sections describe each of the eight steps of the drug-use process. Along with the descriptions are discussions of reported incidents documenting suboptimal drug therapy and identifying opportunities for pharmacists to improve therapeutic outcomes. It should be kept in mind that errors and failures may occur at any point in the drug-use process and that for the process to function optimally, each step must be completed without problems. For example, if a drug is not administered properly, it matters little that tasks such as selection and dispensing have been carried out properly.[21]

Step One: Perception of the Need for a Drug

The potential risk of undesirable consequences from the misuse of drugs requires health care professionals and patients to be circumspect in their decisions to use drug therapy. Patient needs and alternative therapies must be considered before either prescription or nonprescription drug therapy is initiated. However, evidence shows that physicians are inclined to use pharmacologic forms of treatment even when nonpharmacologic modes of therapy are more advantageous.[22] A classic example of unnecessary and non-indicated use of drug therapy is the prescription of antibiotics to treat the common cold.[23] This unnecessary use of antibiotics may lead to clinical complications, including the development of resistant strains of bacteria, a multitude of untoward health consequences, and an unnecessary increase in the cost of drug therapy.[24]

The need for drug therapy must be carefully evaluated and weighed against the alternatives for every patient. Both health professionals and patients must realize that all illnesses do not necessitate drug therapy. Because of the cost of drugs and the potential for adverse effects, drugs should be used only when indicated. Pharmacists should monitor drug use in all practice settings and assist in establishing guidelines to discourage unnecessary drug use, given that two thirds of all patient visits to physicians result in a prescription; pharmacists should also become directly involved in the decision to use drug therapy.[25] Pharmacists can become involved by documenting important drug-related information in patient profiles or medical charts, establishing positive consultative arrangements with physicians in their practice settings, and providing inservices and other forms of education for medical staff, area physicians or group practices, and patients. In the case of decreasing unnecessary antibiotic use, pharmacists acting as academic detailers to educate physicians have been shown to be an effective component of a strategy that has reduced this prescribing problem by one third.[26]

Step Two: Selection of Drug of Choice

The second step in the drug-use process is the selection of the most appropriate drug for a specific diagnosis or condition. This decision should be based on therapeutic goals, patient variables, and costs.[21] One dilemma for the prescriber at this step can be summarized as follows:

> The basic motivations behind a physician's choice of drug therapy must be considered to be rational. [S]/He would be expected to select the product that would do the most good with the least possible side effects, and perhaps the lowest cost. In most cases of drug [of choice] selection, however, physicians try to make a rational decision under conditions of uncertainty.[27]

A number of factors that foster suboptimal prescribing have been identified. Hutchinson at al.[21] noted that some of the most common factors are the rapid rate of new drug introductions to the market, the profusion of promotional product information, failure to keep abreast of current drug topics, careless evaluation of drug information, and the underestimation of the true cost and toxicity of drugs. A review of the literature by Valuck[28] also identified medical practice fads, office or clinic location (e.g., urban versus rural), and a variety of physician characteristics as being correlated with irrational prescribing. A high frequency of suboptimal prescribing practices has been reported in the literature over the past 20 years.[28–30]

One plausible explanation for the frequency of suboptimal prescribing, pointed out by Hutchinson et al.[21] is that, while a significant amount of time and effort is required to understand drugs and their actions, physicians have limited time available for reading and understanding the medical and pharmaceutical literature. The American College of Physicians reported that continuing education in pharmacology for physicians is largely random and incomplete.[31] New information on available drug therapy is reported at an unbelievably rapid pace. It is quite optimistic to suggest that health care professionals in general and physicians in particular have the time to keep up with this information.

When given the opportunity to influence selection of drugs of choice, pharmacists have demonstrated their ability to improve drug prescribing. Pharmacists have targeted specific drugs that were subject to suboptimal prescribing and successfully changed patterns of use.[27]

In an age of rapid technological advancement, maintaining expert knowledge of every aspect of health care is beyond the scope of any single profession, let alone individual practitioners. One societal solution to the exponential growth in drug-related information may be to sanction experts in each field and to follow a professional team approach in ensuring optimal health care delivery.[21] Empirical evidence supports the contentions that pharmacists make sound therapeutic recommendations when given therapeutic objectives and physicians are willing to accept such recommendations.[32,33]

Step Three: Selection of Drug Regimen

The third step of the drug-use process is the selection of a specific drug regimen. A drug regimen includes the dose, dosage form, route, frequency of administration, and duration of drug therapy. In this step, the most appropriate regimen should be selected for accomplishing the desired goals based on patient-specific variables.[21]

Problems in this step exist and deviations from acceptable standards have been cited many times over the years. In an earlier study, nearly 90% of 87 patients monitored received theophylline doses that exceeded recommended guidelines, and more than 81% of these patients experienced toxicity.[34] In more recent studies, pharmacists have shown competence and skill in the selection of the drug regimen and has great potential for reducing costs and increasing the proper and safe use of medications. For example, pharmacists are able to adjust anticoagulant therapy as well as experienced physicians[35,36]; are able to avert dose-related toxicities from digoxin therapy[37]; and are able to apply their knowledge of pharmacokinetics to customize aminoglycoside antibiotic dosage regimens in hospitalized patients.[38]

Step Four: Provision of Drug Product

The fourth step of the drug-use process is the preparation and dispensing of the drug product. Historically, pharmacists have spent the majority of their time compounding and dispensing prescriptions. This step of the drug-use process has received the most attention in pharmacy literature since Barker and McConnell[39] reported that one dose in six was given in error at a large university hospital. In fact, in terms of systems improvement, the unit-dose method of distributing pharmaceuticals has been successful in decreasing both medication errors and the total cost of drug distribution and administration.[40]

Improving the system of drug distribution without implementing changes in the overall drug-use process does not necessarily ensure sound drug therapy. If this were the case, one would not expect problems with drug therapy in hospitals using the unit-dose system. While this system ensures correct dispensing, it does not necessarily ensure that the medication selected is appropriate or that nurses administer the drug to the patient on time or at all. The system employed by most hospitals for dispensing and administering medications allows neither the pharmacists nor the nurses to assume full control for coordinating these two steps. Hence, medication errors continue to be reported.[41]

In the community, drug administration is in the hands of patients, their family members, and their caregivers, and correct administration becomes a function of the individual's understanding of the need for drug therapy, as well as the patient's willingness to abide by the instructions given. Because of these variables, any drug distribution system, regardless of setting, must have supportive clinical services to ensure proper drug use.

In the 21st century, pharmacists need to understand technological advances and incorporate them into their daily practices. Not only can technologies, such as automation and robotics help minimize nonprofessional tasks, they can also offer the opportunity to develop distribution systems that will provide continuous care to patients when they move from one setting to another (i.e., inpatient to outpatient). This is of particular concern given the existing financial pressure for the early discharge of patients from hospitals. Once discharged, patients are expected to seek services from community pharmacies. Community pharmacists are in most cases faced with assessing these patients' needs based on incomplete information. Existing technology can be applied to this problem in useful ways. At least one newly contemplated health care program for the nation is, in fact, centered around the use of smart cards to link services with patient demographic and clinical data. It remains, however, the responsibility of pharmacists to help define the information needed to ensure appropriate care and to be the conduit for the delivery of patient-oriented pharmaceutical care.

Step Five: Consumption or Administration

The fifth step of the drug-use process is the consumption (in the community) or administration (in the inpatient setting) of medication. Problems in drug administration exist due to the lack of effective coordination between those responsible for prescription, distribution, and administration.

Recently reported medication administration errors are no different from those reported in the early 1960's.[39,42] In hospital settings, medication errors are often linked to nursing services regardless of the origin of the error. Moreover, nurses, as professionals, are questioning the wisdom of continuing to assume responsibility for non-nursing tasks.[43] Nursing time devoted to drug administration has not been thoroughly studied.[44] However, it seems reasonable that it is not cost-effective for these health care professionals to continue to perform technical tasks.

Some institutions have approached the identified problems in this step with a pharmacy-coordinated drug dispensing and administering system. Pharmacy-coordinated drug administration teams have been shown to have a positive impact by decreasing the amount of error and human suffering, as well as by decreasing the direct and indirect costs associated with medication administration. However, this positive impact does not necessarily ensure the continuation of such a program, as both pharmacy and nursing staff continue to think of steps four and five in the drug-use process as independent processes in terms of both cost to their departments and consequences on patient care.

Consumption of drugs in the outpatient or community setting is complicated by patient non-compliance as well as the apparent lack of formal systems or processes to ensure that drugs are consumed appropriately.

Step Six: Monitoring Effects of Drug

In the sixth step of the drug-use process, drug therapy is monitored for effectiveness and adverse effects. This step is crucial, given that inappropriate medication monitoring may lead to prolonged illness and to increased resource consumption.

There are many established methods and parameters for monitoring the effectiveness of drug therapy, especially in inpatient settings.[45] Pharmacokinetic monitoring of drug therapy has been an important advancement and is especially valuable with drugs that have narrow therapeutic indices and are sensitive to patient-specific variables. However, determinations of serum drug concentrations represent additional health care resource consumption and must be used efficiently and effectively. Pharmacists have repeatedly been shown to be the most effective health care professionals in providing pharmacokinetic services in hospitals.[38,40]

Opportunities for application of pharmacokinetic skills to patient care are present for pharmacists outside institutional settings as well. Guidelines for drug therapy monitoring, which were developed in collaboration with physicians, provide pharmacists practicing in home health care, nursing homes, community care, and other settings with the chance to positively impact therapeutic outcomes in this step of the drug-use process. Measuring blood pressure and other clinical endpoints, and monitoring patient compliance are two examples of tasks pharmacists can take on and thereby play a key role in improving drug-therapy monitoring in a community setting. There is also tremendous need and opportunity to monitor and measure overall outcomes of therapy—such as patients' health status, satisfaction, and quality of life—things that are extremely important to patients but not routinely monitored by anyone.

Proper monitoring of drug therapy also entails the prevention (or early detection) of adverse drug reactions (ADRs). Although some ADRs are severe and may result in death, the literature has emphasized morbidity, drug-related hospital admissions, increased hospital stays, and related costs.[5,6,46] In addition to their impact upon patients' quality of life, ADRs needlessly increase resource consumption. In one study, patients with one or more ADRs stayed in hospitals an average of 13.7 days more than patients with no ADRs.[47]

Appropriate monitoring is pivotal and of most concern for medications that are highly potent and possess narrow therapeutic indices. Monitoring for drug-related complications or adverse events is rather complicated, however, since drugs are not frequently identified as the cause of patients' problems. In this regard, pharmacists appear more apt to suspect drugs as the source of problems than physicians or nurses, particularly in inpatient settings where these teams of providers more typically work side by side.[48] Pharmacists have both an opportunity and a responsibility, however, to minimize the incidence of ADRs regardless of practice setting.

Step Seven: Patient Education

The seventh step in the drug-use process is patient education. In this step patients are educated about their drugs to assist in compliance with the prescribed regimen and the early detection and reporting of drug-related adverse events.

An investigation by the Office of the Inspector General (OIG) for Health and Human Services, which described the effects of patient noncompliance, placed particular emphasis on the ambulatory elderly population. In this population, it was estimated that 55% of patients do not follow their prescribed regimens.[49] The OIG report concluded that noncompliance with medication regimens increases the use of such resources as hospitals, nursing homes, and clinics and results in unnecessary treatments. Noncompliance can also lead to therapeutic failure, which in some instances results in serious complications or death. Moreover, the report points out that educating patients is the best way to improve compliance with drug therapy and emphasizes that patient education should not be construed to mean simply repeating directions or handing out printed materials. Rather, patient education is a process entailing gathering data, individualizing instructions, prompting and supporting the patient, and following up on and evaluating the patient's response to therapy to determine the success of the treatment in improving patient outcomes.[50] Opportunities abound for pharmacists to overcome traditional obstacles; to use their knowledge and expertise to improve patient understanding, compliance, and clinical outcomes through counseling and education; and to enhance their professional standing as they conform with the OBRA 1990 mandates.

Step Eight: Evaluation and Follow-up

The eighth and final step of the drug-use process is the evaluation of drug therapy effectiveness in light of therapeutic objectives and observed patient outcomes. As with any process where goals and objectives have been set, it is important to monitor the patient's response as compared to desired endpoints. Having such information in hand will facilitate the optimal use of medications.

Perspectives on the Drug-Use Process

The use of drugs in the United States is strongly influenced by a variety of factors that define our society, its culture, and its norms. These factors include, but are not limited to, trends in demography, epidemiology, technology, social structure and function, economics and politics. As Manasse notes

> In our pluralistic, individualistic, and competitive society, our collective drug-use behavior reflects a phenomenon that is unique to the United States but parallels pharmaceutical consumption trends in other parts of the developed world. In short, we are a drug-taking society whose outlook centers on the general view that every malady has a treatment solution and that this solution lies mainly in the use of medicinal agents. Within this set of broader forces, a variety of collective "actors"— each with unique interests, strengths, and limitations—bring differing demands and expectations to the drug-use process.

Forces Precipitating Change

Understanding the drug-use process of the future requires an assessment of the major trends that are influencing health care and pharmacy practice today. Each trend holds within it threats and opportunities for the profession of pharmacy in general and for its practitioners in particular.

Demographic Factors

Demographic data clearly show that the population of the U.S. is growing older. The Bureau of Census projections of 1996 anticipate that the elderly population is expected to increase by 17% from 33.5 million in 1995 to 39.4 million in 2010.[51] In the period between 2010 to 2030, the population aged 65 and older is expected to grow by 75% to over 69 million.[51] The growth in the number of the oldest old (aged 85 and over) is of greater public concern. During 1995 to 2010, this population is expected to grow by 56% as compared with a 13% growth of the population aged 65 to 84.[51] This means that a large share of the elderly population will be over 85. The rapid rise of the aging population presents challenges in providing health services, particularly in the area of medication use.

Few pharmacists would argue that the elderly offer challenging opportunities for pharmaceutical services, but few have been successful in devising practice models that meet the needs of the elderly population and satisfy the professional goals in economically efficient ways. However, efforts are being made by pharmacists to identify and address the unique medication needs of the elderly population. For example, community pharmacists participating in the Pharmaceutical Care Research and Education Project (PREP) documented 559 drug related problems in a sample of 159 elderly patients (a mean of 3.9 problems per patient) whose mean age was 74 years using pharmacy records.[52] Counseling, preventive consultations, and clinical monitoring represented 40% of their recommendations that resulted in improved outcomes for 83% of the sample. With the rapid increases in the elderly population over the next few decades, the profession will now have an opportunity to take a primary role in providing pharmaceutical care services to this therapeutically complex population.

Another changing trend is the ethnic composition of the American population over the next few decades. Between 2010 and 2030, the numbers of African Americans, Asians and Pacific Islanders, and Hispanics will increase dramatically.[51] The rates of growth for these ethnic groups are projected to exceed those of Caucasians. For example, by the year 2010 Hispanics are expected to grow by 52.7%, African Americans by 21%, and Caucasians only by 10%.[51] Other racial groups, including Native Americans as well as Asians and Pacific Islanders will increase by 55.4%.[51] These demographic changes are important for pharmacists to consider in providing pharmaceutical care as differences in cultural, environmental, and genetic factors influence patient beliefs and responses to medications.[53]

For example, differences in the relationship between health beliefs and the use of both prescribed medications among African American and Caucasian hypertensive patients has been documented.[54] Also, variations in response to specific medications have been observed. The ACE inhibitor, carvedilol, reduces the risk of worsening heart failure to a greater degree in black patients compared to nonblack individuals.[55] Similarly, Chinese patients may have a better response to morphine used in pain management than whites.[56] Health beliefs about medications are influenced by ethnicity. Hispanic patients are more likely to use home herbal medications that non-Hispanic whites.[57] Ethnic differences are in part responsible for the variations in health behavior, health beliefs, and perceptions about the role of prescription medications in contemporary society. Pharmacists should attempt to embrace the ethnic and racial composition of their patient populations by understanding their differences and issues unique to their health care beliefs. In doing so, pharmacists will be able to provide optimal pharmaceutical care for these populations.

Epidemiological Factors

A gradual but definite change has occurred in the nature of the illnesses afflicting the U.S. population. The pattern of illness in industrialized nations has shifted from one of mostly acute diseases to one in which chronic conditions predominate.[58] Although these diseases may shorten life expectancy, it is more likely that the diseases will lead to dysfunction and decreased well being.[58] Subsequently there is a growing recognition among providers that the quality of life should be an important consideration in deciding how to treat a patient. The emphasis on quality of life has led to a new group of therapies commonly referred to as lifestyle or quality-of-life medications.[59] These drugs refer to products that are intended to treat a problem that falls into the broader zone between the medical and social definitions of health and often include products used to treat diseases that result from an individual's lifestyle choices.[59] Examples of these products include those for erectile/sexual dysfunction, contraception, baldness, weight loss, smoking cessation, and cognition enhancement.

Consumers are now actively seeking information about these lifestyle products to enhance their quality of life, and these efforts are fuelled by the advertisement medications from the pharmaceutical company directly to the consumer.[60] Pharmacists are now in an advantageous position to serve as credible sources of information for consumers who are both seeking this information or who may benefit from having knowledge about these medications. Given the shift from acute to chronic illness to quality-of-life therapies in the United States, the importance of understanding the entire drug-use process is even more apparent. In order for long-term drug therapy regimens to remain optimal, to be modified as necessary, or to be supplemented with medications that enhance an individual's daily living, constant and careful monitoring of all steps of the drug-use process must be maintained.

Technological Factors

The rapid development of software and hardware applications for pharmacy will allow a redefinition of the future roles of pharmacists: technology will allow them to replace some current functions and fulfill other expanded roles. Information technology can facilitate the prescribing process, distribution and dispensing of medications, monitor medication use, and educate providers and patients about medications.[61] For prescribers, computer-based order entry is a central innovation towards improving the drug-use process. These central systems can also be useful in disseminating information to providers about formularies and practice-specific treatment guidelines on a regular basis.

Technology has also revolutionized the distribution of medications with systems such as Pyxis Medstation that decentralize the distribution of medications in hospitals, managed care, and long-term-care facilities.[62] These computer-controlled medication management systems maintain stocking levels, update inventory, and allow new prescription orders to be transmitted electronically thereby reducing pharmacists' time needed to run these pharmacy operations and allowing them to devote their efforts to providing pharmaceutical care.[62] Another form of technology, bar codes on prescription labels, has great potential to reduce medication errors by using technology to oversee the dispensing process especially when pharmacy technicians often dispense medications under the supervision of the pharmacist.[62]

Decision support databases allow providers to keep abreast with new drug developments and provide clinically based criteria to evaluate the appropriateness of drug therapy and monitor medication use. Drug use review criteria software available through the United States Pharmacopeia and other organizations can compare an individual patient's prescription profile with clinically determined standards that screen for appropriateness of therapy, drug–drug interactions, and drug–disease contraindications.[63]

Finally, the Internet has the capacity to serve as an important educational tool to patients and providers alike. Patients have access to numerous sites, such as www.drugstore.com or www.webmd.com, which provide information about medications. For providers, most journals of medicine and pharmacy can be accessed online thereby providing instant access to the most current information about medications. Thus pharmacists may use information technology to automate processes that free up time, reduce errors, and allow more effective functioning as pharmaceutical care providers.

Social Factors

One of the most prominent changes in the way health care is delivered today is the role that patients or consumers play in the medical decision-making process. Consumers have made it clear that they want to play a more active role in their health care decisions and are becoming increasingly knowledgeable about their medical conditions and the therapeutic alternatives that are available to them.[64] The increased availability of information has empowered consumers to participate in decisions concerning their health care.

An important factor driving this rise in consumerism is direct-to-consumer (DTC) advertising efforts by the pharmaceutical companies. Currently $2 billion a year is spent on DTC.[65] Proponents of DTC believe that consumers will have improved access to information about drug therapies, will be more aware of new and generic or therapeutic equivalents, will be encouraged to undertake preventive health measures, and even help protect themselves from underinformed practitioners.[66] Opponents of DTC argue that the quality of information available through DTC is questionable and consumers are not equipped to handle this medical information which could result in consumers being misinformed about the benefits and risks of medications.[67]

Whether DTC is beneficial or detrimental to consumers, in the process of reacting to DTC, consumers will seek to develop interactive relationships with health professionals. When consumers desire the freedom to self-diagnose and self-medicate (that is, to make their own health care decisions), they also demand accurate, personal, and available information resources.[68] Pharmacists are therefore in an excellent position to meet this unique demand and serve as an information source to consumers by guiding and educating them about the pros and cons of advertised medications.

Changing the status of drugs from prescription to over-the-counter availability (OTC) has also influenced the participation of consumers in their own health care. OTC status for prescription products can increase consumer access to effective medications, decrease their frequency of visits to physicians, lower health care costs, and increase consumer autonomy and education.[69] There are potential concerns in making prescription drugs available over the counter. Inaccurate self-diagnosis can cause harmful effects. The issue of suboptimal care resulting from the improper use of OTC medications for which there are more effective prescription medications can delay treatment for serious conditions.[69]

With the increased emphasis on consumers as active purchasers of health care, whether it be a result of DTC advertising or making prescription medications available OTC, pharmacists can play a pivotal role in providing appropriate care to consumers regarding their medication choices.

Economic Factors

The escalation of prescription drug expenditures in the United States over the past 20 to 30 years has caused concern among patients, providers, and payers alike. It is anticipated that prescription costs will continue to increase at a rate of 11–15% during this decade and sales may reach $243 billion by 2008; this amounts to 12.6% of total health care spending, compared with 8.1% in 1999.[70] The rising costs of pharmaceuticals have spawned a new generation of evaluation in the area of economic assessments for medications, as well as the services provided by pharmacists.

Economic analysis of medications involves cost-effectiveness, cost–benefit or cost–utility analysis of new drug therapies, comparison of competing drug therapies in a drug class, and the evaluation of different drug classes.[71,72] However, there is an increasing recognition among the pharmacy community that pharmacists play an important role in controlling the spiraling costs of health care. In the last decade there has been a growing emphasis on demonstrating the economic value of pharmaceutical care services provided by pharmacists. An examination of the economic impact of pharmaceutical care in ambulatory care settings on drug related morbidity and mortality estimated that negative therapeutic outcomes would be reduced by 53–63%, avoiding $45.6 billion in direct health care costs.[46] Pharmacist-led interventions have consistently shown improved health outcomes, decreased overall health care resource utilization, and reduced health care and pharmacy costs.[73–75] Pharmacists have a responsibility, therefore, to continue identifying ways in which the value of the services they provide can be documented and translated to better patient outcomes and cost savings to third-party payers and the institutions they serve.

Political Factors

As mentioned earlier, there are a number of relevant actors in the drug-use process (i.e., drug consumers, makers, distributors, prescribers, payers, regulators, and policymakers). Each of these groups has a unique set of interests, demands, and resources that they bring to bear on issues relating to drugs and public policy. It is therefore inevitable that the interests of such a wide variety of actors conflict at times and converge at others.

The interplay of economic, social, and institutional forces affects the political domain and vice versa. Ultimately, the confluence of social, political, and economic forces determines the success or failure of drug-use-related political decision-making.[6] The influence of a myriad of political forces in developing a health policy issue can be seen in the efforts directed towards creating a prescription drug benefit for Medicare. The debate on how to develop an optimal model for prescription drug coverage continues to rage in the nation today. The players that have important stakes in this endeavor include

(a) consumer interest groups, such as the American Association of Retired Persons, whose goal is to make prescription medications available to all seniors;

(b) the federal government, which is running out of funds to continue to implement Medicare in the future;

(c) the pharmaceutical industry, which is opposed to any proposals that impose price controls on medications or result in significant discount on medications to seniors; and

(d) private insurers, who are grappling with increasing prescription costs in their general populations and for whom the Medicare managed care experience resulted in large financial losses.

The debate over the creation of an outpatient Medicare prescription drug benefit is relevant to the profession of pharmacy and will be settled in the political arena. Therefore, an understanding of policymaking within the U.S. political system would be useful to pharmacists to fully understand both the nature and impact of any legislation that might arise from these proposals. Not only are the provisions of particular public policies or decisions relevant, but the genesis, formulation, implementation, and evaluation of those policies are crucial for those towards whom the policies are directed. In the case of a Medicare prescription drug benefit, concern that the expense of such a program would primarily be borne by pharmacy providers has been troublesome to practicing pharmacists and pharmacy providers.

Finally, within health care reform and the role of pharmacists in a newly reformed health care system, there are political issues of concern to the public at large. Pharmacists have the responsibility to make both the public and policymakers aware of their role and their contributions to optimal pharmaceutical care. This role is based upon the extensive training that pharmacists receive, their accessibility in most communities, and their patient-centered philosophy of practice.

Divergent Perspectives on Drug Use

As described above, the wide range of actors involved in the drug-use process all have particular interests and perspectives regarding what constitutes the rational use of prescription medications in our society.

For example, patients have a right to expect safe and effective drug therapy when it is indicated and also have a right to safe and appropriate handling and dispensing of prescribed medicines. Patients do, however, contribute to suboptimal drug therapy outcomes by not getting prescriptions filled, by not getting prescriptions refilled when extended use is indicated, by combining the use of prescription medications with other substances or foods that are contraindicated, by storing medications improperly, and by using medications intended for use by other persons.[6]

From another perspective, physicians have broad cultural, social, and legal authority to prescribe as they see fit for any patient in any context. Professional organizations representing prescribers defend this broad authority through legal and professional means.[6]

Providers of alternative medical therapies also affect the drug-use process. For example, homeopaths, herbalists, and advocates of megavitamin therapy or macrobiotic diets are gaining popularity in the United States; it has been estimated that approximately 10% of the U.S. population used one of these forms of alternative medical therapy in 1990.[76] This statistic has implications for pharmacists relating to the role of traditional prescription drugs vis-à-vis these medicines, herbs, vitamins, or foods; the role of the pharmacist vis-à-vis alternative medical providers; and the effects of increasing use of different types and numbers of providers on the health care delivery system.

Pharmaceutical manufacturers are affected by the policies and actions of health professionals. Thus, it is in manufacturers' best interests to involve themselves in professional policy development (e.g., therapeutic interchange, prescribing privileges). Drug manufacturers have lobbied extensively at the state and federal levels to inhibit certain professional practices or regulatory mandates that impinge upon their market definitions.[77]

The distribution of prescription drugs takes place in a number of ways. Most commonly, community pharmacies, hospitals, ambulatory care centers, correctional facilities, military installations, home health care agencies, and nursing homes are the source of prescribed medicines for patients. Other outlets for prescription drugs include mail order pharmacies and dispensing physicians. Each of these distributors has an interest in retaining and expanding market share, creating debates over the most appropriate channels for distributing prescribed drugs to the U.S. population. Similar debates take place over the control of nonprescription medicines, or those drugs that have the potential for switching from prescription to nonprescription status. In most cases, such debates are settled by the political interaction of lobbyists, scientists, regulators, and policymakers.

Finally, third-party payers have an interest in minimizing expenditures and maximizing the health status of their subscriber populations. As a result, many third-party payers incorporate the concepts of cost-sharing (deductibles, copayments, etc.) into their prescription drug benefit plans, along with an array of more complex administrative mechanisms, such as generic or therapeutic interchange, drug utilization review, and the use of drug formularies.

Convergent Perspectives on Drug Use

Despite the number of interested actors and the differences in their perspectives on the drug-use process, there exists a growing body of support from a variety of sources for an increased role for pharmacists in preventing drug misadventures:

- The U.S. Office of the Inspector General (OIG) has concluded that clinical pharmacy services add value to patient care and reduce health care costs.[78] The OIG recommended that the Center for Medicare and Medicaid Services (CMS) facilitate the process of providing pharmaceutical care.

- The Public Health Service's *Healthy People 2000* objectives endorse the role of pharmacotherapy in primary and secondary prevention of disease (i.e., primary prevention via vaccination and secondary prevention via management of chronic conditions).[79] The Public Health Service further recommended that by the year 2000 75% of pharmacies establish linked systems to provide drug reaction or interaction alerts for medications dispensed from different sources.

- The Joint Commission on the Accreditation of Healthcare Organizations has incorporated the concept of pharmaceutical care into its hospital and home care pharmacy standards, thus recognizing the value of pharmacists in the provision of quality health care.[80,81]

- Third-party payers have begun to notice the value of pharmacists in achieving cost-containment objectives, thus providing economic justification for the expansion of pharmaceutical care in managed care settings.[82]

These examples are only a fraction of the growing base of evidence that the concept of pharmaceutical care is receiving support from providers, consumers, regulators, and payers across the United States.

Pharmaceutical Care: A Model to Optimize the Drug-Use Process

We believe that, as a result of a myriad of forces and actors impacting the drug-use process, there exists no single professional group or strategy sufficient for the optimization of the drug-use process. As a result, competing interests often influence patient care. These interests disagree about what constitutes optimal drug therapy and who should be in control, thus increasing the risk of drug misadventuring.

We further contend that there is a significant amount of agreement from a wide variety of sources that pharmacy practitioners, adopting the care model for delivering pharmaceutical services, are in a unique position to help their public realize optimal drug therapy by turning challenges and obstacles into opportunities. Pharmacists should assume the lead role in guiding the drug-use process in a positive direction, that is, towards a coordinated, multidisciplinary drug-use system aimed at achieving optimal drug therapy for the public.

Summary

Rational drug therapy has traditionally been viewed as the right drug, in the right dose, at the right time, for the right patient. Today, the emphasis on cost containment has added an extra dimension: cost-effectiveness of therapeutic regimens.

Most steps of the drug-use process have not been extensively studied. Evidence to date shows duplication of efforts and suboptimal decisions, with little concerted effort to identify means for improvements that may have a favorable impact on costs and patient outcomes. The increasing cost and complexity of drugs, along with the inconsistencies that exist in drug use, demonstrate a need for a complete review of the drug-use process.

The drug-use process, as it currently operates in the United States, is not conducive to the provision of a systematic approach to therapy. The steps in this process are often carried out independent of each other and are poorly performed by a variety of health professionals.[21]

The development of strategies for increased provision of optimal drug therapy through the use of pharmacists as drug therapy experts is both relevant and possible. Indeed it is the basis of and reason for pharmaceutical care. The profession of pharmacy is in a prime position. The adoption of pharmaceutical care will allow for a better coordination of the entire drug-use process. The needs are apparent, the skills of pharmacists are well documented, and the opportunity awaits.

References

1. Miller W. Functional elements of clinical pharmacy practice. In: Ray MD, ed. Basic skills in clinical pharmacy practice. Chapel Hill, NC: Universal Printing and Publishing; 1983.
2. Task Force on Prescription Drugs. Final Report. Washington, DC: U.S. Department of Health, Education, and Welfare, 1969.
3. Rucker TD. Pursuing rational drug therapy: a macro view a la the USA. *J Soc Admin Pharm.* 1989; 5:78–86.
4. Brushwood DB, Catizone CA, Coster JM. OBRA 90: what it means to your practice. *U.S. Pharm.* 1992; 17:47–52.
5. Manasse HR. Medication use in an imperfect world: drug misadventuring as an issue of public policy, part 1. *Am J Hosp Pharm.* 1989; 46:929–44.
6. Manasse HR. Medication use in an imperfect world: drug misadventuring as an issue of public policy, part 2. *Am J Hosp Pharm.* 1989; 46:114–52.
7. Ernst FR, Grizzle AJ. Drug-related morbidity and mortality: Updating the cost-of-illness model. *J Am Pharm Assoc.* 2001; 41:156–7.
8. Hepler CD. Regulating for outcome as a systems response to the problem of drug related morbidity. *J Am Pharm Assoc.* 2001; 141:108–15.
9. Strand LM, et al. Drug-related problems: their structure and function. *DICP Ann Pharmacother.* 1990; 24:1093–7.
10. Brodie DC. Drug-use control: keystone to pharmaceutical service. *Drug Intell Clin Pharm.* 1967; 1:63–5.
11. Mrtek RG. 1940 to 1960: the rise of commercialism. *Drug Topics.* 1982; 126:1124.
12. American Association of Colleges of Pharmacy. Pharmacists for the future. The Report of the Study Commission on Pharmacy. Ann Arbor: Health Administration Press; 1975.
13. Brodie DC, McGhan WF, Lindon J. The theoretical base of pharmacy. *Am J Hosp Pharm.* 1991; 48:536–40.
14. Hepler CD, Strand LM. Opportunities and responsibilities in pharmaceutical care. *Am J Hosp Pharm.* 1990; 47:533–43.

15. Hepler CD. Issues in implementing pharmaceutical care. *Am J Hosp Pharm.* 1993; 50:1635–41.

16. Grainger-Rousseau TJ, Miralles MA, Hepler CD et al. Therapeutic outcomes monitoring: application of pharmaceutical care guidelines to community pharmacy. *J Am Pharm Assoc* 1997; NS37:647–61.

17. Odedina FT, Hepler CD, Segal R et al. Pharmacists' implementation of pharmaceutical care (PIPC) model. *Pharm Research.* 1997; 14:135–44.

18. Knapp DA, Knapp DE, Brandon BM et al. Development and application of criteria in drug use review programs. *Am J Hosp Pharm.* 1974; 31:648–56.

19. Hutchinson RA, Witte K. How to get started—planning clinical pharmacy services. In: Ray MD, ed. Basic skills in clinical pharmacy practice. Chapel Hill, NC: Universal Printing and Publishing; 1983.

20. Kirking DM. Drug utilization review: a component of drug quality assurance. In: Final Report of the APHA Pharmacy Commission on Third Party Programs. Washington, DC: American Pharmaceutical Association; 1986.

21. Hutchinson RA, Lewis RK, Hatoum HT. Inconsistencies in the drug use process. *DICP Ann Pharmacother.* 1990; 24:633–6.

22. Manning PR, Lee PV, Clintnorth WA et al. Changing prescribing practices through individual continuing education. *JAMA.* 1986; 256:230–2.

23. Gonzales R, Bartlett JG, Besser RE et al. Principles of appropriate antibiotic use for treatment of acute respiratory tract infections in adults: background, specific aims, and methods. *Ann Intern Med* 2001; 134:479–86.

24. Mattei MP, Valuck RJ, Barrett PH et al. Decreasing antibiotic use in ambulatory practice: impact and cost. *Pharmacoeconomics: Infectious Diseases.* 1999; 3:4–5.

25. Koch H. Drug utilization in office-based practice: a summary of findings, *National Ambulatory Medical Care Survey—National Health Survey Series.* Hyattsville, MD: National Center for Health Statistics; 1982.

26. Gonzales R, Steiner JF, Lum A et al. Decreasing antibiotic use in ambulatory practice: impact of a multidimensional intervention on the treatment of uncomplicated acute bronchitis in adults. *JAMA* 1999; 281:1512–9.

27. Avorn J, Soumerai SB. Improving drug-therapy decisions through educational outreach: a randomized controlled trial of academically based "detailing." *N Engl J Med.* 1983; 308:1457–63.

28. Valuck RJ. Macro-level screening criteria to identify suboptimal prescribers of controlled substances. Master's thesis, University of Illinois at Chicago; 1992.

29. Davis NM, Cohen MR. Medication errors: causes and prevention. Philadelphia: George F. Stickley; 1981.

30. Baum C et al. Drug use and expenditures in 1982. *JAMA.* 1985; 253:382–6.

31. Meyer BR. Improving medical education in therapeutics. Health and public policy committee, American College of Physicians. *Ann Intern Med.* 1988; 108:145–7.

32. Lobas NH, Lepinski PW, Abramowitz PW. Effects of pharmaceutical care on medication cost and quality of patient care in an ambulatory-care clinic. *Am J Hosp Pharm.* 1992; 49:1681–8.

33. Hatoum HT, Akhras K. 1993 bibliography: a 32-year literature review on the value and acceptance of ambulatory care provided by pharmacists. *Ann Pharmacother.* 1993; 27:1106–19.

34. Burkle WS, Gwizdala CJ. Evaluation of "toxic" serum theophylline concentrations. *Am J Hosp Pharm.* 1981; 38:1164–6.

35. Holden J, Holden K. Comparative effectiveness of general practitioner versus pharmacist dosing of patients requiring anticoagulation in the community. *J Clin Pharm Ther.* 2000; 25:49–54.

36. Farnsworth FA, Kim KY, Jacobs MR et al. Centralized, pharmacist managed anticoagulation service for a university based health system. *Am J Health-Syst Pharm.* 2001; 58:77–8.

37. Ibrahim OM, Bawazir SA, Al-Khamis K et al. Evaluation of clinical pharmacy service impact on therapeutic drug monitoring of digoxin at a teaching hospital. Paper presented at the ASHP Annual Meeting. Baltimore, MD; 1998.

38. Barnett TS, Peck EC, Self RM et al. Pharmacy managed extended-interval aminoglycoside program in a community hospital. *Am J Health-Syst Pharm.* 1998; 55:397–8.

39. Barker KN, McConnnell WE. The problems of detecting medication errors in hospitals. *Am J Hosp Pharm.* 1962; 19:360–9.

40. Crawford SY, Myers CE. ASHP national survey of hospital-based pharmaceutical services—1992. *Am J Hosp Pharm.* 1993; 50:1371–404.

41. Davis NM, Cohen MR. Is your medication error rate acceptable? *Hosp Pharm.* 1994; 29:980,3.

42. Cousins DD, Phillips M, Leape LL et al. National efforts aimed at medication error reduction. Paper presented at ASHP Midyear Clinical Meeting. Las Vegas, NV; 1998 December.

43. Nichols B. Standardized education for nursing. *Am J Hosp Pharm.* 1981; 38:1455–8.

44. Hatoum HT. Megatrends a la pharmacy: potential and promise. *Hosp Pharm.* 1990; 25:825–8, 36.

45. Elenbaas RM. When to monitor blood drug levels. *Hosp Ther.* 1986; 27–7.

46. Johnson JA, Bootman JL. Drug related morbidity and mortality and the economic impact of pharmaceutical care. *Am J Health-Syst Pharm.* 1997; 54:554–8.

47. Spino M, Sellers EM, Kaplan HL. Effect of adverse drug reactions on the length of hospitalization. *Am J Hosp Pharm.* 1978; 35:1060–4.

48. Wong WM, Ignoffo RJ. If there are expert systems and dose checks, why do we still need the clinical pharmacist? *Pharm Pract Man Quarterly.* 1996; 16:50–8.

49. Office of the Inspector General. Medication regimens—causes of noncompliance. Washington, DC: U.S. Department of Health and Human Services, Publication OAI04-89-89121; 1990.

50. Hatoum HT, Hutchinson RA, Lambert BL. OBRA 90: Patient counseling—enhancing patient outcomes. *U.S. Pharmacist.* 1993; 18:38–45.

51. Administration on aging. Growth of the elderly population. Race groups and Hispanics. Washington, DC: U.S. Bureau of Census; 1996. www.aoa.dhhs.gov/aoa/stats/aging21/demography. Accessed 2001 October 29.

52. Kassam R, Farris KB, Burback L et al. Pharmaceutical care research and education project: pharmacists' interventions. *J Am Pharm Assoc* 2001; 41:401–10.

53. Levy RA. Ethnic and racial differences in response to medicines: preserving individualized therapy in managed pharmaceutical programs. *Pharm Med.* 1993; 7:139–5.

54. Brown CM, Segal R. Effects of health and treatment perceptions on the use of pre-scribed medication and home remedies among African American and white American hypertensives. *Soc Sci Med.* 1996; 43:903–17.

55. Yancy CW, Fowler MB, Colucci WS et al. Race and the response to adrenergic block-ade with carvedilol in patients with chronic heart failure. *N Engl J Med.* 2001; 344:1358–65.

56. Zhou HH, Sheller JR, Nu H et al. Ethnic differences in response to morphine. *Clin Pharm Ther.* 1993; 54:507–13.

57. Dole EJ, Rhyne RL, Zeilmann CA et al. Influence of ethnicity on use of herbal remedies in elderly Hispanics and non-Hispanic whites. *J Am Pharm Assoc.* 2000; 40:359–65.

58. Coons SJ, Motheral BR. Quality-of-life drugs? *Clin Ther.* 2000; 22:773–4.

59. Lexchin J. Lifestyle drugs: issues for debate. *Can Med Assoc J.* 2001; 164:1449–51.

60. IMS Health reports U.S. pharmaceutical promotional spending reached record $13.9 billion in 1999. Westport CT: IMS Health Incorporated; 2000. www.imshealth.com/ public/structure/dispcontent/1 2779,1009-1009-75077,00.htm. Accessed 2001 March 19.

61. Murray MD. Information technology: infrastructure for improvements to the medi-cation use process. *Am J Health-Syst Pharm.* 2000; 57:565–71.

62. Felkey BG, Barker KN. Technology and automation in pharmaceutical care. *J Am Pharm Asso.* 1996; NS36:309–14.

63. Thompson CA. USP issues first report from medication errors database. *Am J Health-Syst Pharm.* 2001; 58:106–7.

64. Hibbard JH, Weeks EC. Consumerism in health care: prevalence and predictors. *Med Care.* 1987; 11:1019–32.

65. DTC ads controls emerging as collateral issue from prices, Medicare. *FDC Reports.* 2000; 62:11–2.

66. Perri M, Shinde S, Banavali R. Past, present, and future of direct to consumer pre-scription drug advertising. *Clin Ther.* 1999; 21:1798–1811.

67. Wilkes MS, Bell RA, Kravitz RL. Direct to consumer prescription drug advertising: trends, impact, and implications. *Health Affairs.* 2000; 19:110–26.

68. Penna RP. Creating our futures. Paper read at Indiana Pharmacy Consensus-Building Conference. Indianapolis, Indiana; 1991 May 31.

69. Brass EP. Changing the status of drugs from prescription to over-the-counter avail-ability. *N Engl J Med.* 2001; 345:810–6.

70. Mehl B, Santell J. Projecting future drug expenditures—2001. *Am J Health-Syst Pharm.* 2001; 58:125–33.

71. Johnson JA, Bootman JL. Drug-related morbidity and mortality: a cost-of-illness model. *Arch Intern Med.* 1995; 155(18):1949–56.

72. Dean BB, Siddique RM, Yamashita BD et al. Cost effectiveness of proton pump inhibitors for maintenance therapy of erosive reflux esophagitis. *Am J Health-Syst Pharm.* 2001; 58:1338–46.

73. Malone DC, Carter BL, Billups SJ et al. Economic analysis of a randomized, con-trolled, multicenter study of clinical pharmacist interventions for high risk veterans: the IMPROVE study. *Pharmacother.* 2000; 20:1149–58.

74. Simpson SH, Johnson JA, Tsuyuki, RT. Economic impact of community pharmacist intervention in cholesterol risk management: evaluation of the study of cardiovascular risk intervention by pharmacists. *Pharmacother.* 2001; 21:627–35.

75. Nesbit TW, Shermock KM, Bobek MB et al. Implementation and pharmacoeconomic analysis of a clinical staff pharmacist practice model. *Am J Health-Syst Pharm.* 2001; 58:784–90.

76. Wood AJ, Zhou HH. Ethnic differences in drug disposition and I responsiveness. *Clin Pharmacokinet.* 1991; 20:350–73.

77. Victor K. New kids on the block. *National J.* 1987; Oct 31: 2726–30.

78. Office of the Inspector General. The Clinical Role of the Community Pharmacist. Washington, DC: U.S. Department of Health and Human Services, Publication OAI01-89-89020, 1990.

79. Public Health Service. Healthy people 2000: national health promotion and disease prevention objectives. Washington, DC: U.S. Department of Health and Human Services; 1990.

80. Joint Commission on Accreditation of Healthcare Organizations. 1991 Accreditation manual for hospitals. Chicago: JCAHO Publications; 1991.

81. Joint Commission on Accreditation of Healthcare Organizations. 1991 Accreditation Manual for Home Care. Chicago: JCAHO Publications; 1991.

82. Myers M. Thirty-party programs. In: Effective pharmacy management, 4th ed. Kansas City, MO: Marion Labs; 1987.

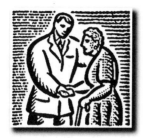

Chapter 6: The Nature and Extent of Drug-Related Problems in the United States

Henri R. Manasse, Jr., Ph.D., Sc.D.
Kasey K. Thompson, Pharm.D.

Introduction

In late 1994, Betsy Lehman, a health reporter for the *Boston Globe*, died after receiving four times the intended daily dose of cyclophosphamide for four consecutive days while undergoing chemotherapy for breast cancer.[1] The investigation into Ms. Lehman's death, its personal and professional effects on her care providers, and the public furor that accompanied her case and others like it, helped propel the rarely addressed problem of medication error to the forefront of public awareness.

In 1999, the Institute of Medicine of the National Academy of Sciences published its report, *To Err Is Human: Building a Safer Health System*.[2] The IOM report shed sobering light on the prevalence and preventability of medical errors in the United States. IOM estimated that between 44,000 and 98,000 deaths occurring in U.S. hospitals each year result from preventable errors in the provision of medical care. Approximately 7,000 of these occur in the prescribing and administration of medications. Even the lower figure of 44,000 deaths per year, the report stated, would rank medical errors as the eighth leading cause of death annually in the U.S.—above motor vehicle accidents, breast cancer, and AIDS.[2]

Just as important as these statistics, though, are the lessons to be learned from reports of adverse medical events and near misses. Perhaps the most crucial lesson is the imperative to move beyond individual blame and institutional damage control. Modern discoveries in human cognitive psychology and human factors engineering demand that we focus instead on the systems, processes, and cultures involved in the provision of health care. In this chapter we examine how these concepts will drive our profession's continual progress toward a fail-safe medication-use system. Pharmacists, by nature of their expertise and training, play an increasingly vital role in this process. We will illustrate that role and demonstrate the intrinsic linkages between the safe use of medications and the philosophy of pharmaceutical care.

Why Do Accidents Happen? Moving Beyond Blame

The reader is probably familiar with such landmark accidents as the Space Shuttle Challenger explosion and the nuclear reactor disasters at Three Mile Island in the U.S. and Chernobyl in the former Soviet Union. Hearing stories like these in the media, we are tempted to assign blame to the individuals steering those situations at the time of the accidents—the reactor operators or mission control staff, for example. Likewise, in the case of Ms. Lehman's death, we may blame the hospital employees who transmitted, transcribed, or administered the incorrect dosages. However, minimal analysis makes clear that all of these accidents occurred within broader contexts. A rocket, a reactor, or an oncology unit can exist and function only through the coordinated efforts of the multiple operators—human and automated—that make up a system. James Reason defines a system as "a set of interdependent elements interacting to achieve a common aim. The elements may be both human and non-human (equipment, technologies, etc.)."[3]

Accidents of the magnitude described above, occurring within systems, are typically shown to involve a number of isolated, often undetected, or latent errors. These errors can originate with any—or many—system elements, at any number of different locations and times. Gradually these errors align and accumulate to cause the unfortunate accident about which we hear or read. Shortly we will discuss the most common types and causes of errors found in systems, but first let us demonstrate how systems concepts apply to several manufacturing industries and to the provision of health care services.

Errors in a System Setting

It is not difficult to discern elements of systems at work in modern industries. In aviation and space travel, system elements include design engineers, manufacturing machinery and personnel, quality and safety regulators, accountants, flight control personnel and computers, and the crew who operate the aircraft or spacecraft. Similarly, a system for energy production incorporates various human and electronic elements responsible for mining and transporting raw materials and for operating reactors and refineries continuously and safely. As with aviation or space travel, this system involves personnel assigned to monitor compliance with standards of practice, laws, and regulations mandating safety and environmental requirements. These and other industries invest substantial resources in the continual refinement of system performance, using findings from past accidents as well as research in cognitive psychology and human factors to optimize their systems for efficiency and safety. Moreover, such industries operationalize safety requirements as "mission one."

Clearly, providing contemporary health care services is a sufficiently complex endeavor to necessitate a systems approach. The processes of admitting, monitoring, treating, and discharging patients; securing payment for their care; and maintaining and improving medical facilities and equipment all require multiple, complex interactions of personnel and technology. Our discussion will sharpen the focus on the issue of whether medication-use processes, in particular, are by design reflective of true systems. If a system exists to accomplish a specific aim or goal, then the goal of a true medication-use system could be achieving the "five rights," as stated by the National Coordinating Council for Medication Error Reporting and Prevention: the right medication, in the right dose, to the right person, by the right route, at the right time.[4]

On the contrary, the absence of a system results in a series of disconnected people, machines, and processes, which lack clearly understood, agreed upon, and recognized goals and responsibilities. The concepts and tools described in the next sections will equip the reader to both understand and help improve the systems and system elements currently at work in the medication-use process in his or her practice setting.

The words accident and error are commonly used in our vernacular but not clearly defined. The following definitions are useful in discussing these terms in a systems context. An accident is an unplanned, unexpected, and undesired event, usually with an adverse consequence. Error can be defined as an unintended act, either of omission (omitting a correct step in a process) or commission (performing an incorrect act or an act that does not achieve its intended outcome).[5,6] Errors within systems can generally be classified as either active errors, which occur at the level of the frontline operator (e.g., a pilot or a nurse) and whose effects are felt almost immediately; or latent errors, which are typically removed from the control of the operator and can include factors such as poor design, incorrect installation, faulty maintenance, bad management decisions, and poorly structured organizations.[2] Latent errors are often buried in computer program language, routine processes, erroneous or old information, or organizational structure or policy. They can be very difficult to detect and therefore very dangerous, as they may escape notice during initial design or even during an accident investigation.

Sharp End and Blunt End: The Organizational Hierarchy

A complex system, or an organization with some system characteristics, can be visualized as an isosceles triangle with a sharp end (the point) and a blunt end (the base). At the sharp end are the aforementioned frontline operators—in the medication-use process these are pharmacists, physicians, nurses, and other medical technical specialists. The working conditions and available resources that surround and influence the sharp end are largely determined at the blunt end. Blunt-end operators—hospital or health-system administrators, department managers, government regulators, and insurance companies—make decisions that govern the direction and priorities of the whole organization. These decisions are driven by myriad, often competing, factors—financial constraints, legal and regulatory requirements, community demands, human resources, and even political considerations. When blunt-end operators work in "silos"—lacking adequate communication and coordination with the rest of the organization—then organizational integrity and the system itself begin to weaken.

Because any organization has limited resources to draw on in achieving its objectives, some aspects of its services will inevitably be compromised. These compromises are sometimes buffered by chance or by defenses built into the system. Even these defenses are likely compromised to some degree, so they possess certain flaws. When the flawed defenses, or gaps, align such that errors latent in the system pass unhindered from blunt end to sharp end, then an accident is likely to result—particularly if any kind of active error is occurring simultaneously at the sharp end. Examples of latent errors that originate with blunt-end actions can include poorly lit work spaces; too few or too many warning screens on a medication order entry system or computerized prescriber order entry interface; insufficient personnel to perform multiple checks of a prescription order; or excessive workload or shift length, resulting in fatigue and distraction. Personal stress and drugs or chemicals taken to combat stress or fatigue can also heighten the likelihood for error. The potential for accumulation of error in a complex set of processes can be largely offset by designing systems with standards, buffers, and redundancies that prevent a single operator's error from causing an accident.[7–9]

Error Is Inevitable

Reason sub-categorizes human error into "slips," "lapses," and "mistakes." A slip and a lapse are very similar, both describe an action that is not the intended action. A slip, however, is observable—for example, a prescriber intends to write down "1 mg" for an appropriate medication, but writes down "10 mg" instead. A lapse is an unobservable error, such as the inability to correctly recall information from memory on a certain medication or dose. A mistake is an action that proceeds as planned but does not achieve the correct outcome, because the intention behind the act was incorrect. For example, a prescriber may misdiagnose a patient, then intentionally and correctly order a medication that turns out to be inappropriate because the patient was misdiagnosed. It is very important to understand that human error is unavoidable and is not a de facto indicator of incompetence or negligence. Several studies have found that the cognitive processes that allow errors to happen stem from the same mental capabilities that allow us to quickly perform routine tasks and solve unique problems.[3] The mental processes that prompt us to misplace our car keys or date a check "2001" instead of "2002" also cause prescribers to misplace a decimal point or pharmacists to reach for the wrong container. Accidents may be caused by one or more errors, by uncontrollable external forces (e.g., "acts of God"), or a combination.[10]

Errors in Medicine

Studies conducted over the past two decades indicate that medical errors are widespread and cause significant injury and death in the United States. Two major studies cited in the 1999 IOM report used data gathered in New York in 1984 and data from Colorado and Utah in 1992, to show that 3.7% and 2.9% of hospital admissions, respectively, resulted from adverse events. Of these, 13.6% led to death in the 1984 New York study; in the Colorado and Utah study, 6.6% of adverse events were fatal. The Harvard Medical Practice Study, which conducted the New York hospital research, defines an adverse event as "an injury caused by medical management rather than by the underlying disease or condition of the patient." The New York data indicated that 58% of adverse events were attributable to error and therefore could have been prevented; similarly, 53% of the adverse events documented in the Colorado and Utah study were found to be preventable. The IOM extrapolated these two studies' findings to determine their estimate of 44,000–98,000 deaths per year in inpatient settings from preventable medical errors. Comparing these figures to those for other leading causes of death in the U.S. (43,458 for motor vehicle accidents; 42,297 for breast cancer; and 16,516 for AIDS) illustrates the urgency of improving safety and quality of care in our health systems.[2,11,12] A number of private and public sector initiatives have been organized to address this serious challenge to U.S. health care.[13,14]

Of particular concern to our profession is the Harvard Study's finding that adverse drug events (ADEs) caused 19% of the adverse events—more than any other single factor. Forty-five percent of these ADEs were due to errors and thus were preventable.[9] In a 1993 study at two Massachusetts hospitals, Bates, Cullen, Laird et al.[15] identified the stage at which various ADEs originated in the drug delivery process. Forty-nine percent originated during prescription ordering, 11% during transcription, 14% in dispensing, and 26% occurred in administration of medications. Cohen[16] cites the following as common causes of medication errors:

1. Failed communication, such as unclear prescriber handwriting, ambiguous orders, confusion of drug names, misplaced or misread zeroes or decimal points, and faulty conversion between metric and apothecary dosing systems;

2. Poor drug distribution practices, such as similarly packaged or labeled containers or syringes, insufficient checks and verifications, and insufficiently trained personnel granted access to medications;

3. Dose miscalculations, especially with pediatric patients and with intravenously administered medications;

4. Problems related to drugs and drug devices, such as packaging that makes labels difficult to see or read clearly, the misprogramming of automatic drug dispensing devices, and the lack of fail-safe clamps in some devices that allow free-flow infusion;

5. Incorrect drug administration, including mix-ups in patient identification and route of drug administration (e.g., intravenous administration of enteral feeding supplements or bladder irrigations, topical medications swallowed); and

6. Lack of patient education, failure to ensure that the patient understands the function and appropriate use of his or her medications, or failure to encourage the patient to ask questions.

Pharmacists are in a unique position to identify, and often to intercept, situations such as these before patients are harmed. However, there are not enough pharmacists to catch every potential error before it causes an accident. A properly designed system of medication delivery could augment defenses against these gaps and remove some of the burden of hyper-vigilance from individual shoulders.

Social and Economic Costs of Inappropriate Medication Use

The social and economic costs associated with inappropriate medication use are substantial. Pharmacists and health care professionals have a moral and ethical duty to help people make the best use of medicines. As if the burden of illness weren't enough for our patients, their concerns are compounded by the high potential for suffering from preventable adverse events due to drug therapy.

Bates and colleagues[15] found that almost 2% of hospital admissions experienced a preventable adverse drug event. This resulted in an average increase in length of stay of 4.6 days and a $4700 increase in hospital costs per admission. A landmark study by

Johnson and Bootman[17] estimated the annual cost of drug-related illness and death in the United States to be approximately $76 billion. Of this amount, hospitalizations accounted for $47 billion. In a 1997 follow-up study published in the *American Journal of Health-System Pharmacy*, Johnson and Bootman[18] noted that pharmacist intervention could reduce this amount by over $30 billion. The Alliance for Aging in 1998 estimated that for every dollar spent on medications, another dollar is spent to treat new health problems caused by medications.[19] In 2001 Ernst and Grizzle[20] updated Johnson and Bootman's cost-of-illness model to estimate that drug-related morbidity and mortality cost over $177 billion in the year 2000.

Fail-Safe Medication Use As the Professional Ideal: Designing Safe Systems for Health Care

We have stated that human error is unavoidable. Therefore, because even the best-designed systems begin with and rely on human action, accidents will happen. However, we owe our patients the assurance that their safety is our primary objective. We must think not in terms of "acceptable" rates of injury or death—even one is too many—but simply in terms of preventing harm. We may never be completely free from failure, but we must strive to use the considerable knowledge and tools available to us in designing systems to compensate for our innate imperfections. Our duty is to design processes and systems that prevent, as often as possible, human error from causing accidents, injury, or death.

Certain military and industry organizations have attained admirably low accident rates by adopting what are called high reliability principles. Simply stated, high reliability organizations are characterized by an organizational commitment to safety, redundancies built into safety and personnel processes, and a culture that supports learning and willingness to change.[21,22] Leaders in patient safety have begun to apply high reliability principles in proposing models for safer health care systems. The following are five Principles for the Design of Safety Systems in Health Care Organizations, proposed by the Institute of Medicine in the 1999 report *To Err is Human: Building a Safer Health System*.[2]

1. *Provide Leadership*

    • Make patient safety a priority corporate objective. Boards of directors, management, and clinical leadership must state explicit safety goals and initiate monitoring processes to ensure goal achievement.

    • Make patient safety everyone's responsibility. All personnel should be empowered and expected to participate in improving safety performance. Leaders should convey this message clearly and consistently to all levels of health personnel. Guaranteeing immunity from punishment for reporting potential and actual errors is a vital step in establishing a culture of safety.

    • Make clear assignments for and expectations of safety oversight. Meaningful safety programs would include senior-level leadership, defined program objectives and plans, personnel, budget, data collection and analysis, and regular progress monitoring by reporting to the board of directors.

    • Provide human and financial resources for error analysis and systems redesign. The IOM suggests considering putting the entire medication-use process, including safety system analysis and improvement, under the oversight of one clinician, allocating at least 50% of that person's time to those responsibilities.

• Develop effective mechanisms for identifying and dealing with unsafe practitioners. Rarely does a health care professional wake up one morning and decide to intentionally injure or kill a patient under his or her care. The evidence is so overwhelming on the systemic causes of error that little time need be taken here discussing issues of negligence and intent to harm. Intent to harm is a legal issue, not an issue of designing better medication-use systems. However, health care facilities must have reliable systems in place to identify and prevent individuals with criminal backgrounds and those with the potential to harm patients from working in or providing services to their facilities. Beyond those who intend to do harm, a very few will be intentionally negligent, capricious and careless, or fundamentally incompetent. A comprehensive safety program should have a means to rapidly identify those few individuals and take immediate corrective actions.

2. *Respect Human Limits in Process Design.* This principle applies the precepts of human factors engineering (HFE). HFE integrates knowledge about humans' intrinsic abilities and limitations into the design of job functions, working conditions, and machines—from shift lengths to lighting conditions, from buttons on consoles to software screen layout. Institutions should be accountable for employing the expertise of human factors experts in implementing these steps, then testing designs thoroughly with actual sharp-end personnel.[23]

• Design jobs for safety. Work hours and workloads should be designed, to the greatest degree possible, to reduce fatigue and accommodate the natural rhythms and capabilities of the human mind and body. Specific time periods and work areas should be set aside for more complex tasks, such as calculating doses and mixing i.v. solutions.

• Avoid reliance on memory. Checklists, protocols, drug-interaction software, and dosing cards are useful tools to lessen demands on memory and reduce risk of error. Continual updates and improvements to protocols should be encouraged and expected.

• Use constraints and forcing functions. These can be process steps that signal or warn the user of a potentially hazardous or irreversible upcoming decision, such as in automated drug-distribution systems. Forcing functions can also include the removal of hazardous options from an array of available choices, such as removing potassium chloride from patient floor stock, programming automated drug-distribution devices to default to the safest settings, and installing clamps to prevent free-flow.

• Avoid reliance on vigilance. Processes must not be over-automated to the point where human action is only sporadically called upon. The mind cannot remain vigilant, or at a heightened state of attention or readiness, over long periods of inactivity; a certain level of arousal must be maintained.[5] Warnings issued by automated systems should not be so frequent that overriding them becomes habitual. Checklists, variation of duties, and reasonable shift lengths are important.

• Simplify key processes. Minimize hand-offs and duplication of tasks between personnel, e.g., order processing and data entry. Centralize data storage instead of keeping multiple databases or files. Ensure easy access to frequently used medications. Consider reducing the choices of drugs and strengths available in pharmacies and reducing the number of daily drug administrations.

• Standardize work processes. Wherever possible, apply systemwide consistency of design and provide clear instructions to key processes and machine functions. Use standard drug order forms and abbreviations, apply standard protocols for complex medication administration, and standardize placement and labeling of drug products in pharmacy facilities, including necessary extra labeling or bright colored tape on potential look-alike products.

3. *Promote Effective Team Functioning*

• Train in teams those who are expected to work in teams. Health systems can adapt relevant elements of the Crew Resource Management (CRM) approach used by airlines.[24] Team members, especially those from diverse health disciplines, need to train together in order to communicate effectively, to defuse conflicts of personal style or professional stature, to collaboratively use available tools and technologies, and to learn how their respective specialized skills complement the team. Simulations of emergency situations are part of this approach.[25]

• Include the patient in safety design and the process of care. For better or worse, today's patients possess unprecedented access to a universe of health information. Consequently they are demanding a greater role in their own care decisions. In *To Err Is Human* and in the 2001 follow-up report, *Crossing the Quality Chasm: A New Health System for the 21st Century*, the IOM urges health systems to adopt a fully patient-centered mindset, to welcome patients as members of the health care team. Health systems are urged to tailor care to patients' priorities, to disclose organizational performance statistics, and to promptly admit error.[26]

4. *Anticipate the Unexpected*

• Adopt a proactive approach. Examine processes of care for threats to safety and redesign them before accidents occur. Systems designers can use failure mode effects analysis (FMEA), another concept borrowed from engineering and industry, to assess and correct flaws in medication-use systems before they cause accidents. A multidisciplinary team identifies as many failure modes—opportunities for error—as they can find in the existing system (e.g., potentially lethal drugs stored in floor stock, dosage or flow rate miscalculations, patient misidentification, outdated drug references). Each failure mode is examined for its root cause(s), then system improvements or "error traps" are developed on the basis of these assessments to reduce the severity and likelihood of each.[27] Error traps can include real-time alerts in an automated drug control system that alert for contraindications or patient incompatibilities with medications; bar coding on patient wristbands, files, and medication packaging; "hear-backs" or having pharmacists repeat phone orders back to the physician or patient; and monitoring lab results and other vital signs for patients receiving hazardous drugs. This proactive, prevention-oriented approach to safety design helps to allay the difficulties inherent in retrospective investigations. Blame, shame, conflicting recollections, and hindsight bias (the way our impression of how we acted or would have acted changes when we learn the outcome of an event) are the effects of compromises in safety.[28]

• Design for recovery. Concurrently with error prevention, system designers should plan for ways to mitigate the effects of errors when they do occur. Examples include keeping adequate stock and easy access to antidotes for high-risk drugs, developing and training staff on procedures for responding to adverse events, using equipment that defaults to the safest setting in emergencies, and applying simulation training as used in airline CRM activities.

• Improve access to accurate, timely information. The most up-to-date information on the patient, relevant medications, and alternate therapies should be available at the point of care. Means to achieve this include pharmacist participation in rounds, networked electronic clinical and lab data, relevant data and protocols accessible from the patient's bedside, accelerated completion of lab reports, and regular tracking and reporting of errors and near misses.

5. *Create a Learning Environment*

• Use simulations whenever possible. Simulating various situations, especially accidents or near misses, will help teach personnel an awareness of the potential sources, results, and prevention of error.

• Encourage reporting of errors and hazardous conditions. Reporting of errors and near misses is absolutely vital if system designs and safety performance are to be improved in our health systems. Unreported system weaknesses are accidents waiting to happen. The IOM advocates for confidential and voluntary reporting programs within health organizations to provide needed data for safety enhancement. They also recommend state-run mandatory reporting programs for the public's information, which provide incentives for health systems to invest continually in quality improvement. Finally, hospitals and practitioners should commit to openly and honestly discussing errors with affected patients and families. Full disclosure eases the emotional suffering of both families and practitioners, saves considerable public-relations damage, and has been shown to reduce settlement costs.[29] In its Statement on Reporting Medical Errors, ASHP asserts, "The fundamental purpose of reporting systems for medical errors is to learn how to improve the health care delivery process to prevent these errors."[30] ASHP recommends the following steps toward establishing a national solution to the problem of underreporting: (1) the establishment of a standardized, uniform nationwide system of mandatory reporting of adverse medical events that cause death or serious harm; (2) continued development and strengthening of systems for voluntary reporting of medical errors; and (3) strengthening efforts to implement process changes that reduce the risk of future errors and improve patient care.

• Ensure no reprisals for reporting of errors. Practitioners are often reluctant— or afraid—to report errors or near misses in which they have been involved, for fear of the consequences. Traditional medical education has imposed unrealistic expectations of error-free practitioner performance, which social attitudes and the specter of litigation serve to reinforce. A professional culture of blame has thus evolved, where accountability for accidents is too often ascribed to the suspected personal incompetence or carelessness of one "bad apple," rather than to a combination of latent system flaws. The bad apple is disciplined and left to bear the burdens of shame, censure, and self-doubt, while other personnel are admonished to be more careful and possibly retrained in protocols and procedures. System flaws remain unstudied and unchanged, positioned for a repeat incident. The only way to improve this reality is by putting in place non-punitive reporting systems that welcome—and reward—the open, honest exchange of information among workers and levels of authority and across institutional and geographic borders. Studies show that as few as 5% of known medical errors have traditionally been reported—yet when punishment disappears from the equation, reporting increases dramatically.[5] It cannot be stated strongly enough: Health delivery systems must be designed to compensate for the innate fallibilities of humans under suboptimal working conditions and often superhuman demands.[31] We cannot hope to reduce errors until we free ourselves from the fear of reporting them.

• Develop a working culture in which communication flows freely regardless of the authority or power gradient. This is another challenging but necessary shift. Personnel should feel comfortable sharing important observations or suggestions about safety improvements with any coworker, regardless of any differences in seniority, power, or professional discipline.

• Implement mechanisms of feedback and learning from error. IOM identifies five phases to improving safety: reporting events in a richly detailed story style, understanding and clarifying the meaning of the story, developing recommendations for improvement, implementing those recommendations, and tracking changes to monitor for any potential new problems. Appropriate policies and procedures should be implemented, their progress monitored, and needed financial and human resources allocated to ensure improvement. Technical expertise in human factors engineering, systems analysis, and other disciplines should be employed as needed.

The Role of Pharmacists in Reducing Errors and Improving Safety

Where does pharmacy fit amidst the rapidly changing culture, science, and practice of health care services? There are many answers. First, the window is open for our profession to apply our knowledge and offer our expertise in the quest to make our health systems safer places for people. This means it is the personal and professional obligation of pharmacists to move to the forefront and offer our expertise to administrators who are under fire to respond to the call for making their institutions safer. As Zellmer[32] states, "…when medication tragedies occur and no one thinks to find out what the pharmacist has to say, we have a profound credibility problem." We must apply our knowledge of how to make medication processes more effective and must push with renewed vision for a systems approach through the reengineering and redesign of antiquated, unsafe systems.

Secondly, we must assume new roles and responsibilities in patient care. As advocates of pharmaceutical care and collaborative drug therapy management, we serve an integral role within the multidisciplinary health care team. In fulfilling that role we must assume responsibility and accountability for leading interdisciplinary problem solving. All health care professions possess valuable expertise and training. With our background in assessing and resolving medication-use system deficiencies, we are in the unique position of being appropriate initiators of a collaborative interdisciplinary dialog. Without collaboration, change cannot occur. We can lead the team into a mutual commitment of resources and expertise to create and implement a change. We can reach out to engage patients and their families as partners in our safety efforts by ensuring that they are well informed as advocates for their own safety. They must be part of the risk–benefit equation, as well as eyes and ears for safe medication use.

Where do you start as initiator of collaborative problem solving? Pharmacists can start by initiating discussions across professional lines. There are a number of opportunities for pharmacists to lead:

- Share the pharmacy literature on building effective systems that reduce error with your colleagues in other health professions. This helps problem-solving groups to avoid re-inventing the wheel. ASHP's Web site (www.ashp.org) houses a Center on Patient Safety that offers an extensive review of the pharmacy literature on medical error. The National Patient Safety Foundation Clearinghouse bibliography (www.npsf.org) can also supplement your literature review.

- Build relationships of respect and exchange ideas with your colleagues across professional lines. Find champions for safety in other disciplines and divisions within your organization, and present your administration with a shared view of the acuity of the problems of health care delivery in your health system. Point out specific examples of systems defects, problems with hand-offs, etc.

- Invite your senior management to spend a day at the sharp end where the administrators can witness the challenges of patient care and how it is impaired by unwieldy prescription order entry systems, understaffing, and overabundant hand-offs.

- Make contact with your colleagues in other practice settings that have error reduction systems in place and glean from them how they make their processes work.

- Encourage your senior management to meet with other leaders that employ effective error reduction systems.

- Arrange for experts from other high-risk industries such as aviation, chemical manufacturing, and nuclear power to come and speak to your organization about how they have created systems that anticipate and account for error.

Third, we cannot be leaders outside our profession if we do not follow our own advice. In order to practice what we preach, we must work on issues within our own practice. Consider the implications for pharmacists of the error types discussed above—errors in planning (mistakes), and errors in execution (slips or lapses). Pharmacists who contribute medication expertise to prescribing decisions minimize the possibility of errors in planning. Pharmacists who conscientiously prepare, distribute, monitor, and evaluate the results of medication therapy minimize the possibility of errors of execution.

The one sure way to ensure that practitioners play their part in reducing medical error is to assume personal responsibility and accountability for all aspects of patients' medication therapy so that we cannot live with ourselves unless we do. Pharmacy's culture must change so that no pharmacists could live with themselves if they knowingly did not ensure that patients' initial medication therapies were optimal and safe and that those patients are carefully monitored to ensure efficacy, effectiveness, and safety. Failure to equip for and assume this additional responsibility should equate in the mind of the practitioner with knowingly putting patients in harm's way.

There are several steps you can take today to reduce medication error in your organization.

- Implement what is already known and apply the *ASHP Best Practices for Health-System Pharmacy* guidelines relating to safe medication use.[30]

- Ensure that pharmacists are an integral part of the patient care team: insert yourself into the clinical decision-making process and its follow-up.

- Recognize that change in the practice of pharmacy, often significant, is inevitable in a pharmacy department that commits to elimination of medication error. Facilitating change in practice among professionals is a complicated skill that goes far beyond traditional managerial approaches to workplace change. Commit to learning how to maximize the possibility that your colleagues will choose and effect change. ASHP's Practice Change Model is an example of a tool for developing an individualized plan for changing the outlook and practice patterns of your colleagues.[33,34]

These are steps that you can take now, but persistence is required to change systems and cultures. Highly visible activity by pharmacists on this issue will enhance public awareness of the patient care role of our profession. The most critical function is that as a profession, we take advantage of this opportunity to take action: to share the scope of our knowledge and to work with our colleagues to make change at a time when the public demands a re-thinking of the present health care system.[26]

Error Reporting

As discussed earlier, health care providers and institutions must have the opportunity to learn from mistakes. As simple as this sounds, it is one of the most difficult problems in the new era of patient safety. Punitive systems have been a major inhibitory factor in allowing us to learn from mistakes. Voluntary (learning) reporting systems do exist in many private institutions and public agencies, but debate persists regarding the access to the information residing in them. The data reported and stored in these systems describe events that did not cause harm to patients. Such reports typically fall into the category of near misses. Trend data are of special value for us in learning and in improving systems to prevent near misses from transforming into harmful accidents. For practitioners and health care organizations to feel comfortable reporting such non-harmful near misses, they must be assured that their reports will not be used against them in disciplinary or court proceedings. Such assurances are not the norm today. However, legislation has been introduced to the 106th and 107th Congresses that would extend the confidentiality of peer review protections to data reported to voluntary reporting systems.[35] Mounting external pressures from legislation, regulation, and public policy may accelerate the gradual cultural shifts that are needed to achieve safer systems.

Patient Safety: The New Science

In the same sense that the 1990's marked the beginning of the modern era for dialog on the topic of patient safety, the 1999 release of the IOM's *To Err is Human: Building a Safer Health System* ignited the beginning of a new era for patient safety research. This is illustrated by the fact that, by the end of the 2001 fiscal year, the Agency for Healthcare Research and Quality (AHRQ) had awarded $50 million in new grants for patient safety research, making it the world's largest sponsor of research funding on the topic.[36] Although unprecedented amounts of funding from the federal government became available over what seems a relatively short period of time, it should be recognized that a decade of studies throughout the 1990's provided the spark that resulted in the formation of the IOM Committee on Quality of Health Care in America, which produced the now famous report.

A major event in 1996 was the formation by the American Medical Association of the National Patient Safety Foundation, whose mission is primarily to disseminate knowledge about patient safety and to foster public awareness and professional receptivity to a change in culture toward safer health care.[37] Several national conferences on patient safety also stimulated dialog and public policy interest.[38–41] If the 1990's saw the spark that ignited a new era, then it can also be said that the pharmacy profession's work to advocate for and design safer medication-use systems over the last 50 years,[42–45] as well as anesthesiology's accomplishments over the last 20 years in equipment redesign and research in human error,[46] held the match.

The new science of patient safety is nothing if not complex. Research in patient safety combines all the traditional qualitative sciences well known to health care professionals with other non-health care related areas of study, such as human factors and ergonomics, ethnography, sociology, anthropology, psychology, logistical sciences, systems engineering, architecture, law, and numerous others. Many of these areas of study will need to be included to some degree in pharmacy school curricula, but it is most important to recognize that there is a cadre of new scientists with whom pharmacist patient safety researchers should acquaint themselves. Multidisciplinary research teams are working now at centers around the nation to determine how technology can be applied to prevent medical errors, what impact working conditions have on patient safety, and how to best disseminate patient safety research.[47]

The need for pharmacists to assume leadership roles as researchers in patient safety is great. This new science demands a well-rounded pharmacy practitioner who can see beyond the walls of the pharmacy and address the many complex issues of the safety sciences in the entire medication-use system. Beyond a thorough understanding of the complexities of medication use, the new pharmacist will need strong skills in logistics, information technology, human factors, communication and team building, and other skills not currently possessed by most in the pharmacy profession. Addressing these challenges through residency training, continual learning, and a belief in the absolute necessity for multidisciplinary collaboration will provide great opportunities for pharmacists now and in the future.

Medication-Use Safety and Risk as a Matter of Public Policy

The inherent risks associated with medications and the complex settings where they are used provide major challenges for all pharmacy practice settings. In this context, no medication is intrinsically safe. As a matter of public policy the concept of risk as it relates to medication use is neither well understood nor appreciated. Medication use is an invasive process, much like surgery. Individuals respond to medicines in unique and different ways, to their benefit and to their detriment. Genetic research is giving us better insight into this phenomenon.[48] The responsibility for safe medication use is shared by many, including patients and families, various health care providers, pharmaceutical industry, and government. Patients trust providers to offer treatment options based on their expertise and knowledge of the most current scientific evidence. With this information, patients must also accept a level of risk if they choose treatment with medications.[49] The phenomena of patient nonadherence and medicine misuse constitute in large part a failing of the health care system, not of patients.

In the past, paternalistic beliefs that the doctor always knows best have dominated patients' medication-use decisions. As the information age matures it becomes ever clearer that these assumptions are obsolete. Today patients can be armed with reliable information with which to make decisions. The advent of the Internet has spawned a flood of information, making the issue of reliability of information more important than ever. It has been shown that direct-to-consumer advertising affects the behavior of both the patients seeking medications and the physicians prescribing them.[50] With drug costs skyrocketing, basic access to medications for all patients has resurfaced as a major issue of public policy.[51] The issue of ensuring affordable patient access to prescription drugs dominates public policy discussions. However, even more important than ensuring that patients have access is making sure they understand and are educated on the issues of safe and effective use of medications. Pharmacists are a major part of the solution when they take leadership in collaborating with patients and prescribers to make better drug therapy decisions. As drug approvals and complex therapies increase in tandem with one another, and access to medications increases, the time has come for pharmacists to be proactive in demonstrating their value as medication-use experts.

The Role of Professional Organizations in Safety Advocacy

The commitment to continually improving the standard and quality of care should be part of the mission of every professional organization representing pharmacists, pharmacy technicians, and other health care providers. Professional societies can provide leadership in such ways as:

- disseminating practice guidelines, professional policies, and accreditation standards that encourage safety;
- sponsoring and publishing research that helps to identify and resolve vulnerabilities in health delivery systems;

- providing educational programs for members to develop current competencies and knowledge in safe practices;

- advocating to legislative bodies and public agencies for public policy, legislation, and regulations that support higher safety standards;

- advocating to private-sector groups and large employers for business practices and benefits purchasing decisions that reward improved health care safety performance; and

- providing information to the public concerning patient safety that draws upon members' expertise.

It is vital that pharmacy practitioners participate in the professional organizations available to them. By virtue of their size and stature, associations can often accomplish objectives that individuals cannot—but they cannot remain relevant without the driving force of member input and interaction.

Education and Training: Equipping Pharmacists with Contemporary Competencies

In order to ensure that practitioners possess and maintain the education and competencies required to safely engage in all aspects of the medication-use process, better communication is needed between practice sites and the various licensing and credentialing boards that certify these competencies.

IOM states, "Responsibilities for documenting continuing skills are dispersed among licensing bodies, specialty boards and professional groups, and health care organizations with little communication or coordination. In their ongoing assessments, existing licensing, certification and accreditation processes for health professionals should place greater attention on safety and performance skills."

Professional schools do not yet sufficiently provide students with the skills necessary to address issues of patient safety. Furthermore, professional licensing boards do little to assess competence and knowledge of safety practices. Students must be taught early, and continuously throughout their professional education, the principles of patient safety and how those principles will apply throughout their professional careers. Licensing boards must assess and reassess these fundamental patient safety skills. Hospital privileging committees should develop and use criteria to assess whether practitioners possess necessary patient safety skills and are competent in applying them.[52] Community pharmacies must adopt safety standards, and adherence to these standards must be examined by external review processes.

The Safe Use of Technology in Pharmacy

As technological systems and processes grow ever more intricate and interconnected, we entrust and empower them to an ever-greater degree—often with our lives, as in the cases of industries such as energy production, defense, transportation, and health care. But because automated systems can only function in tandem with human design and interaction, the risk of accident due to human error persists. Thus, when an accident occurs in a system that is entrusted with maintaining human life or safety, the outcomes often include injury, death, emotional damage, and financial hardship or ruin.

It is necessary, then, to identify the benefits and liabilities of both human and automated decision-making as we work to implement technology into a medication-use system that approaches the fail-safe ideal. The growing use of robots and other automated systems to perform many of the routine, mundane functions of dispensing medications has freed pharmacists for more complex tasks, such as collaborating in treatment decisions, monitoring patient outcomes, and counseling patients. Maintaining relational databases of drug information, warnings, and interactions helps decrease the pharmacist's and prescriber's reliance on memory. Computerized prescriber order entry, a method gaining popularity in U.S. health systems, has the potential to profoundly reduce medication dispensing errors related to unclear prescriber handwriting or deficiencies in critical technical information. Computerized patient records, identified as an "essential technology" by IOM, would ensure that all providers caring for a patient—regardless of location—would have access to the patient's most current clinical data. This would assist prescribers and pharmacists in determining the safest, most effective treatment regimen for that patient at that point in time.[53] Legitimate concerns for privacy must be considered when implementing these information-sharing networks. The patient should be regarded as the owner of his or her clinical data, and the benefits of sharing that data should never come at the expense of confidentiality. Likewise, data reflecting the prescribing habits of providers or institutions should never be placed where it could be mined or exploited for commercial purposes.

Caution is crucial in integrating technology into the medication-use process. Over-automation can disrupt effective procedures already in place and functioning properly at a site. The power afforded by modern information technology and automation can be wielded to the benefit or the detriment of processes and patients. Although automated systems and devices can prevent many of the errors caused by interpersonal miscommunication and reduce repetitive tasks, it must be remembered that computers are designed, programmed, and run by humans. Automated decisions and actions are not incapable of error. A computer can accurately transmit an inaccurately entered prescription order. A doctor under stress can inadvertently override a drug-interaction warning. These types of errors can best be corrected by placing trained pharmacy professionals at key points in the sequence of events between order and delivery of the drug. Technology in medication distribution and delivery is best viewed as a tool to assist human decision making, not a panacea to replace it.

Conclusion

As we draw to a close this brief introduction to the nature and extent of drug-related problems in the U.S., two themes should resonate clearly in the reader's mind: complexity and change. The issue is complex in that no single topic discussed in this chapter can be viewed as separate, distinct, or unrelated to another. A major problem with health care in the United States is that it is a cottage industry, where the vast majority of services are delivered via loosely connected silos. Ideally, care should be delivered to all patients via interconnected systems that are safe, effective, patient-centered, timely, efficient, and equitable.[26] Change refers to the fact that for substantive improvement to occur, the current health care system needs to be re-engineered from the antiquated structure in which care is currently delivered.

The second and final report of the Institute of Medicine Committee on Quality, entitled *Crossing the Quality Chasm: A New Health System for the 21st Century*, provides a high-level framework for how the ideal health care system should be designed and structured. Safety is a very important aspect, but safety is just the tip of the iceberg as we delve deeper into the broader dimensions of quality and seek to rebuild the system in its entirety from the ground up. The leadership of pharmacists in conceptualizing the specifics of the ideal medication-use system is vital. Dealing with complexity and adapting to rapid changes in the way care is delivered will be the defining characteristics of the successful pharmacy practitioner in the twenty-first century. The status quo is no longer acceptable. It is the responsibility of pharmacists to diligently work in collaboration with other disciplines to draft blueprints for the twenty-first century medication-use system. Defining the role of the pharmacist as a provider of care, not just a provider of product, is an absolute imperative if the pharmacy profession is to avoid becoming a relic of an obsolete health care process.

Acknowledgement

The authors appreciate the contribution of Scott Cowan, Executive Communication Associate, American Society of Health-System Pharmacists, in preparing this chapter.

References

1. Cohen MR, Anderson RW, Attilio RM et al. Preventing medication errors in cancer chemotherapy. *Am J Health-Syst Pharm*. 1996; 53:737–46.
2. Institute of Medicine. To err is human: building a safer health care system. Kohn LT, Corrigan JM, Donaldson MS, eds. Washington, DC: National Academy Press; 2000.
3. Reason JT. Human Error. New York: Cambridge University Press; 1990.
4. National Coordinating Council for Medication Error Reporting and Prevention. Recommendations to reduce errors related to administration of drugs. In: Deffenbaugh JH, ed. Best practices for health-system pharmacy. 2001–2002 ed. Bethesda, MD: American Society of Health-System Pharmacists; 2002.
5. Leape LL. Error in medicine. *JAMA*. 1994; 272:1851–7.
6. Senders JW. Medical devices, medical errors, and medical accidents. In: Bogner MS, ed. Human error in medicine. Hillsdale, NJ: Laurence Erlbaum Associates; 1994.
7. Flynn EA, Barker KN. Medication errors research. In: Cohen MR, ed. Medication errors. 2nd ed. Washington, DC: American Pharmaceutical Association; 1999.
8. Nolan TW. System changes to improve patient safety. *BMJ*. 2000:320; 771–3.
9. Leape LL, Bates DW, Cullen DJ. Systems analysis of adverse drug events. *JAMA*. 1995; 274:35–43.

10. Cook RI, Woods DD. Operating at the sharp end: the complexity of human error. In: Bogner MS, ed. Human error in medicine. Hillsdale, NJ: Laurence Erlbaum Associates; 1994.

11. Brennan TA, Leape LL, Laird NM et al. Incidence of adverse events and negligence in hospitalized patients: results of the Harvard Medical Practice Study I. *N Engl J Med.* 1991; 324:370–6.

12. Leape LL, Brennan TA, Laird NM et al. The nature of adverse events in hospitalized patients: results of the Harvard Medical Practice Study II. *N Engl J Med.* 1991; 324:377–84.

13. American Society of Health-System Pharmacists Center on Patient Safety. http://www.ashp.org/patient_safety/links.html (accessed 2002 Jan 20).

14. The Leapfrog Group for Patient Safety. http://www.leapfroggroup.org (accessed 2002 Jan 20).

15. Bates DW, Cullen DJ, Laird NM et al. Incidence of adverse drug events and potential adverse drug events: implications for prevention. *JAMA.* 1995; 274:29–34.

16. Cohen MR. Causes of medication errors. In: Cohen MR, ed. Medication errors. 2nd ed. Washington, DC: American Pharmaceutical Association; 1999.

17. Johnson JA, Bootman JL. Drug-related morbidity and mortality: a cost-of-illness model. *Arch Intern Med.* 1995; 155:1949–56.

18. Johnson JA, Bootman JL. Drug-related morbidity and mortality and the economic impact of pharmaceutical care. *Am J Health-Syst Pharm.* 1997; 54:554–8.

19. When medication hurts instead of helps. Washington, DC: The Alliance for Aging Research; 1998.

20. Ernst FR, Grizzle AJ. Drug-related morbidity and mortality: updating the cost-of-illness model. *J Am Pharm Assoc.* 2001; 41:192–9.

21. Roberts K. Organizational change and a commitment to safety. Chicago: Enhancing Patient Safety and Reducing Errors in Health Care. National Patient Safety Foundation at the AMA; 1999.

22. Sagan SD. The limits of safety. Princeton, NJ: Princeton University Press; 1993.

23. Bagian JP. Making the best use of your most valuable resource. Saint Paul, MN: Annenberg III Conference on Communicating Risk and Safety in Healthcare; 2001.

24. Agency for Healthcare Research and Quality. Making health care safer: a critical analysis of patient safety practices. Rockville, MD: U.S. Department of Health and Human Services, 2001; AHRQ Publication 01-E058.

25. Simon R. Communicating in the midst of complexity: the MedTeams experience. Saint Paul, MN: Annenberg III Conference on Communicating Risk and Safety in Healthcare; 2001.

26. Institute of Medicine. Crossing the quality chasm: a new health system for the 21st century. Kohn LT, Corrigan JM, Donaldson MS, eds. Washington, DC: National Academy Press; 2001.

27. Cohen MR. One hospital's method of applying failure mode and effects analysis. In: Cohen MR, ed. Medication errors. 2nd ed. Washington, DC: American Pharmaceutical Association; 1999.

28. Hoffrage U, Hertwig R, Gigerenzer G. Hindsight bias: a by-product of knowledge updating? Journal of Experimental Psychology: Learning, Memory and Cognition. 2000; 26:566–81.

29. O'Connell D, Kraman SS. We made a mistake. Saint Paul, MN: Annenberg III Conference on Communicating Risk and Safety in Healthcare; 2001.

30. Deffenbaugh JH, ed. Best practices for health-system pharmacy. 2001–2002 ed. Bethesda, MD: American Society of Health-System Pharmacists; 2002.

31. Cohen MR, Smetzer JL. Risk analysis and treatment. In: Cohen MR, ed. Medication errors. 2nd ed. Washington, DC: American Pharmaceutical Association; 1999.

32. Zellmer WA. The invisible pharmacist. In: The conscience of a pharmacist: essays on vision and leadership for a profession. Bethesda, MD: American Society of Health-System Pharmacists; 2001.

33. Nimmo CM, Holland RW. Transitions in pharmacy practice, parts 1-4. *Am J Health-Syst Pharm.* 1999; 56:1758–64, 1981–7, 2235–41, 2458–62.

34. Nimmo CM, Holland RW. Transitions in pharmacy practice, part 5. *Am J Health-Syst Pharm.* 2000; 57:64–72.

35. American Society of Health-System Pharmacists. ASHP Government Affairs legislative issues summary. http://www.ashp.org/public/proad/legislative/july_2002.html (accessed 2002 Jan 20).

36. Agency for Healthcare Research and Quality. Fiscal year 2001 budget in brief. http://www.ahrq.gov/about/budbrf01.htm (accessed 2002 Jan 20).

37. National Patient Safety Foundation. About the Foundation. http://www.npsf.org/html/about_npsf.html (accessed 2002 Jan 20).

38. Re-engineering the medication-use system: proceedings of a national interdisciplinary conference conducted by the Joint Commission of Pharmacy Practitioners. *Am J Health-Syst Pharm.* 2000; 57:537–601.

39. National Patient Safety Foundation and Annenberg Center for Health Sciences. http://www.mederrors.org (accessed 2002 Jan 20).

40. Proceedings of the Understanding and Preventing Drug Misadventures Conference. http://www.ashp.org/public/proad/mederror/pexsu.html (accessed 2002 Jan 20).

41. Proceedings of the National Summit on Medical Errors and Patient Safety Research. Quality Interagency Task Force; 2000. http://www.quic.gov/summit/summary1.htm (accessed 2002 Jan 20).

42. Barker KN. Effects of an experimental medication system on medication errors and costs. Part one: introduction and errors study. *Am J Hosp Pharm.* 1969;26:324–33.

43. Barker KN, McConnell WE. Problems of detecting medication errors in hospitals. *Am J Hosp Pharm.* 1962; 19:360–9.

44. Manasse HR. Medication use in an imperfect world: drug misadventuring as an issue of public policy, part 1. *Am J Hosp Pharm.* 1989; 46:929–44.

45. Manasse HR. Medication use in an imperfect world: drug misadventuring as an issue of public policy, part 2. *Am J Hosp Pharm.* 1989; 46:1141–52.

46. Gaba DM. Human error in dynamic medical domains. In: Human error in medicine. Boyner MS, ed. Hillsdale NJ: Laurence Erlbaum Associates; 1994.

47. Agency for Healthcare Research and Quality. Patient safety research initiatives: fiscal year 2001. AHRQ publication no. 02-P006. http://www.ahrq.gov/qual/ps2001.htm (accessed 2002 Jan 20).

48. Jaggers LD. Pharmacogenomics: worthy of pharmacy's attention. *Am J Health-Syst Pharm.* 1999; 56:27.

49. Safe Medical Treatments: Everyone Has a Role. Proceedings of a workshop co-sponsored by the Food and Drug Administration and the National Patient Safety Foundation, 2000. http://www.fda.gov/cder/calendar/meeting/npsf2000/summary.pdf (accessed 2002 Jan 20).

50. Zachry WM III, Shepherd MD, Hinich MJ et al. Relationship between direct-to-consumer advertising and physician diagnosing and prescribing. *Am J Health-Syst Pharm.* 2002; 59:33–41.

51. Shah ND, Vermeulen LC, Santell JP. Projecting future drug expenditures—2002. *Am J Health-Syst Pharm.* 2002; 59:131–42.

52. Clause S, Fudin J, Mergner A et al. Prescribing privileges among pharmacists in Veterans Affairs medical centers. *Am J Health-Syst Pharm.* 2001; 58:1143–5.

53. Dick RS, Steen EB, eds. The Computer-Based Patient Record: An Essential Technology for Health Care. Washington, DC: National Academy Press; 1991.

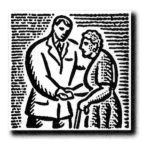

Chapter 7: Sociological Implications of Pharmaceutical Care

Donna E. Dolinsky, M.A., Ph.D.
John M. Lonie, R.Ph., M.A.

The Nature of Our Profession

The profession of pharmacy has never had more prospects for professional growth than it does today. The opportunities are many and varied as the profession continuously changes and redefines its role as a major cog in the health care system. A degree in pharmacy can lead to employment in a rich array of pharmacy practice areas. Such areas include community and chain pharmacy practice, institutional (hospital, long-term care) practice, as well as a host of specialized practice areas. However, along with the great potential for career diversity and fulfillment, there are and have been complex sociological tensions that exist both within and outside the profession.

Very often, where there is change there also exists tension. Change is not new to the profession of pharmacy. The pharmacist's role has continuously adapted to the changing needs of society and health care for hundreds of years. As noted by Zacker and Mucha[1]: "Historically, a pharmacist's function was to convert raw chemicals and plants into finished pharmaceutical dosage forms upon the written orders of physicians. . . . With increasing industrialization after World War II, the large scale manufacturing of pharmaceutical products diminished pharmacists' drug preparation function and left them with a primarily distributive role." In this instance, we see pharmacists having to change and adapt to new professional roles. The change in this case left pharmacists with primarily a distributive function and diminished their drug preparation function. Along with this new role came increased public responsibility as pharmacists were expected to be accurate, efficient, and error-free dispensers of medication.

More recently, within the last 30 years, pharmacy has experienced two other shifts in professional responsibility. First came the clinical pharmacy movement in which pharmacists were being utilized as much for their knowledge about medications and their effects in disease states as they were for their dispensing functions. Ritchey and Sommers[2] commented further on the origins of the clinical pharmacy movement:

"Recognizing the importance of technological and economic changes in hospital prac-

119

tice, pharmacy elites advocated a new 'clinical pharmacy' role which had a norma-
tive dimension—a patient, rather than product, orientation. By the 1970's, clinical
pharmacy assumed the character of a professional movement to boost its professional
status. Pharmacy elites worked on 'credentialing' and accreditation, and cultivated
professional autonomy through control over practice standards and the work envi-
ronment."

The clinical pharmacy movement brought pharmacists out of the basement pharmacy and up to the floors performing rounds with physicians and providing the physicians with valuable medication-related information. This movement toward clinical practice was a result of several factors including changes in the pharmacy school curriculum
from a four-year program to a five-year program. This extra year of study introduces
pharmacy students to practice areas, such as hospital pharmacy, to which they may not
have previously been exposed.

In the early 1990's, the next (and current) wave of change hit the pharmacy profession—pharmaceutical care. Hepler, in 1988, defined pharmaceutical care as ". . . a covenantal relationship between a patient and a pharmacist in which the pharmacist performs drug use control functions (with appropriate knowledge and skill) governed by the
awareness of and commitment to the patient's interest."[3] This definition brings to the fore
a new conceptualization of pharmacy practice—the movement completely away from
dispensing functions to direct patient care functions. It is interesting to compare the pharmacists' role in the era of clinical pharmacy with their role in the era of pharmaceutical
care. The clinical pharmacist of the late 1960's through the mid 1980's was primarily
hospital (institution) based and was considered to be a resource to the physician. The
pharmaceutical care model proposed a strong patient focus with the development of a
direct therapeutic relationship between the pharmacist and the patient, in which both
parties worked together to solve medication-related problems and improve the patient's
health. This new conceptualization of pharmacy practice was independent of practice
site. That is, both community- and institution-based pharmacists were charged with practicing patient-centered pharmaceutical care. In 1990, Hepler and Strand revised the definition of pharmaceutical care to its current foundational meaning: "Pharmaceutical care
is that component of pharmacy practice which entails the direct interaction of the pharmacist with the patient for the purpose of caring for the patient's drug-related needs."[4]

Sociologists call the changes that have occurred in the profession "reprofessionalization." Birenbaum observed, "Traditional sociological analyses of the professions
rarely have considered how, and under what conditions, an established profession seeks to
change its position within a single industry. In the structural–functional perspective an
occupation becomes a profession when granted autonomy and receives recognition from
society for possessing a technical knowledge base, demonstrating effective performance,
developing a lengthy and superior education, and espousing ethical commitments to the
common good."[5]

We saw how the practice of pharmacy changed because of the post-World War II
industrialization, and the changes in pharmacy school curricula caused the clinical
reprofessionalization, and ultimately the current reprofessionalization to pharmaceutical
care. It is important to be aware of how these changes have created sociological tensions
within the profession of pharmacy and precisely what tensions exist for those who prac-

tice pharmacy today. To that end, it is helpful to distinguish between tensions (or forces) within (internal) versus tensions outside (external) the profession, which have an effect on the current practice of pharmaceutical care.

Forces from Within Pharmacy

What are some of the internal forces within pharmacy that affect how pharmaceutical care is practiced in the 21st century? This chapter identifies six major internal forces that can create tension and conflict in pharmacy practice:

- economic factors,
- the "knowing versus doing" dilemma,
- autonomy versus organizational restraints,
- personality versus practice setting/environment,
- the "business versus professional" dilemma (marginality), and
- boundary maintenance.

Economic Factors

Today's pharmacy graduates can expect to be highly compensated as they embark on their new careers. Depending on location (area of the country), some practice areas may be compensated at a higher rate than others. Generally chain pharmacy practice tends to pay a higher starting salary than such practice sites as institutional or independent community pharmacy practice.[6] Moreover, the rapid expansion of chain pharmacies within the last decade has created many new positions and opportunities for pharmacists at the staff, supervisory, and managerial/administrative levels.

Many times the desire to obtain the highest starting salary is the major motivation to young pharmacy students when they are seeking their first employment opportunity after graduation.[6] This may be necessary as the need to begin repaying student loans may be pressing or the desire to start a family causes immediate pressure to obtain the highest starting income possible.

Because of these and other economic pressures, new graduates may initially find themselves in high paying positions but ultimately become discontented as they realize that the decision to accept a higher salary may not have been the best decision in terms of career fulfillment.

The "Knowing versus Doing" Dilemma

The knowing versus doing dilemma exists when pharmacists experience conflict over the fact that they practice a small percentage of what they are trained to do. Because of the advent of the pharmaceutical care philosophy, as well as the mandate of six-year doctor of pharmacy degree programs in all colleges of pharmacy, pharmacists have never been more knowledgeable and prepared to deliver effective, efficient, and patient-centered health care services.

In some instances, however, pharmacists may feel that they are not using their full range of professional knowledge and skills. Problems such as this may be particularly evident in practice sites, such as community (chain or independent) pharmacy, where the pharmaceutical care model has not been successfully implemented. In such cases, the older model of pharmacist as technician or dispenser of prescriptions, predominates. Pharmacists can easily become demoralized or burned-out if they find themselves in these types of situations for an extended period.

Professional Autonomy versus Organizational Constraints

Professional autonomy is the ability to make work-related decisions independent of organizational, political, economic, or social constraints. As highly educated well-trained professionals, pharmacists expect a level of professional autonomy equivalent to most other health professionals. In many practice areas (community and institutional practice), pharmacists are enjoying high levels of professional autonomy. Pharmacists are increasingly showing their worth as the decisions they make have proven to be highly cost effective to organizations. In addition to cost effectiveness, pharmacists make valuable patient care therapeutic decisions that improve health outcomes and quality of life.[7]

However, there may be instances where a pharmacist's professional decision-making ability is compromised by competing organizational values. For example, pharmacists may feel that work policies constrain their ability to practice pharmaceutical care properly.[8] This dilemma is evident in organizations and institutions whose mission requires pharmacist employees to choose between a pharmaceutical care philosophy and improving organizational profits. For example, many chain pharmacies offer incentives to pharmacists if they suggest therapeutic equivalent medications to prescribers. Often these therapeutically equivalent medications are more profitable to the organization or institution. The conflict in this case occurs as pharmacists' personal decision-making ability is, in effect, compromised.

Personality versus Practice Setting

Personality is the relatively stable set of dispositions or traits that tend to persist over time and across different situations.[9] Psychologists generally accept the notion that personality is relatively stable across the life span. This does not mean that people cannot change aspects of themselves with which they are unhappy. Change can occur but it takes commitment and vigilance.

It is important to recognize the potential fit between personality styles and the careers that we choose. Certainly, a person who is easily made anxious and tends to overreact might not be very happy on the bomb squad of a police department. The same is true for many other career choices, including pharmacy. It may be asking a lot for a young person fresh out of pharmacy school to choose the perfect practice setting, but it is important to stress the value of knowing who we are and what type of career position is right for us.

In practice, some pharmacists may find themselves in areas that are not well suited to their personality. For instance, a pharmacist with a personality style that is in conflict with a fast-paced emergency room pharmacy may not be very happy, may become anxious, depressed, and may consider a career change. Alternatively, this same pharmacist may thrive if put in a different practice setting. It is important for pharmacy students to make the most of their experiences in pharmacy school, in order to be able to make well-informed career decisions later on.

Marginality: Business versus Professional Dilemma

Zacker and Mucha comment[1]: "Pharmacy has always had characteristics of both a business and a profession. In the sociology of occupations and professions, this situation is termed professional marginality." The conflict of marginality in pharmacy has traditionally been found mainly in community type practices, where the pressure to maintain a profit was akin to staying in business. However, in recent years, the marginality problem has also affected institutional practice as pharmacy managers and administrators are increasingly asked to obtain business and management degrees rather than clinical or professional degrees.

Zacker and Mucha explain the problem of professional marginality further: "Pharmacy illustrates the problems that can arise from marginality because of a conflict between professional and business norms. The formal education of pharmacists is intended to provide the theoretical study of a body of knowledge that Thorner[10] described as essential to professionalization. The conflict that develops is between these professional norms in which the pharmacist has been trained and the business norms that permeate the work environment. A strong push, either from within pharmacy or from the external environment, could completely professionalize pharmacy or drive it toward a mostly business orientation."

This is not a new problem. As early as 1899 pharmacists asked, "Shall pharmacists become tradesmen?"[11] The problem of professional marginality overflows into other problem areas previously mentioned. For instance, practicing a marginal profession could have an effect on the psyche of the practitioner. Constantly feeling professionally inferior to other heath care professionals can lead to a lowered sense of professional self-esteem accompanied by lower self-expectations and less willingness to engage in professional activities like patient consultation.

Boundary Maintenance

Boundary maintenance in pharmacy deals primarily with how the professional roles of pharmacists intersect with the roles of other health care providers—particularly physicians. Until the beginning of the clinical pharmacy movement, there were little professional boundary problems between physicians and pharmacists. Pharmacists were primarily highly knowledgeable technicians or dispensers of medication, whereas physicians always held the superior social, economic, and intellectual role within medicine.[2]

As pharmacists began taking a more active role in patient care (clinical pharmacy then eventually pharmaceutical care), in addition to having the title of doctor (with the addition of the Pharm.D. degree), some physicians began to feel their professional sovereignty threatened. Ritchey and Sommers[2] explain

> "Physicians may perceive pharmacy expansion as encroachment and use their institutional power to limit it. Moreover, pharmacist control over esoteric tasks can be fleeting because pharmaceutical knowledge is not inherently the domain of pharmacists. In fact, in the 1950's, the opportunity for pharmacists to move toward a clinical role was nearly lost as drug companies and a few medical schools vigorously pushed a medical specialty called clinical pharmacology. Fortunately, for pharmacists, this specialty, which combined clinical medicine with basic pharmacology, had limited appeal to physicians who favored life sciences over physical sciences."

Issues of boundary maintenance and encroachment between pharmacists and physicians and vice versa will continue to be contentious issues within the profession, especially as pharmacist's roles become more patient-centered. Also, as pharmacists complete pharmacy residencies and become board certified in their chosen specialty, the issue of professional boundaries will probably continue to surface from time to time.

How pharmacists deal with boundary issues depends upon a number of factors. These factors include self-confidence, inter-professional self-efficacy, and quality of inter-professional social skills. Self-confidence, in this case, is concerned with the individual pharmacist's confidence in his or her ability to assume a rightful role in the health care team. Inter-professional self-efficacy deals with a pharmacist's ability to effectively handle specific work situations in which other members of the health care team may be involved. Finally, the quality of social skills that a pharmacist develops can significantly determine the outcome of potentially uncomfortable role boundary issues.

Forces from Outside Pharmacy

Just as there are forces from within the profession creating tensions in the field, there are forces from outside the profession that influence how the profession is practiced. The following categories of external forces appear to exert the most influence on pharmaceutical care practice:

- people,
- corporatization and managed care,
- bureaucratization, and
- technical changes.

People

Pharmacy is not practiced in a vacuum. The objective of pharmaceutical care practice is to deliver appropriate, efficient, and effective care to people (patients). In addition, modern pharmaceutical care practice means interacting with a variety of other members of the health care team. Any time people interact, a door is left open for miscommunication or misunderstanding. Individuals outside of the profession—patients, customers, physicians, nurses, or other pharmacists—have profound effects on how pharmaceutical care is practiced.

Corporatization and Managed Care

One of the most influential forces acting on pharmacy today is the increase in corporatization that is and has been occurring in the U.S. health care system throughout the last decade.[1] Corporatization is defined as pressure put on an industry by large or key stakeholders within that industry in order to decrease costs and/or increase bottom line profits. Zacker and Mucha acknowledge[1] "Large insurance purchasers, such as employers, labor unions and private organizations are putting increased competitive and economic pressures on pharmacies and are having a major impact on how pharmacists and other providers are paid." In an attempt to decrease expenditures on pharmaceuticals and increase efficiencies, third-party administrators have negotiated with pharmacists to provide services at reduced rates—essentially reducing the role of pharmacists to one of low-bid contractor.

The advent of managed care has had a profound effect on community and chain pharmacy practice. Managed care organizations use the term disease management to mean control of the types and quantities of medications that are used in their organizations. Managed care has changed the way decisions are made by both pharmacists and physicians. Medical and pharmaceutical decisions are made as much for economic reasons as they are for therapeutic reasons. Community pharmacists have felt economic pressure brought on by them, under the guise of disease state management. Pharmacists need to assess the managed care revolution rationally, not emotionally. Cipolle et al.[12] observe "Disease management has, in contemporary terms, been used by the pharmaceutical industry as a marketing technique. In this framework, the industry develops drug entities, markets the product and advertises it within a particular disease domain so that the value of the product can be managed relative to other entities treating the same disease. Managed care organizations have converted this concept into a cost-accounting system, wherein the cost of the drug entity can be understood relative to other treatments for a particular disease."

Lowered professional fees from third-party payers have forced many independent community pharmacies to expand other less professional areas of their pharmacy in order to stay in business. This expansion can create a professional conflict causing an increase in the gulf between business and profession, therefore causing the perception of marginality within the profession.

Bureaucratization

Bureaucratization is the proliferation of rules, procedures, and paperwork by an organization in order to respond to demands for increased efficiency and profitability.[13] Pharmacy has been called the most regulated of all professions.

These tensions within the profession can be seen because of disparate views of the value, in terms of patient health outcomes and economic benefit, of pharmacists' role. Will they go away because of reprofessionalization and documentation of the outcomes of effective reprofessionalism? Can full reprofessionalism resulting in the delivery of pharmaceutical care reduce drug costs; permit pharmacists to do what they were educated to do; give the pharmacist autonomy; address problems of personality-practice setting conflict; solve the business versus professional dilemma; reduce the ambiguity of boundary maintenance; resolve conflicts between pharmacists and other health professionals, pharmacists, and patients; reduce problems in the corporatization of health care; and reduce bureaucracy? Is there something pharmacists can do to reduce these tensions? We will argue that reprofessionalization, an organizational change, is necessary but not sufficient to reduce professional tensions within pharmacy.

Reprofessionalism to full professionalism will succeed when pharmacists choose to engage in activities that support pharmaceutical care. Pharmacy education has imbued pharmacists with information and skills that may be necessary but not sufficient to deliver pharmaceutical care. Pierpaoli[14] iconoclastically believes that "to elevate the level of pharmacy practice, individual practitioners need will; too much attention has been given to skill. Many new practitioners have earned Pharm.D. degrees but not received enough nurturing from colleagues to develop into innovators who will continue the profession's progress." By "will," Pierpaoli means that pharmacists need to want to be able to deliver pharmaceutical care. Professional skills are necessary but not sufficient for bringing about change. The profession has changed, but the professionals have not. To paraphrase a former president, ask not what pharmacy can do for you, but what you can do for pharmacy.[15]

Reprofessionalization as a Solution to Forces in Pharmacy Practice: What Is My Role?

What is the role of pharmacy students in the midst of reprofessionalization towards pharmaceutical care? How can students cope with the anxieties caused by change? How can students deal with the ambiguity encountered when receiving conflicting messages in practice (reduce medication errors but do not take time to talk to patients) or when practice demands conflict with personal attitudes, beliefs, values, and behaviors? What is reprofessionalization and why does it cause so many problems if it is supposed to bring about solutions? Why do we have to change the way the profession practices? What do students need to know about the process of reprofessionalization and the personal effect of change? What is reprofessionalization?

Reprofessionalization

"Reprofessionalization is the process by which an emerging profession (or deprofessionalized occupation) regains momentum in its professional development. To be deprofessionalized or reprofessionalized, however, there must be evidence that the occupation once met or began to meet criteria for the status of a profession."[16] Pharmacy was called a marginal profession, an evolving profession,[17] and a quasi-profession,[18] because pharmacy before the 1960's did not meet all the criteria for a profession—primarily because of a lack of autonomy and use of a theoretical information base to meet client need. The term marginality referred to potential conflicts between professional and business standards, i.e., serving the client or serving the business. Pharmacy was considered deprofessionalized during the 1950's when community pharmacists 1) were no longer manufacturing medicines, 2) were not allowed to discuss the medication with the patient, and 3) their main function was dispensing. Helpler said, "pharmacy became a channel of distribution for the pharmaceutical industry."[3]

Professionalism developed during the clinical pharmacy movement, in the late 1960's and early 1970's, when drug information services and decentralized pharmacies supported pharmacist consultation with physicians on medication needs of individual patients during hospital rounds.[19] Although the patient was helped by the consultation with the physician, the direct client of the clinical pharmacist was the physician, not the patient. In pharmaceutical care, the direct recipient of services is the patient—hence an additional criterion of a profession had been met. For pharmaceutical care to happen nationwide in every type of pharmacy practice, all pharmacists had to be educated as clinical pharmacists. This organizational change within pharmacy, in response to differential levels of knowledge, skill, attitude, and behavior was an example of reprofessionalization.[5] The practitioners, whose skills were not at the level of clinical pharmacists, were expected to upgrade their skills. All new members of the professions had to be trained as clinical pharmacists, and all had to have Pharm.D. degrees.

When innovators within a profession mandate change, all members are expected to change and upgrade their level of practice. Practitioners may not be asked if they believe change should occur or if they would like to change or be excused from change if they do not like the change. The voices advocating professional change are often the intellectual elite, rather than practitioner groups, clients, or interested parties. There was a need that pharmacists could have fulfilled that was driven not by elite members of the profession, but by patients. Patients were asking for medication information and help in making decisions about if and how to use medicines, since they were not receiving this information from their physicians. They were, however, not necessarily asking pharmacists, but pharmacy had a chance to meet this need, which it rejected.[20] Within one month of pharmacy's rejection of the provision of Patient Package Inserts, the American Medical Association provided Physician Medication Information to the public.

When people are asked to change their behavior and do not want to, one can feel loss of control and frustration that can lead to resistance, anger, dissatisfaction, depression, and subsequent defiance and immobility. For example, a change-adverse pharmacist may say, "You can legislate patient counseling but you can't make me do it or want to do it." In the last section of this chapter, the authors will address how students can cope with their reactions to the changes brought about by reprofessionalism.

Why Reprofessionalize?

Why did pharmacy need to reprofessionalize to embrace pharmaceutical care? What was broken that needed to be fixed? Were we moving from something deficient about the profession or towards better patient outcomes, profession development and respect, or reducing the cost of health care? Birenbaum[5] suggested that the reprofessionalism in pharmacy was driven not by altruistic goals of enhancing patient outcomes but rather by structural forces within the health care system and within pharmacy. Some of the forces that threatened pharmacy follow:

- Decline of independent pharmacies because of competition from corporate pharmacies, which meant that many pharmacists could not run their own businesses.

- Managed care, which limited the reimbursement that pharmacies received.

- Automation, which meant fewer pharmacists would be needed for dispensing functions.

- Physician extenders, who could prescribe medications either alone or under standing orders of a physician, such as physician assistants, nurse practitioners, and a small cohort of psychologists. These practitioners, some with fewer years of education than pharmacists, were getting paid for something that many pharmacists believed they could do (and do better) but were not permitted to do.

- Increased communication within the profession, which allowed pharmacists to discuss their dissatisfaction and fears of being dispossessed.

It could be inferred that if pharmacy did not find a new niche, it could become deprofessionalized.

Conversely, Penna[21] believed that reprofessionalism occurred to meet the unmet needs of patients—needs for information, help in making decisions, and self-management. Whether reprofessionalism occurred to save the profession or to meet patient needs, change is occurring. To survive professionally and personally, students will need to manage the conflicts that change may cause in practice.

What do students need to know about the process of reprofessionalization and the effects of change? Reprofessionalism brings about changes in expectations of the way students will practice.

Process of Reprofessionalization

Reprofessionalism has occurred in many professions including law, counseling, social work, occupational therapy, the military, engineering, architecture, optometry, chiropractic, and physical therapy. These changes occurred primarily through forces from professional organizations and mandatory increased educational requirements, with some practitioners not wanting the change. In almost every case, reprofessionalization in these professions was towards greater client service through advanced education for practitioners and increased adherence to the professional role by all members of the profession. Professional associations united to champion the change, rewarded adapters, and admonished laggards. Reprofessionalization in physical therapy included expanded diagnostic and treatment modalities to meet client needs that arose from an increase in "car crash victims, the elderly, and the growth of sports medicine."[2] Rehabilitation counseling, a specialty in which people with disabilities are helped, went through a reprofessionalization process during which ethical standards were readdressed and unified as well as sincere concern for the well-being and interests of clients.[17] As in any change, there were the innovators, the early adapters, the late adapters, and the laggards.[22]

Change and Its Side Effects

"It should be borne in mind that there is nothing more difficult to arrange, more doubtful of success and more dangerous to carry through than initiating change. The innovator makes enemies of all those who prospered under the old order, and only lukewarm support is forthcoming from those who would prosper under the new."[23] Many pharmacists have prospered financially and emotionally through the old order of counting, pouring, licking, and sticking. Many individuals entered the profession because they did not want to take responsibility for the provision of drug therapy for the purpose of achieving definite outcomes that improve a patient's quality of life. They did not want to talk about drugs—certainly not with patients—or have to monitor patients. They definitely did not want those things. Pharmacy was about drugs, not people. Now the profession is advocating change towards pharmaceutical care, which is about drugs, how people use drugs, and the outcomes of drugs on people.

What happens to people when they are expected to change and they choose not to, are not ready to change, or are not capable of change? Some common reactions are

- Fear of failure, such as not being able to answer a patient's questions or not being able to deal with an angry patient.

- Fear of the unknown, such as not knowing what practice will be like in three years, when dispensing functions will be taken over by non-professional personnel using technology.

- Anxiety over ambiguity, such as being asked to fill many prescriptions and counsel at the same time.

- Frustration, such as not being able to use all your knowledge, which can lead to anger.[24]
- Depression over feeling out of control in the pharmacy, because there is too much going on and not enough time to do it all or do it well.

We know there are drugs to reduce fear, anxiety, frustration, anger, and depression. There are also behavioral and social ways to reduce these negative emotions. Let's look at how people change and see if we can translate these developments into strategies.

How Does Change Occur? How Can I Cope with Change?

"That the carriers of the ideas of clinical pharmacy may influence a new generation of graduates of colleges of pharmacies, there can be no doubt. Whether they will produce the results they intend may have more to do with their way of solving problems of adoption in a stressful environment"[5] Holland and Nimmo, a Dean of a College of Pharmacy and a Director of Educational Resources in the American Society of Heath-System Pharmacists, have investigated means of solving problems or change and adopting new pharmacy practice patterns.[25] In response to reported failures to persuade pharmacists to adopt and to expand their role to clinical pharmacy and pharmaceutical care functions, the authors wrote a five-part series of articles on transitions in pharmacy in which they present a model of change. The model and its strategies for change will be summarized here.

Holland and Nimmo posit that there are five practices of pharmacy, all needed to support patient health outcomes. This model, called Total Pharmacy Care, combines drug information, self-care, clinical pharmacy, pharmaceutical care, and distribution. To practice in all of these models, the pharmacist needs professional competencies of cognitive and psychomotor skills, professional socialization into pharmacy with appropriate patient care attitudes and values, and professional judgment.[26] Based upon theories of change, which are beyond the scope of this chapter, Zacker and Mucha[1] suggested that two levels of pharmacy, not five, have evolved and are needed: the distributive and the drug therapy models. They infer that pharmacy functions in response to market needs, and that the profession should remain flexible and address these needs. An analysis of this argument suggests that we rename pharmacy practice to pharmacy practices. Changing the name of something influences how we perceive it and react to it, including greater flexibility in understanding a phenomenon of change.

To effect a change in pharmacy practice, Holland and Nimmo believe that all of three conditions must exist: an appropriate practice environment, learning resources to help the pharmacist learn new knowledge, and skills and motivational strategies to develop pharmacists.[27] To create an appropriate practice environment, all parties involved in the professional practice need to work together to design a plan for the clearly defined change—an individual working alone is not likely to be effective. When people decide together, they are more likely to "buy in" and go along with a change. The cost of the change must be determined and resources set aside to support the change. Job descriptions need to be written and possibly some older jobs need to be re-engineered. Communications among personnel, resources, the ability to plan, and the flexibility to negotiate are all needed.

Decisions about learning resources should be based upon very clear job descriptions and patient needs, not just what is available from professional organizations or pharmacy websites. If the change involves a pharmacist counseling low literacy patients, for example, the learning resources may include a distance-learning course through the Internet on identifying, assessing, and addressing the needs of low literacy patients.[28] Lastly, even with an appropriate practice environment and educational resources, change will not occur without human energy and direction, which means motivation. *Movere*, the Latin word for "to move," is the root for the word motivation. Individual needs and choice, as well as external incentives, can cause a human to move.

A pharmacist's willingness to change is a function of both "personality and . . . current state of professional socialization."[29] Personality, "the unique psychological qualities of an individual that influence a variety of characteristic behavior patterns (both overt and covert) across different situations and over time,"[30] is relatively stable, but professional socialization and the development of attitudes, values, and beliefs about oneself within a profession can change over time. Nimmo and Holland suggest that some pharmacists may be resistant to change to newer practice models because of certain personality characteristics held commonly by segments of pharmacists, e.g., avoiding communication. They concluded   ". . . We have within the profession today a large proportion of individuals whose personalities matched well with pharmacy when distribution was the primary model. However, when these same individuals are asked to deal directly with patients, work on clinical problems in the context of a teach approach, or solve problems having no clear right or wrong answer, they experience incongruity with their personality."[1] While it may not be possible to change a pharmacist's personality, it may be possible to enhance professional attitudes, values, and beliefs through professional socialization.

In the last article in their series, Nimmo and Holland[31] explained a developmental plan, described below, to help managers help change pharmacists' attitudes towards the delivery of pharmaceutical care (including clinical pharmacy and drug information services), if pharmacists choose to change. A pharmacy student or pharmacist can use the same model to develop his or her own professional socialization, that is, attitudes, values, beliefs, and behaviors towards the delivery of pharmaceutical care, if *chosen*. A pharmacy student can do this by enlisting the help of the pharmacy faculty who are teaching this course and the rest of one's courses in pharmacy school. To master this process, it is recommended that one should read, think, and talk about the entire series on Transitions in Pharmacy Practice, and create, track, and evaluate a personal developmental plan. The model below is outlined, with definitions, examples, and strategies.

The model incorporated, among other evidence-based developmental theories, Krathwohl's et al. hierarchical model of attitude and value change,[32] based upon intrinsic or internal motivation and not external motivation, and Prochaska's developmental plan for changing one's own health behavior.[33] Each of the five stages in the model can be used by individual students and practitioners to develop their own attitudes and behaviors towards their role in the delivery of pharmaceutical care. Our discussion will be based upon the readers helping themselves to change their own values and attitudes towards the delivery of pharmaceutical care.

In the Krathwohl hierarchy, it is assumed that lower levels of the hierarchy must be achieved before advancing to the next level. These levels, supported with descriptions, strategies and examples, are presented in **Table 7.1**. Examples of Krathwohl's levels will be applied to the development of attitude change about provision of pharmaceutical care.

Table 7.1. Krathwohl and Prochaska Developmental Levels of Change[32,33]

Krathwohl Levels	Receiving	Responding	Valuing	Organization	Value Complex
Definition	Receiving and paying attention to information on PC.[a]	Trying out PC behaviors.	Changing perception of worth of PC.	Committing to delivering PC.	PC becomes part of professional identification.
Example	Attending a workshop on PC.	Counseling a patient for 1 minute and thinking about the outcome	Writing about PC from personal experience	Having a plan for education and practice	Delivering PC automatically and naturally.
Strategy	"Recognize a different way of practice, PC inter-lectures, guided discussion, lead by "near peer compare and contrast old ideas with PC, real life examples, principles, not facts, not lecture."[40]	Doing something, even a small step; Receiving feedback and deriving satisfaction; Addressing barriers.	"Arrange to be in places where PC can be practiced successfully" "Talk to other people about your new beliefs."[40]	Engage in discussion and collaboration with co-workers who deliver PC Identify and obtain additional training and other necessary resources.	

Prochaska Stages of Change	Precontemplation	Contemplation	Preparation	Action	Maintenance
Definition	Aware of need to exercise, not ready to do much about it. Not convinced that cost outweigh benefits.	Considering changing within near future. Thinking about change.	Thinking how to change, planning.	Beginning to change.	Aware of possible relapse, but continuing changed behavior.
Strategy	Consciousness raising and inspecting reasons for not exercising.	Seeking information from people and resources	Focus on attitude and plan or how and when to exercise.	Deciding to exercise working in small steps, like exercising for 15 minutes, telling people about my exercise, "own" plan.	Starting to exercise. Structuring the environment to help me exercise, like buying a treadmill. Finding people to exercise with. Having a plan to begin exercising if I stop. Seeing myself as an athlete.

[a] PC = pharmaceutical care.

Examples of the Prochaska stages of change will be applied to the development of stages in beginning to exercise, maintaining appropriate weight, and reducing stress. The second example is given as something that may be familiar as a common health problem and can help one understand how to apply similar change strategies to implementation of pharmaceutical care.

In the first stage of the Krathwohl hierarchy, one would receive information about pharmaceutical care, possibly through a workshop. It is important that the workshop be interactive, as learning occurs when you think about what you are learning and relate it to what you already know. Kolb[34] described learning as involving the receipt of information, thinking about it, forming a hypothesis, testing the hypothesis, and relating the outcome to what is already known. Learning about pharmaceutical care requires thinking about it and testing ideas about it, not memorizing Hepler and Strand's definition. At this stage of attitude change, one needs to discuss pharmaceutical care ideas with peers who have more positive attitudes, as well as with experts. One needs to see living examples of pharmaceutical care. In the responding stage, one should try out a pharmaceutical care function, get some feedback from one's actions, and think about what happened. In this stage, it is also important to address barriers to pharmaceutical care, such as the forces discussed in the first part of this chapter, and find ways to overcome them. These forces were

- economic factors,
- the "knowing versus doing" dilemma,
- autonomy versus organizational restraints,
- personality versus practice setting/environment,
- the "business versus professional" dilemma (marginality),
- boundary maintenance,
- people, and
- corporatization and managed care.

One should not get stuck at this step but be flexible and see occurrences of phenomena on a continuum, not as a dichotomy (i.e., you can either deliver pharmaceutical care or you cannot; there is no in-between stage). There are many in-between stages, and when making changes, one often progresses systematically. In the valuing stage, it may be useful for one to write or speak about thoughts, feelings, beliefs, and behaviors regarding pharmaceutical care. "We write to find out what we know and what we want to say . . . writing . . . clarified half-formed ideas."[35] One can write to learn about attitudes and values. In the organization stage, one begins to commit to the delivery of pharmaceutical care by having a plan for getting the resources needed and a plan for beginning to change. In the last stage, value complex, one sees him- or herself as a pharmaceutical care professional, naturally and automatically delivering pharmaceutical care.

The Prochaska stages of change were developed from an analysis and synthesis of existing models of change, as in therapy, and from interviewing people who were successful in changing their own attitudes, beliefs, values, and behavior. These stages are presented below using an exercise program as the example. The same stages would apply to beginning to change one's attitudes, beliefs, value, and behavior about pharmaceutical care.

The first stage is called precontemplation. At this stage, there is an awareness of the need to exercise, but one has not really thought of doing it. Information on exercise may be sought. This stage is like the first stage in the Krathwohl series: receiving. In the second stage, contemplation, one considers changing and begins to think about how to do it. In the preparation stage, one actually plans a strategy, tries out pieces of it, and often tells people that he or she is beginning to exercise. Making change public is very important, because it indicates a "buy in" to the change. In the action stage, one is engaged fully in the change, changing the environment to support change, perhaps joining a gym. In the fifth stage, maintenance, one sees him- or herself as an athlete, or at least as a person who exercises and has plans for continuing the new behavior if there is a potential to become derailed by one's environment or self.

While there is not a one-to-one correspondence between Prochaska's and Krathwohl's models, they parallel each other in that they show change as development from thinking to doing and receiving feedback, to attitude change (as a function of behavior), to believing and valuing, to commitment to new behaviors, and finally to seeing oneself differently.

Summary

Societal impediments to professionalism in pharmacy were described and explained, as well as common deleterious emotional and behavioral responses of professionals and future professionals to conflict and change. This was followed with a description of directives towards reprofessionalization, in pharmacy and other professions, primarily through an increased emphasis upon meeting client needs. Finally, the Nimmo and Holland practice change model was described and examples were provided. The model is a developmental system of professional socialization for practitioners and pharmacy students that showed how attitudes towards practice could change through behavioral change.

What all this means is that pharmacy students, given a supportive work environment with educational resources, can be the change agents that reprofessionalize pharmacy towards the delivery of pharmaceutical care.

References

1. Zacker C, Mucha L. Institutional and contingency approaches to the reprofessionalization in pharmacy. *Am J Health-Syst Pharm.* 1998; 55:1302–5.
2. Richey FJ, Sommers DG. Medical rationalization and professional boundary maintenance: physicians and clinical pharmacists research in the sociology of health care. *Resr Soc Hlth Care.*1998; 10:117–39.
3. Hepler CD. The third wave in pharmaceutical education and the clinical movement. *Am J Pharm Ed.* 1987; 51:369–85.
4. Hepler CD, Strand LM. Opportunities and responsibilities in pharmaceutical care. *Am J Pharm Ed.* 1990; 53(winter suppl): 75–155.
5. Birenbaum A. Reprofessionalization in pharmacy. *Soc Sci Med.* 1982; 16:871–8.
6. Ukens C. Up, up, and away. *Drug-Top 2001.* 2001; 145:25–35.
7. Brodie DD, Parish PA, Poston JW. Decisions pharmacists make. *Am J Pharm Educ.* 1980; 44:40–3.

8. Weiss MC, Scott D. Clinical decision making-application of judgment analysis and its potential for pharmacy. *Int J Pharm Pract.* 2000; 8:33–41.

9. McCrae RR, Costa PT. Personality in adulthood. New York: Guilford Press; 1990.

10. Thorner I. Pharmacy: the functional significance of an institutional pattern. *Soc Forces.* 1942; 20:321–8.

11. Seabury GJ. Shall pharmacists become tradesman? New York: George J. Seabury; 1989.

12. Cipolle RJ, Strand LM, Morley PC. Pharmaceutical care practice. New York: McGraw-Hill, 1998.

13. Montgomery K. Professional dominance and the threat of corporatization. Current Research on Occupations and Professions, 1992; 52:1763–70.

14. Pierpaoli PG. An iconoclastic perspective on progress in pharmacy practice. *Am J Health-Syst Pharm.* 1995; 52:1763-70.

15. Kennedy JF.

16. Emener WG, Rocco Cottone RR. Professionalization, deprofessionalization, and reprofessionalization of rehabilitation counseling according to criteria of professions. *J Couns Dev.* 1989; 67:576–81.

17. Gosselin RA, Robbins J. Inside pharmacy. The anatomy of a profession. Lancaster, PA: Technomic; 1999.

18. Shuval JT. The pharmacist. In: Pharmacy practice. 2nd ed. Wertheimer AI, Smith MC, eds. Baltimore: University Park Press; 1981.

19. Higby GJ. From compounding to caring: an abridged history of American pharmacy. In: Pharmacy practice. 2nd ed. Wertheimer AI, Smith MC, eds. Baltimore: University Park Press; 1981.

20. Food and Drug Administration (September 12, 1980). Title 21-Food and Drug. Federal Register, 45 (171) 60754–60817.

21. Penna R. Pharmaceutical care: pharmacy's mission for the 1990s. *Am J Hosp Pharm.* 1990; 47:543–9.

22. Rogers EM. Diffusion of innovations. 4th ed. New York: Free Press; 1995.

23. The changing face of pharmaceutical education: the management of change. AACP/ICI Pharmaceuticals Group Symposium. Washington, DC: February 28–March 2, 1991.

24. AACP/ICI: 4.

25. Holland RW, Nimmo CM. Transitions, part 1: beyond pharmaceutical care. *Am J Health-Syst Pharm.* 1999; 56:1758–4.

26. Nimmo CM, Holland RW. Transitions in pharmacy practice, part 2: who does what and why. *Am J Health-Syst Pharm.* 1999; 56:1981–7.

27. Holland RW, Nimmo CM. Transitions in pharmacy practice, part 3: effecting change—the three-ring circus. *Am J Health-Syst Pharm.* 1999; 56:2235–41.

28. Lonie JM, Dolinsky D, Thakkar B. Counseling patients with low health literacy: an education intervention. *J Manage Pharm Care.* In press.

29. Nimmo CM, Holland RW. Transitions in pharmacy practice, part 4: can a leopard change its spots? *Am J Health-Syst Pharm.* 1999; 56:2458–62.

30. Zimbardo P, Gerrig R. Psychology and life. 14th ed. New York: HarperCollins College Publishers; 1996.

31. Nimmo CM, Holland RW. Transitions in pharmacy practice, part 5: walking the tightrope of change. *Am J Health-Syst Pharm.* 2000; 57:64–72.

32. Krathwohl DR, Bloom BS, Masia BB. Taxonomy of educational objectives; the classification of educational goals, handbook II: affective domain. White Plains, NY: Longman; 1964.

33. Prochaska JO, Norcross JC, DiClimente CC. Changing for good. New York: Avon Books; 1994.

34. Kolb DA. Experiential learning: experience as the source of learning and development. Englewood Cliffs, NJ: Prentice Hall; 1984.

35. Zissner W. Writing to learn. New York: Harper and Row; 1988.

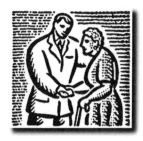

Chapter 8: Public Policy Impact on Pharmaceutical Care

Susan C. Winckler, R.Ph., J.D.

Impact of Public Policy: Regulator and Payor

Perhaps more than any other industry, public policy has a significant effect on health care, including pharmaceutical care, stemming from two primary roles of the government: as a regulator of the profession and as a payor of services. Pharmacy is a regulated health profession. Health care providers are regulated to protect the public's health, safety, and welfare—to establish standards that protect consumers from incompetent practitioners.[1] Regulation typically involves issuance of a license and accompanying authorization to engage in a defined scope of activity. Such license procedures, administered by authorities competent to judge licensure requirements, provide consumers an assurance that certain qualifications have been met.[2]

Regulation of the pharmacy profession creates a "can" versus "cannot" situation: if the state practice act[a] does not allow pharmacist administration of medications, pursuing such activity subjects the practitioner to claims of malpractice and licensure sanctions. This chapter will discuss the impact of regulation—when regulation facilitates pharmaceutical care and when it creates barriers—and will evaluate both federal and state regulations.

The impact of public policy on the government's role as a payor of pharmaceutical care is also significant. A common lament of pharmacists is that they are not recognized as "providers" under the Social Security Act.[3] As such, the Centers for Medicare and Medicaid Services (CMS), the administrator for the Medicare program, is not required to pay for pharmacist services, including pharmaceutical care.[b] This limitation does not, however, mean that pharmacists are not health care providers or are somehow prohibited from performing certain functions—what a pharmacist can or cannot do is a function of law and regulations of practice, not payor policy. Whether or not a service is paid by third parties is important, however, in determining what happens in pharmacy practice. If payment for a service is denied or limited, adoption and expansion of that service is often limited.[4] As noted by a committee of the Institute of Medicine, "Even among health professionals motivated to provide the best care possible, the structure of payment incentives may not facilitate the actions needed to systematically improve the quality of care, and may even prevent such actions." This chapter will discuss the impact of federal and state payor policy and the opportunities and barriers created for pharmaceutical care.

The Regulatory Role

Regulations can limit a pharmacist's ability to provide pharmaceutical care, and many regulations at both the state and federal level must be considered when discussing pharmacy practice. At the same time, misperceptions of those regulations can be just as paralyzing—a pharmacist who believes that certain activities are prohibited will not perform such functions, regardless of the actual content of the practice act and regulations.

The primary regulator of pharmacy practice is the state board of pharmacy, which is responsible for implementing the state pharmacy practice act.[5] The state pharmacy practice act outlines the regulation of the practice of pharmacy, including the licensure of pharmacists; the registration of pharmacy technicians; and the licensure of all sites or persons that distribute, manufacture, or sell drugs.[6] Federal regulations are also important, but unfortunately are not contained in one primary source of authorizing legislation. The impact of various federal regulations will be discussed later in this chapter.

Incorporation of pharmaceutical care into state practice acts and regulations varies widely. When interpreting a pharmacist's scope of practice, some state regulators appear to operate from the position that a state practice act or regulation must refer to the specific phrase "pharmaceutical care" to authorize performance of specific functions. Other state regulators seem to prefer the articulation of all activities encompassed in providing pharmaceutical care, and may not even mention pharmaceutical care.[7] For example, "The Iowa Pharmacy Practice Act does not contain the phrase 'pharmaceutical care,' but authorizes a wide range of activities including performing skin punctures for patient training, measuring blood pressure, and administration of adult immunizations. At least 20 states include the phrase "pharmaceutical care" in the practice act or regulations (see **Table 8.1**).[8] The effect of that phrase varies widely, however, ranging from merely referring to pharmaceutical care as a component of pharmacy practice[9] to articulating the components of pharmaceutical care required of nuclear pharmacists.[10]

Table 8.1. State Pharmacy Practice Act or Regulations Including the Phrase "Pharmaceutical Care"

Connecticut	New Mexico
Florida	North Carolina
Guam	North Dakota
Illinois	Oregon
Indiana	Rhode Island
Louisiana	South Dakota
Maryland	Tennessee
Minnesota	Texas
Mississippi	West Virginia
Nebraska	Wyoming
Nevada	

It is important for pharmacists to understand the philosophy of their state board and the scope of authorized practice. Without understanding this orientation, pharmacists may perceive a more limited scope of practice than truly exists, believing that they are prohibited from a certain activity because it has not been a component of their traditional practice, or because a specific phrase does not appear in the governing act or regulations. When in doubt, requesting an opinion from the state regulator (e.g., the state board of pharmacy) about a specific practice may clarify any question about performing specific functions and improve compliance with requirements for conducting such functions.

Many states follow the guidance provided by the National Association of Boards of Pharmacy (NABP) when advancing changes or interpreting existing authority. These recommendations are encompassed in the Model State Pharmacy Act and Model Rules of the NABP. Within the Model Act, pharmaceutical care is defined as "the provision of drug therapy and other patient care services intended to achieve outcomes related to the cure or prevention of a disease, elimination or reduction of a patient's symptoms, or arresting or slowing of a disease process as defined in the rules of the board."[11]

Inclusion of such broad language in a state pharmacy practice act could authorize a wide-ranging scope of activities required to complete this responsibility. This approach is common in medical practice acts, where nearly all health care services are included within the practice scope. Accompanying regulations are often very broad and authorize all activity required to carry out that responsibility.[12] In contrast, most pharmacy practice acts are more narrowly drawn and specifically articulate the approved activities and the conditions under which such activities may be performed. This limits the services within the pharmacist's scope of practice to an articulated inventory that only allows for performing certain monitoring tests, such as taking blood pressure, performing drug utilization review activities, etc. In Texas, for example, authorized pharmaceutical care activities are specified to include services that "shall" be provided and those that "may" be provided (see Table 8.2).[13] In this structure, a minimum standard for such practice is established: if a pharmacist chooses to provide "pharmaceutical care," that activity must involve certain functions—the "shall" requirements. Importantly, though, the "may" activities expand the authorized activities and authorize additional pharmacist activity under the rubric of pharmaceutical care.

Table 8.2. Texas—Core Definition of Pharmaceutical Care Services

Pharmaceutical care services. *(The "shall" pharmaceutical care services.)*

A. Drug regimen review.

(i) For the purpose of promoting therapeutic appropriateness, a pharmacist shall at the time of dispensing a prescription drug order, review the patient's medication record. Such review shall at a minimum identify clinically significant:

    (I)   known allergies;

    (II)   rational therapy–contraindications;

    (III)   reasonable dose and route of administration;

    (IV)   reasonable directions for use;

    (V)   duplication of therapy;

    (VI)   drug–drug interactions;

    (VII)   drug–food interactions;

(VIII)   drug–disease interactions;

(IX)   adverse drug reactions; and

(X)   proper utilization, including overutilization or underutilization.

(ii) Upon identifying any clinically significant conditions, situations, or items listed in clause (i)of this subparagraph, the pharmacist shall take appropriate steps to avoid or resolve the problem including consultation with the prescribing practitioner. The pharmacist shall document such occurrences.

Authorized Pharmaceutical Care Services *(The "may" pharmaceutical care services.)*

B. Other pharmaceutical care services which may be provided by pharmacists include, but are not limited to, the following:

(i) managing drug therapy as delegated by a practitioner as allowed under the provisions of the Medical Practices;

(ii) administering immunizations and vaccinations under written protocol of a physician;

(iii) managing patient compliance programs;

(iv) providing preventative health care services; and

(v) providing case management of patients who are being treated with high-risk or high-cost drugs, or who are considered "high risk" due to their age, medical condition, family history, or related concern.

Ensuring compliance with state practice acts and regulations is vital. Failure to comply with these requirements can result in suspension, revocation, denial, or refusal to renew a license.[c] Boards may also establish probationary periods, censure or reprimand a licentiate, and assess fines or civil penalties.[14]

The Pharmacist and the Pharmacy

Unique to pharmacy is the regulation of the profession at two levels: the pharmacist (the professional) and the pharmacy (the place of practice).[d] This creates a more complex regulatory structure than that of most other health care professions. (By contrast, physicians are licensed to practice medicine, but their primary place of practice—the physician's office—is not.)[15] This dual system of regulation can create challenges for implementing pharmaceutical care, particularly when the pharmacist and pharmacy are regulated by separate state boards.

In the District of Columbia, for example, the board of pharmacy implements the portions of the pharmacy practice act relevant to pharmacist licensure and practice. Oversight of the pharmacy is managed by a separate process: pharmacy licenses are issued by the Mayor.[16] This structure can be cumbersome, particularly when determining where a proposed change in the practice act would be implemented and overseen.

Regulation of the pharmacist and the practice facility can create further complexities. For example, the authority to adjust drug therapy regimens according to a protocol with a prescriber (a practice often called collaborative drug therapy management [CDTM]) is important to the provision of pharmaceutical care. Although 38 states authorize collaborative drug therapy management in some way, a few limit the practice to pharmacists who work in specific settings. Until a statutory amendment passed in 2002, pharmacists in Hawaii may adjust the dosage of a patient's drug regimen pursuant to a physician's only if they practice in a licensed acute care hospital.[17] Should the same pharmacist leave practice in the hospital to work with patients in a community setting, their scope of practice would contract with that change in work site.

Although it may be arguable that the dual regulation of the profession is responsible for this limitation based on place of practice, it is a plausible explanation. With different requirements for various practice settings, a perception of enhanced prescriber oversight in one practice setting over another may exist. In evaluating the provision of such services, then, the professional must evaluate not only the personnel requirements but also the requirements and, potentially, limitations for the practice setting.

Another important component of pharmaceutical care is ongoing monitoring and management of drug therapy; various laboratory tests are vital to this monitoring activity. Having the authority to conduct such testing can be helpful to advance pharmaceutical care. Whether or not these laboratory tests can be conducted depends on the authority of the pharmacist and requirements for facilities where such tests may be conducted.

In North Dakota, a pharmacist can conduct a blood glucose monitoring test after completing a board-approved continuing-education program,[18] but that authority can only be exercised in an appropriate environment. If that environment is a pharmacy, the pharmacy must have a proper registration, meet Clinical Laboratory Improvements Act requirements,[e] and must notify the board of pharmacy that such a certificate has been obtained. If the pharmacist is conducting these tests in a facility other than a pharmacy—a facility not licensed by the board of pharmacy—one might assume that no additional requirements existed. Nonetheless, the board extends oversight to the non-pharmacy facility through the pharmacist license. In this situation, the pharmacist must notify the board that such a certificate has been obtained for the nonpharmacy facility. Notifications must be made before conducting any tests, specifying the types of tests to be performed.[19] Requirements for the facility, in addition to the involved professional, do not always constitute barriers to pharmaceutical care, but must be considered in providing services.

Other State Regulators

In addition to the board of pharmacy, other state regulators affect the implementation of pharmaceutical care. As pharmacists expand their practice beyond core dispensing activities, those activities are sometimes subject to oversight from other entities, such as state health departments, and occasionally, regulators of other professions, such as the board of medicine or nursing.

Some state health departments have the authority to inspect certain facilities, including pharmacies.[f] Pharmacists may be required to report certain activities to health departments. For example, pharmacists who administer immunizations in Nevada must notify, among others, a county health department and state regulators.[20] In other states such as Iowa, state health departments are involved in the initial licensing of pharmacies; detailed floor plans for a nuclear pharmacy must be submitted to the board of pharmacy examiners and the state health department before a license for the facility can be approved.[21]

Requirements to report to state health departments may increase as the threat of bioterrorism increases. A model law addressing bioterrorism would require pharmacists to serve as an early warning system, reporting specific symptoms or the sale of certain medications.[22] Under the proposal, pharmacists would be required to report to the state public health authority (within 24 hours) "any unusual or increased prescription rates, unusual types of prescription, or unusual trends in pharmacy visits that may be caused by bioterrorism, epidemic or pandemic disease, or novel and highly fatal infectious agents or biological toxins." This reporting, in itself, may not affect the provision of pharmaceutical care, but will constitute another layer of administrative requirements.

While these regulations often create additional hurdles to implement pharmaceutical care, occasionally, other state regulators also provide mechanisms to advance the adoption of pharmaceutical care. In North Carolina, for example, the expansion of the pharmacist's scope of practice to allow collaborative drug therapy management[g] by clinical pharmacist practitioners is part of the medical practice act.[23] The medical practice act confirms that CDTM, when performed within certain parameters,[h] is not the practice of medicine and thus may be performed by pharmacists. The pharmacy practice act has limited language relating to the clinical pharmacist practitioner (CPP): a definition of the CPP as "a licensed pharmacist who meets the guidelines and criteria for such title established by the joint subcommittee of the North Carolina Medical Board and the North Carolina Board of Pharmacy and is authorized to enter into drug therapy management agreements with physicians in accordance with the provisions of . . . [the medical practice act]."[24]

Federal Law and Impact on Pharmaceutical Care

The regulation of pharmacy practice and subsequent impact on pharmaceutical care from the Federal level comes from more diverse sources than at the state level, including the Food and Drug Administration through the Federal Food, Drug and Cosmetic Act; CMS through the Clinical Laboratory Improvement Amendments of 1988; the Occupational Safety and Health Administration (OSHA) from the Occupational Safety and Health Act; and the Drug Enforcement Administration (DEA) through the Controlled Substances Act. In 2003, the Department of Health and Human Services Office of Civil Rights will be responsible for implementing the patient privacy provisions of the Health Insurance Portability and Accountability Act and will also impact pharmacy practice.

FDA's impact on pharmaceutical care is most drastic when the agency prohibits pharmacists from dispensing certain drug products, erecting barriers to pharmaceutical care activities with those patients. While the provision of pharmaceutical care does not require concurrent provision of the medication itself, actions by FDA to preclude pharmacist involvement with specific products disrupts the pharmacist's role.

FDA occasionally imposes restricted distribution as a condition of approving use and marketing of a drug product in the United States.[i] In December 1999, FDA granted marketing approval for Tikosyn (dofetilide) to treat atrial fibrillation and limited the distribution to "those hospitals and other appropriate institutions confirmed to have received applicable dosing and treatment initiation education programs."[25] Distribution limitations were required because the product may induce a different type of irregular heartbeat in attempting to control atrial fibrillation, thus treatment may be initiated only in a hospital setting where such effects are closely monitored and corrected.[26]

In practice, however, Tikosyn is available for inpatient use only at hospitals choosing to comply with education and training requirements. For outpatient dispensing (providing product for patient use upon release from the hospital), this drug is available from only one mail-service facility.[27] It is unclear in this situation if FDA explicitly required the manufacturer to limit non-hospital dispensing to one pharmacy. The FDA-approved labeling requires distribution to hospitals "and other appropriate institutions"[28] to ensure compliance with efforts to limit drug-induced arrhythmia, but the manufacturer's implementation plan limits dispensing to one pharmacy to "facilitate this process."[29] At the least, it appears that FDA approved this extreme distribution restriction.

Such restrictions disrupt the provision of pharmaceutical care. Disrupting access to medication therapy and monitoring for drug interactions can result in negative patient outcomes. Some medications impact the safety and/or effectiveness of other medications and should not be used concurrently. For example, the use of erythromycin with the non-sedating antihistamine Seldane (terfenadine) occasionally resulted in severe cardiac arrythmias.[30] By moving one component of a patient's drug therapy to a different pharmacy or other dispenser, the ability to check for interactions at the primary pharmacy of record is substantially limited. Requiring the patient to use more than one pharmacy because one medication is available only from another distributor disrupts this system and requires the patient to inform both providers of pharmacy services about full medication therapy. A pharmaceutical care provider must access both sets of medication records. This can be difficult and creates risks for patients.

When pharmaceutical care involves laboratory testing or administration of certain medications, three federal agencies become involved. CMS, in collaboration with FDA and CDC, oversee the implementation of the requirements within the Clinical Laboratory Improvements Amendments (CLIA) of 1988. When pharmacists choose to provide onsite laboratory testing, a number of federal and state laws apply to that practice. The state practice act must be reviewed to ensure conducting such tests is within the scope of practice, then any testing must be conducted in compliance with CLIA and applicable requirements of OSHA. (Additionally, CLIA and OSHA permit states to establish stricter requirements taking precedence over federal standards.[j])

CLIA was intended to improve the quality of laboratory practice and protect patients by ensuring that lab equipment functions as intended.[31] Most pharmacists will provide "waived" laboratory testing services, working with tests often designed for use by patients at home.[32] To establish a waived laboratory, a pharmacist must apply for a CLIA certificate of waiver and comply with requirements for good laboratory practice and personnel.[33] Meeting these requirements is not particularly challenging, and pharmacists in more than 40 states are securing this certification.[34]

Applicable OSHA requirements include the Bloodborne Pathogens Standard[35] and the Occupational Exposure to Hazardous Chemicals in the Laboratory.[36] These regulations focus on ensuring workplace safety and that the pharmacy personnel understand how to work with blood products and chemicals in the laboratory, including how to minimize exposure. With these requirements, all personnel involved with the practice should be familiar with and follow the plans. These regulations provide guidance for the implementation of certain pharmaceutical care activities.

The Drug Enforcement Administration's effect on the practice of pharmaceutical care emanates from enforcement of the Controlled Substances Act.[37] The federal regulations for controlled substances, in combination with controlled substance regulation at the state level, monitor the movement of controlled substances from manufacturer to patient. The structure is intended to ensure that controlled substances are available for legitimate medical purposes and are not used for illicit reasons.[k] Pharmacists ensure that controlled substances are dispensed for a legitimate medical purpose, or risk prosecution along with the prescriber. This is a felony offense and may result in the loss of one's pharmacy registration or professional license.[38]

Most controlled substance regulation involves tracking and reporting the movement of controlled substances. In some states, copies of controlled substance prescriptions are filed with the state, in others, records of dispensing are filed in electronic databases.[39] These programs have an immediate impact on the prescribing practices of physicians, substantially reducing the prescribing of schedule II medications.[40] For example, a Texas study showed that after a triplicate prescription program began in 1982, prescriptions for schedule II narcotics decreased, but prescriptions for pain medications that were not subject to additional regulatory oversight increased.[41]

Such oversight also affects pharmacist's willingness to stock such products in their pharmacies,[42] and potentially their willingness to recommend sufficient dose amounts to support pain management. In a randomly selected sample of 30 percent of New York City pharmacies, 51 percent did not have sufficient supplies of opioids to treat patients with severe pain. Only 25 percent of pharmacies in predominantly nonwhite neighborhoods had opioid supplies that were sufficient to treat patients in severe pain, as compared with 72 percent of pharmacies in predominantly white neighborhoods. Primary reasons cited for not stocking such products were lack of demand, fear of theft, and regulatory burden.

The "chilling effect" of controlled substance regulation—decreasing the prescribing and dispensing of these products because of fear of regulatory oversight—is an example of the effect the perceptions of regulation can have on pharmaceutical care. While the number of actions by the DEA against health care providers is moderate, practitioners' fear of the potential for such oversight is significant, and it affects their practice.[l] Pharmacist fears are compounded by the ramifications against the pharmacy facility. The pharmacy is the registrant with the DEA,[43] so action against that registration would preclude pharmacies from stocking controlled substances, a significant problem for the practice. These fears affect pharmacists' provision of pharmaceutical care: a tendency to shy away from use of controlled substances may negatively impact pain management and the pharmacist's role in optimizing medication use.[44] In a survey of Wisconsin pharmacists about knowledge of and attitudes toward opioid pain medications in relation to federal and state policies, most respondents were knowledgeable about the issues. There were, however, important exceptions. Not all pharmacists knew what constitutes legitimate dispensing practices for controlled substances under federal or state policy in emergencies or for patients with terminal illnesses. Many respondents did not view the chronic prescribing/dispensing of opioids for more than several months to patients with chronic pain of malignant or nonmalignant origin as a lawful and acceptable medical practice; this was especially true when the patient had a history of opioid abuse. The authors concluded that the incorrect knowledge and inappropriate attitudes of some pharmacists could contribute to a failure to dispense valid prescriptions for opioid analgesics to patients in pain.

In 2003, another federal regulatory agency will become involved in pharmacy practice and affect the implementation and provision of pharmaceutical care. The Health Insurance Portability and Accountability Act (HIPAA) established guidelines for health insurance and included a section on administrative simplification to promote the use of electronic health insurance billing systems and decrease the complexity of those systems.[45] With the encouraged expansion of electronic billing systems, Congress also included a provision requiring the development of standards to protect the privacy of health information.[46] These standards must be implemented by health care providers, including pharmacists, in 2003, and compliance will be enforced by the U.S. Department of Health and Human Services Office of Civil Rights.[47]

The effect of the privacy regulations on pharmaceutical care could be dramatic. As issued in December 2000, the regulations require pharmacists to secure consent from patients before using their protected health information[m] for treatment, payment, or health care operations.[48] (Substantial revisions to the consent requirement were proposed by the Bush Administration in 2002. Whether or not these changes would be incorporated in the regulation was not resolved by the time this book was published.) Securing this consent, and providing the patient with a notice of the pharmacist's privacy practices will become a requirement for pharmacists engaged in any pharmacy practice, including the provision of pharmaceutical care. But an accurate and complete description of this activity for the patient may be positive and may help patients better understand how pharmacists use their information to provide pharmaceutical care. Pharmacists will need to accurately describe their use of protected health information when they secure the patient's consent.[n] A poorly crafted consent could preclude pharmacists from providing pharmaceutical care, because they do not have the patient's approval to use his or her health information in that manner.[49]

Another component of the HIPAA privacy regulations requires pharmacists and other health care providers to limit the amount of protected health information disclosed when submitting bills for payment or conducting health care operations.[49] Required to use the minimum amount of information necessary to accomplish these activities, these requirements will change most current billing practices. An important exception to the minimum necessary requirement, however, is treatment. When providing treatment, pharmacists and other health care providers do not have to worry about establishing a threshold limiting the amount of information shared—important for the communication among pharmacists and prescribers integral to pharmaceutical care.

Another policy issue affecting pharmaceutical care is any expansion of liability when implementing these services. Generally, however, this is an unfounded concern. Although performing additional services does carry additional liability, most professional liability policies cover activities encompassed within the pharmacist's scope of practice.[50] For example, a description of professional liability coverage notes "Pharmacy is a rapidly changing profession which goes beyond the traditional dispensing function into areas of patient consultation, drug product selection, and patient profiles. The pharmacist of today is a dispenser of drug information as well as drug products. These new and challenging areas of practice bring a proportional increase in professional liability exposure. Our professional policy meets the needs of today's pharmacists." Liability coverage does not equate, however, with protection from litigation. In a malpractice action, the plaintiff must show that (1) the pharmacist owed a duty of reasonable care in providing treatment to the patient, (2) breached his duty by failing to exercise reasonable care, (3) proximately caused the patient's injury because of the breach of duty, and (4) the plaintiff suffered damages as a result of the pharmacist's negligence.[51] The threshold issue in malpractice litigation is establishing the standard of care. Courts in health professional malpractice actions have delegated this task to the affected medical profession and hold health professionals responsible for adhering to customary practices of the profession.[52]

While courts have universally held that a physician owes a rather broad legal duty of care to his patient,[53] the same is not true for pharmacists in providing pharmaceutical care.[54] Pharmacists have been seen to meet their legal duty by "properly filling legal prescriptions that contain no apparent discrepancies on their face."[55] This activity is far short of working with patients to ensure appropriate medication use. But a trend to hold pharmacists legally responsible for more than accurate dispensing—and closer to responsible to providing pharmaceutical care—is emerging in the courts. In 1999, the Missouri Court of Appeals held that pharmacists have a duty to do more than accurately fill prescriptions.[56] Specifically, the court held that the pharmacist's duty may extend to protecting patients "from risks which pharmacists can reasonably foresee."[57]

Should this legal duty expand even further into a duty to perform pharmaceutical care, the competent, conscientious pharmacist should not be deterred from providing this service. In such a situation, pharmacists would be required to meet the customary standard of a "reasonable pharmacist" providing pharmaceutical care. Exercising sufficient care and ensuring compliance with state practice acts and regulations and federal requirements would be a significant step towards meeting that duty.

Pharmacy practice regulation affects the provision of pharmaceutical care, but familiarity with applicable requirements and diligence in tracking changes to those requirements minimizes the disruption. As pharmaceutical care becomes more widespread and recognition of pharmacist contributions to medication use increase, some limitations on practice setting may be removed. Any pharmaceutical care implementation and compliance plan should include an initial evaluation of applicable state and federal requirements, with a periodic assessment for conformity.

The Payor Role

When state and federal governments choose to pay for pharmaceutical care, pharmacists face another challenge: meeting the payors' payment requirements. A now common component of health care are the standards set for third-party payment, such as mandatory second opinions for non-emergency surgery. In pharmacy, such policies include limitations in covered services or in the frequency of providing such services. In the provision of pharmaceutical care, the payor impact is substantial. From restricted networks that limit pharmacist participation in patient care to limits on payable services, payor policy shapes pharmacist activity.

Importantly, however, payor policy (even when the payor is a government program such as Medicare or Medicaid) does not prohibit certain pharmacist activity—it merely limits the availability of third-party payment. Payment denial can limit services, when affected patients are unable to pay for the services themselves. And some payor policies, particularly Medicare, prohibit charging for services that are not covered, requiring the provider to forgo providing such services or provide them at no cost.°

The majority of government involvement in health care in pharmacy is through the Medicaid program, the state–federal partnership that provides health care services to the indigent and disabled.[58] Although an optional component of the Medicaid benefits package, 50 states and the District of Columbia pay for outpatient medications.[59] The majority of these programs pay for medications in a traditional fee-for-service model, with compensation based on an estimate of product cost and a dispensing fee.[60] This compensation structure pays for the dispensed medication, prospective drug utilization review, and an offer to counsel.[61]

In a few states, however, the Medicaid programs have been expanded to include payment for more advanced services by pharmacists. In Wisconsin, pharmacists may secure additional payment for specific services, including, for example, intervening on late refills to improve patient compliance or recommending lower cost medications.[62] In Mississippi, specially trained pharmacists are eligible for disease state management payments.[63] In Iowa, certain pharmacists and collaborating physicians are eligible for case management services when provided to identified at-risk patients.[64]

CMS has outlined the parameters for approving Medicaid plans to pay for additional pharmacist services.[65] CMS will reimburse states for what they call "cognitive" or "disease management" services under the "Other Licensed Practitioners" category of the federal regulations, but will not pay for those services as an add-on to the dispensing fee.[66] To secure CMS payment, the state must amend its Medicaid plan and describe, among other things, the practitioners providing the service, the specific services to be provided, the state law(s) authorizing the provision of such services, training or certification requirements, the unit of service (e.g., 15 minutes), average length of the service envisioned, and procedures for communication with the patient's primary care provider to ensure coordination of care.[67]

In the Medicare program, payments to pharmacists are much more limited. With few exceptions, the Medicare program does not pay for medications used in the outpatient setting.[p] The exclusion of coverage for pharmacist services in the Medicare program is often described as a failure to "recognize pharmacists as providers."[68] The translation of this phrase means that pharmacist services are not included in the Social Security Act's list of Medicare-payable services, and thus CMS is not required to pay pharmacists for their services, including pharmaceutical care. Nothing in current Medicare law, however, would prohibit pharmacists from providing these services to Medicare beneficiaries and charging them cash. (When these services are associated with the few medications covered under Medicare, limits on service charges exist.)

Pharmacists are eligible for payment from Medicare for a few discrete services, if quality parameters are met. Specifically, pharmacists may secure payment for administering immunizations[69] and, with the appropriate program, a pharmacy may secure payment for providing diabetes self-management education services.[70]

The Medicare program pays for a few medications directly, primarily those associated with hospice care, those required by transplant patients, chemotherapy regimens, and medications used in conjunction with durable medical equipment.[q] "The term "hospice care" means the following items and services provided to a terminally ill individual by, or by others under arrangements made by, a hospice program under a written plan (for providing such care to such individual) established and periodically reviewed by the individual's attending physician… (E) medical supplies (including drugs and biologicals) and the use of medical appliances, while under such a plan…" In hospice care, payor policy affects pharmaceutical care via the limits on available funds: hospice care is funded by a per diem fee and must cover medications and all other services.[71] In many situations, this per diem is insufficient to cover medication costs alone, and must also be used to cover other care as well.[72] "For a patient pain-stabilized with significant amounts of morphine, paying out of pocket for the morphine would cost more than $325 per day. This figure is for the morphine only—and does not include medications for other problems." In this situation, patients are denied access to necessary medications, directly thwarting any efforts to optimize drug use through pharmaceutical care. Similar situations exist in the infusion therapy environment.[73]

Occasionally, payor policy also promotes the use of one product over another, or preference for one delivery mechanism. As noted previously in the outpatient setting, Medicare pays for a limited number of medications, primarily chemotherapy and associated medications and other products delivered through durable medical equipment. Specifically, Medicare Part B covers the cost of supplies necessary for the effective use of durable medical equipment (DME), including drugs and biologicals that require DME for administration. To qualify for coverage, the ordering physician's medical records must contain information that supports the medical necessity for all DME and related supplies. For patients requiring medication for respiratory disorders, this creates a dilemma: albuterol delivered through a metered dose inhaler is not covered by Medicare, but the same medication delivered through a nebulizer is payable.[74] If a patient is unable to afford the medication, the nebulizer treatment will likely be prescribed—even if the MDI delivery would be therapeutically preferable. If the choice is between a sub-standard delivery mode and no medication, the choice is easy.

Revision of the Medicare system to add coverage for outpatient medications is a popular topic among policy makers, and will be essential for improving the delivery of pharmaceutical care to the nation's seniors. A poorly designed program, however, such as the existing system, could pose additional problems. Payor policy does guide care delivery, and the impact of such decisions must be considered in the design of new programs.

Conclusion

The impact of public policy on pharmaceutical care can be substantial, primarily in the breach. If a pharmacist pursues expanding practice without first investigating the applicable statutes and regulations, fines and licensure sanctions may follow. Due diligence in evaluating practice parameters from both federal and state regulators can limit this exposure.

Due diligence in evaluating payment policies of public payors is also important, particularly when explaining services to patients and the opportunity for Medicare or Medicaid payment. While payor policy does not preclude specific activity, it can create barriers for individual patients to access important services.

Endnotes

1. Pew Health Professions Comm'n, *Reforming Health Care Workforce Regulation: Policy Considerations for the 21st Century*, i (December 1995) (Report of the Taskforce on Health Care Workforce Regulation).
2. Dent v. West Virginia, 129 US 114 (1889)
3. "Coalition to Secure Pharmacist Provider Status Patients to Benefit from Pharmacist Services Under Medicare," Press Release of the American College of Clinical Pharmacists, March 6, 2001, http://capwiz.com/accp/issues/alert/?alertid=17378 &type=CO.
4. "Even among health professionals motivated to provide the best care possible, the structure of payment incentives may not facilitate the actions needed to systematically improve the quality of care, and may even prevent such actions." "Aligning Payment Policies with Quality Improvement," *Crossing the Quality Chasm: A New Health System for the 21st Century*, Committee on Quality of Health Care in America, Institute of Medicine, p. 181.
5. "'Board of Pharmacy' or 'Board' means the governmental regulatory body empowered to regulate pharmaceutical practices including granting and disciplining licenses of individuals and companies." The Model State Pharmacy Act and Model Rules of the National Association of Boards of Pharmacy, Article 1 Title, Purpose and Definitions, Section 105, Fall 2000.
6. The Model State Pharmacy Act and Model Rules of the National Association of Boards of Pharmacy, Article 1 Title, Purpose and Definitions, Fall 2000.
7. The Iowa Pharmacy Practice Act does not contain the phrase "pharmaceutical care," but authorizes a wide range of activities including performing skin punctures for patient training, measuring blood pressure, and administration of adult immunizations. Iowa Practice Act Chapter 155A Pharmacy Practice Act.
8. Compiled from NABLAW, National Association of Boards of Pharmacy, Version 3.2A, Spring 2001.
9. "'Pharmaceutical care,' also referred to as 'pharmaceutical services' means the care or services afforded by the licensed pharmacist or licensed pharmacy to the resident that is required by practice standards, laws, regulations, and guidelines." Maryland Board Regulations, Subtitle 34 Board of Pharmacy, Chapter 23 Pharmaceutical Services to Residents in Long Term Care Facilities, .02 Definitions.
10. "The following minimum level of pharmaceutical care services shall be provided whenever a therapeutic prescription drug order is dispensed and, when in the professional judgement of the pharmacist dispensing a diagnostic prescription drug order, the services are necessary to protect the patient s health while striving to produce positive patient outcomes. When it is determined that the following services are necessary, the dispensing pharmacist shall assure that efforts are made to gather the information necessary to properly perform the services…" Texas Board Regulations 22 TAC, Part XV, Chapter 291 Pharmacies, Subchapter C, nuclear pharmacy (class B) § 291.54 Operational Standards.
11. The Model State Pharmacy Act and Model Rules of the National Association of Boards of Pharmacy, Article 1 Title, Purpose and Definitions, Section 105 (rr) Definitions, Fall 2000.

12. Pew Health Professions Comm'n, *Reforming Health Care Workforce Regulation: Policy Considerations for the 21st Century*, 23 (December 1995) (Report of the Taskforce on Health Care Workforce Regulation).

13. (a) The following pharmaceutical care services shall be provided by pharmacists of the pharmacy... (b) Other pharmaceutical care services which may be provided by pharmacists include, but are not limited to,...". Texas Pharmacy Rules, Chapter 291 Pharmacies, Subchapter B Community Pharmacy (Class A), § 291.36.

14. The Model State Pharmacy Act and Model Rules of the National Association of Boards of Pharmacy, Article IV Discipline, Section 402 Grounds, Penalties and Reinstatement, Fall 2000.

15. A Guide to the Essentials of a Modern Medical Practice Act, Ninth Edition, Federation of State Medical Boards of the United States, Inc., April 2000.

16. District of Columbia Pharmacy Practice Act, Section 4 General Prohibitions, 4(d).

17. "Practice of Pharmacy. Definitions." Hawaii Pharmacy Practice Act, Chapter 461: Pharmacists and Pharmacies, 461-1 Definitions.

18. Practice act authorizes the pharmacist to conduct tests approved for in-home use if they complete a Board approved course of study that incorporates principles of general laboratory procedures. ND BReg Chapter 61-04-10 CLIA WAIVED LABORATORY TESTS, ND BReg 61-04-10-02. Education Requirements for pharmacists to perform CLIA waived laboratory tests.

19. ND BReg Chapter 61-04-10 CLIA WAIVED LABORATORY TESTS, ND BReg 61-04-10-05. Notification of the Board of Pharmacy.

20. Nevada State Board of Pharmacy Regulations, Chapter 639, Regulations Regarding the Administration of Immunizations by Pharmacists, Section 7.

21. Iowa Board of Pharmacy Regulations, 657 Iowa Administrative Code, Chapter 16 Nuclear Pharmacy, 16.3 General requirements for pharmacies providing radiopharmaceutical services.

22. The Model State Emergency Health Powers Act, Developed by the Center for Law an the Public's Health at Georgetown and Johns Hopkins Universities, October 2001.

23. North Carolina General Statutes, Chapter 90 Medicine and Allied Occupations, § 90-18(c)(3a), Practicing without license; practicing defined; penalties.

24. North Carolina General Statutes, Chapter 90, Medicine and Allied Occupations, § 85.3 Definitions.

25. Pfizer U.S. Pharmaceuticals, Tikosyn Prescribing Information (1999) at 17.

26. Id. at 1.

27. "Dear Pharmacist" letter from Pfizer Labs, Pharmacy Today, May 2000.

28. Tikosyn Prescribing Information, *supra* note 25, at 17.

29. "Dear Pharmacist" letter from Pfizer Labs, Pharmacy Today, May 2000.

30. Hecht M, *Drug Options Pushed Seldane Off the Shelf*, The times-Picayune, July 31, 1999, at E7.

31. Munroe Rosenthal W, "Pharmacy-Based Laboratory Services: A New Dimension in Pharmacy Practice," The Dynamics of Pharmaceutical Care: Enriching Patient Health, American Pharmaceutical Association, Monograph 13, p. 2.

32. Id.

33. Id., p.3.
34. Id., p.6.
35. Code Of Federal Regulations, Title 29—Labor Subtitle B—Regulations Relating To Labor Chapter Xvii—Occupational Safety And Health Administration, Department Of Labor Part 1910—Occupational Safety And Health Standards Subpart Z—Toxic And Hazardous Substances, § 1910.1030.
36. Code Of Federal Regulations, Title 29—Labor, Subtitle B—Regulations Relating To Labor, Chapter Xvii—Occupational Safety And Health Administration, Department Of Labor, Part 1910—Occupational Safety And Health Standards, Subpart Z—Toxic And Hazardous Substances, § 1910.1450.
37. See Controlled Substances Act, Public Law 91-513, 84 Stat. 1242, codified as 21 U.S.C. § 801 et seq. (1970).
38. Pharmacist's Manual, U.S. Department of Justice Drug Enforcement Administration, Office of Diversion Control, March 2001.
39. Joranson DE, Gilson AM, Ryan KM et al. "States with Prescription Monitoring Programs," Table 1, Achieving Balance in Federal and State Pain Policy: A Guide to Evaluation. The Pain & Policy Studies Group, University of Wisconsin Comprehensive Cancer Center. Madison, Wisconsin, 2000.
40. Cooper JM et al. Prescription Drug Diversion Control and Medical Practice, 268 JAMA 1306, 1307 (1992) (noting same results, and questioning clinical implications for patients); Joranson DE, Federal and State Regulation of Opioids, 5 J. Pain & Symptom MGMT. S12 at S12-23 (discussing results documented from evaluation of programs); Weintraub M et al., Consequences of the 1989 New York State Triplicate Benzodiazepine Prescription Regulations, 266 JAMA 2392, 2392-97 (1991) (noting dramatic decrease in benzodiazepine prescriptions one year after enactment). •
41. Sigler KA et al. Effect of a Triplicate Prescription Law on Prescribing of Schedule II Drugs (60.4% decrease in Schedule II prescriptions in 1,200 bed teaching hospital one year after enactment), 41 Am. J. Hosp. Pharmacy 108, 109-10 (1984).
42. Morrison RS, Wallenstein S et al. "We don't carry that"—failure of pharmacies in predominantly nonwhite neighborhoods to stock opioid analgesics. *New England Journal of Medicine* 342(14):1023.
43. "The Attorney General shall register practitioners (including pharmacies, as distinguished from pharmacists) to dispense, or conduct research with, controlled substances in schedule II, III, IV, or V." 21 U.S.C. § 823(f).
44. Joranson DE, Gilson AM. Pharmacists' Knowledge and Attitudes Toward Opioid Pain Medication in Relation to Federal and State Policies, *J Am Pharm Assoc.* 2001;41:213-20.
45. Health Insurance Portability and Accountability Act of 1996, Public Law 104-191, § 261.
46. Health Insurance Portability and Accountability Act of 1996, Public Law 104-191, § 264(b).
47. Department Of Health and Human Services Office Of The Secretary, Office For Civil Rights; Statement Of Delegation Of Authority, *Federal Register,* Vol. 65, No. 250, December 28, 2000, 82381.

48. Consent for uses or disclosures to carry out treatment, payment, and health care operations. 45 CFR Subtitle A, § 164.506.

49. "Minimum necessary disclosures of protected health information." 45 CFR Subtitle A, § 164.514(d)(3).

50. Description of professional liability coverage, Pharmacist's Mutual, http://www.pharmacistsmutual.com/Web.nsf.

51. Keeton WP et al. Prosser and Keeton on the law of torts § 30, at 164-68 (5th ed. 1984) and Restatement (Second) of Torts § 281 (1965).

52. Keeton WP et al. Prosser and Keeton on the law of torts § 32 at 189, 5th ed. (1984).

53. McCoid AH. The Care Required of Medical Practitioners, 12 Vand. L. Rev. 549, 553-55 (1959).

54. Hornish ML. "Just What the Doctor Ordered—Or Was It?: Missouri Pharmacists' Duty of Care in the 21st Century" 65 Mo L Rev 1075 (Fall 2000).

55. Kampe v. Howard Stark Prof'l Pharmacy, Inc., 841 S.W. 2d 223, 227 (Mo. Ct. App. 1992).

56. Horner v. Spalitto, 1 S.W. 3d 519, 522 (Mo. Ct. App. 1999).

57. Id.

58. "For the purpose of enabling each State…to furnish (1) medical assistance on behalf of families with dependent children and of aged, blind, or disabled individuals, whose income and resources are insufficient to meet the costs of necessary medical services…," 42 U.S.C. 1396 (2001).

59. National Pharmaceutical Council, *Pharmaceutical Benefits under State Medical Assistance Programs*, Section 4: Medicaid and Pharmacy Program Characteristics, December 1998, p.4-17.

60. Id. at 4-43.

61. Id. at 4-32.

62. Hogue M, Whitmore S. *The History of the Wisconsin Medicaid Pharmaceutical Care Project: Part II*, Wisconsin Pharmacist, March/April 1997.

63. Carlson B. "Others Await Promise of Mississippi's Experiment With Pharmaceutical Care," *Managed Care*, March 1999.

64. Iowa Medicaid Pharmaceutical Case Management initiative, http://www.iarx.org.

65. Correspondence from Eugene A. Gasser, Division of Medicaid and State Operations with the Centers for Medicare and Medicaid Services, to Bob Sharpe, Deputy Secretary for Florida Medicaid, October 12, 2001.

66. Id., paragraph 3, 4.

67. Id., paragraph 5.

68. "Coalition to Secure Pharmacist Provider Status Patients to Benefit from Pharmacist Services Under Medicare," Press Release of the American College of Clinical Pharmacists, March 6, 2001, http://capwiz.com/accp/issues/alert/?alertid=17378&type=CO.

69. "How to Bill Medicare for Influenza and Pneumococcal Vaccinations," Centers for Medicare and Medicaid Services, http://www.hcfa.gov/quality/3g8.htm.

70. "Expanded Coverage of Diabetes outpatient Self-Management Training," Program Memorandum Carriers, Transmittal B-01-40, Centers for Medicare and Medicaid Services, http://www.hcfa.gov/pubforms/transmit/B0140.pdf

71. Definitions of Services, Institutions, Etc. for the Medicare Program, 42 USCA § 1395x(dd).

72. Excerpt from Testimony of the American Pharmaceutical Association to the Senate Health, Education, Labor and Pensions Committee on the hearing Regarding Pain Management and End-of-Life Care, October 13, 1999.

73. National Home Infusion Association Definition of Per Diem, developed by the Legislative/Regulatory Committee Approved by the NHIA Board of Directors, June 2001, http://www.nhianet.org/perdiemfinal.htm.

74. In a 2001 study of payments in Region C, 287 claims had insufficient documentation in the suppliers' records or the physicians' medical records to determine whether the prescriber considered the use of a metered dose inhaler prior to prescribing inhalation drugs. *Review of Payments for Inhalation Drugs Make by Region C Durable Medical Equipment Regional Carrier*, Department of Health and Human Services Office of Inspector General, Report A-06-00-00053, October 2001.

Footnotes

[a] The parameters of pharmacy practice regulation vary from State to State. To facilitate discussion, this chapter will use the Model State Pharmacy Act developed by the National Association of Boards of Pharmacy (NABP) as a sample practice act. Specific practice acts will be used to illustrate variation among the States.

[b] Title XVIII and XIX of the Social Security Act establish the parameters of the Medicare program. The Centers for Medicare and Medicaid Services (CMS) implements those parameters.

[c] A portion of the licensing section of the Model State Pharmacy Act notes: "c) The Board may suspend, revoke, deny, or refuse to renew the license of any Person, Pharmacy, or Pharmacy Benefits Manager on any of the following grounds:

(1) The finding by the Board of violations of any Federal, State, or local laws relating to the Practice of Pharmacy, Drug samples, Wholesale or retail Drug or Device Distribution, or Distribution of controlled substances;

(2) Any felony convictions under Federal, State, or local laws;

(3) The furnishing of false or fraudulent material in any application made in connection with Drug or Device Manufacturing or Distribution . . .

[d] A portion of the licensing section of the Model State Pharmacy Act notes: "(a) The following Persons located within this State, and the following Persons located outside this State that provide services to patients within this State, shall be licensed by the Board of Pharmacy and shall annually renew their license with the Board:

(1) Persons engaged in the Practice of Pharmacy;

(2) Persons engaged in the Manufacture, production, sale, or Distribution of Drugs or Devices;

(3) Pharmacies where Drugs or Devices are Dispensed, or Pharmaceutical Care is provided; and

(4) Pharmacy Benefits Managers." The Model State Pharmacy Act and Model Rules of the National Association of Boards of Pharmacy, Article V Licensing of Facilities, Section 501 Licensing, Fall 2000.

[e] Discussion of specific requirements of the CLIA process appears in the discussion of applicable Federal regulations.

[f] Boards of Pharmacy are often organized within the State Department of Health. This discussion is limited to those situations where the State Health Departments exercise authority independent of that delegated to the specific pharmacy regulatory body.

[g] Collaborative drug therapy management is a coordinated approach to care. CDTM authorizes physicians to enter into agreements with pharmacists to jointly manage a patient's drug therapy. Activity includes: Selecting, initiating, modifying, continuing, discontinuing, and monitoring a patient's drug therapy; Ordering, performing, and interpreting medication-related laboratory tests; Assessing patient response to therapy; Counseling and educating a patient on medications; and Administering medication. Alliance for Pharmaceutical Care materials, "Pharmacists Finding Solutions through Collaboration," http://www.aphanet.org/PHARMCARE/AllianceCollaboration.pdf.

[h] "(a) Any pharmacist who is approved under the provisions of G.S. 90-18(c)(3a) to perform medical acts, tasks, and functions may use the title "clinical pharmacist practitioner." Any other person who uses the title in any form or holds himself or herself out to be a clinical pharmacist practitioner or to be so licensed shall be deemed to be in violation of this Article.

(b) Clinical pharmacist practitioners are authorized to implement predetermined drug therapy, which includes diagnosis and product selection by the patient's physician, modify prescribed drug dosages, dosage forms, and dosage schedules, and to order laboratory tests pursuant to a drug therapy management agreement that is physician, pharmacist, patient, and disease specific under the following conditions…" North Carolina General Statutes, Chapter 90 Medicine and Allied Occupations, § 90-18.4. Limitations on clinical pharmacist practitioners.

[i] The legal authority of the FDA to impose such restrictions is a source of continuing debate.

[j] Most states do not have additional regulatory restrictions. The following state regulations impose some requirement beyond the federal threshold: Alabama, Arizona, California, Maine, Maryland, Massachusetts, New Jersey, New York, North Dakota, Oregon, Pennsylvania, Rhode Island, Tennessee, and Nevada. Compilation from Ben Bluml, Senior Director, American Pharmaceutical Association Foundation.

[k] "(1) Many of the drugs included within this title have a useful and legitimate medical purpose and are necessary to maintain the health and general welfare of the American people. (2) The illegal importation, manufacture, distribution, and improper use of controlled substances have a substantial and detrimental effect on the health and general welfare of the American people." 21 U.S.C. § 801.

[l] Controlled substance laws may obstruct good care, due to specific provisions or fear and misunderstanding surrounding legal requirements. "Pain-prescribing laws stand out in this regard and, in the view of the committee, *warrant revisions to minimize discouragement of effective pain management.*" [Emphasis supplied] National Academy of Sciences, Institute of Medicine, 1997. "Approaching Death: Improving Care at the End of Life."

[m] "Protected health information" is individually identifiable health information... that is: (i) Transmitted by electronic media; (ii) Maintained in any medium described in the definition of *electronic media* ...; or (iii) Transmitted or maintained in any other form or medium. 45 CFR Subtitle A, § 164.501 Definitions.

[n] "A consent under this section must be in plain language and: (1) Inform the individual that protected health information may be used and disclosed to carry out treatment, payment, or health care operations; (2) Refer the individual to the notice required by § 164.520 for a more complete description of such uses and disclosures and state that the individual has the right to review the notice prior to signing the consent..." 45 CFR Subtitle A, § 164.506(c).

[o] With enactment of the Benefits Improvement and Protection Act of 2000 (effective after Feb 1, 2001), all drugs and biologicals covered under Medicare Part B must be submitted on an assigned basis regardless of the physician's provider agreement with Medicare.

[p] Medicare Part B includes coverage for medications used in conjunction with durable medical equipment (such as chemotherapy and some inhalation and infusion products) and for immunosuppressive medications for patients with transplants. 42 U.S.C. 1395m.

[q] The only outpatient prescription drugs covered by Medicare are: a) Immunosuppressive for a Medicare covered organ transplant; b) Erythropoetin for the treatment of anemia for persons with chronic renal failure who are on dialysis; c) Oral anticancer agents used in chemotherapy if they have the same ingredients and are used for the same indications as those covered as non-self-administered drugs; d) Hemophilia clotting factors for hemophilia patients who are able to use such factors to control bleeding without medical supervision; e) Injectable osteoporosis drug approved for treatment of post-menopausal osteoporosis; f) Supplies (which include drugs) necessary for the effective use of covered durable medical equipment; g) Hepatitis B vaccine for those beneficiaries at high or intermediate risk of contracting hepatitis B; h) diabetes testing supplies. Definitions of Services, Institutions, Etc. for the Medicare Program, 42 USCA § 1395x.

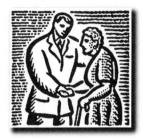

Chapter 9: Outcomes of Drug Therapy

Charles D. Hepler, Ph.D.

Every health profession claims to serve the public interest. People can judge the validity of such claims by considering three interrelated issues: cost, access, and quality. Outcomes directly affect cost and quality of care and indirectly affect accessibility. Therefore, developing and maintaining demand for pharmaceutical care may depend greatly on pharmacists' ability to influence accessibility, cost, or quality of health care.

To most people (and their families), the outcome of care is by far the most important aspect of quality; more important, than, say, the organization and processes of care. Some definitions of quality of care reflect this perspective by including outcomes. For example, according to the Institute of Medicine, quality of care is "the degree to which health services for individuals and populations increase the likelihood of desired health outcomes and are consistent with current professional knowledge."[1] The U.S. Office of Technology Assessment has defined quality health care as "the degree to which the process of care increases the probability of outcomes desired by patients and reduces the probability of undesired outcomes given the current state of knowledge."[2]

Pharmaceutical care is outcome oriented. One definition of pharmaceutical care includes the phrase "definite outcomes intended to improve a patient's quality of life."[3] Hepler and Strand then enumerate four outcomes:

1. cure of a disease,

2. elimination or reduction of a patient's symptomatology,

3. arresting or slowing of a disease process, and

4. preventing a disease or symptomatology.

This chapter will explore patient outcomes from both the clinical and evaluative perspectives: ways to think about outcomes, how patients may experience them, and how professionals may recognize them. Finally, it will describe an approach to the continual improvement of the outcomes of drug therapy.

Outcomes, Outputs, Therapeutic Objectives, and Patient Progress

If a cure, control of symptoms, and retardation or prevention of diseases are outcomes, and if a patient's quality of life is also an outcome, the definition of pharmaceutical care involves patient outcomes on at least two levels of complexity. This may appear to be mainly a problem of terminology. However, vague terminology often conceals real problems with conceptual clarity. In such cases, professional purpose may be blurred and performance reduced.

To begin from a broad perspective, a person's life can be understood as comprising many processes (e.g., working, playing, eating, resting) that occur in one or more structures (e.g., the society within which the person lives, its cultures, institutions, and organizations). In this framework, health care is one group of processes occurring in one group of structures within the larger socioeconomic environments. In health care, as in life, every outcome (e.g., hyperglycemia as an "outcome" of diabetes) seems to give way to another outcome (e.g., renal damage). An outcome is defined in plain English as "the final result of complex or conflicting causes or forces."[4]

Avedis Donabedian[5] has defined an outcome of health care as a change in state or condition attributable to antecedent health care. He includes changes in health status, changes in knowledge or behavior pertinent to future health status, and satisfaction with health care (expressed as opinion or inferred from behavior).

Neither definition is specific enough to help the clinician decide which events in the course of pharmaceutical care should be called outcomes. An outcome is somewhat easier to define in acute diseases than in chronic diseases, because therapy within an acute episode usually has a clear end. Consider, for example, a patient receiving five days of norfloxacin for the treatment of a urinary tract infection (UTI). Cure of the UTI (i.e., no pathogens in urine after the end of therapy) would be an outcome according to both definitions, a change in status which is the *result* of antecedent health care. Remission of symptoms or disappearance of bacteriuria during therapy satisfies Donabedian's definition, but not the common definition, because symptoms and bacteriuria can return if treatment is too short, so such an outcome would not be final in any sense.

Outcomes are harder to define for chronic diseases. Consider for example Mr. A and Mr. B, who have been receiving drug therapy for hypertension for six months. Both have mean diastolic blood pressures of 95. Mr. A is on a diet and exercise program, and his diastolic blood pressure is slowly falling. Mr. B's diastolic blood pressure has been approximately constant for the last three months. Should either person's blood pressure after a certain period of therapy be called an outcome? Shall we say, according to the common definition, that Mr. B's blood pressure is an outcome because it is a stable result, but A's outcome is still in the future because his diastolic blood pressure is still changing? Or, shall we say, according to Donabedian's definition, that Mr. A's blood pressure is an outcome because it has changed since his last visit, but Mr. B.'s is not an outcome because it has not changed? Furthermore, although we may be justified in assuming that drug therapy has lowered both men's blood pressures, how shall we know whether A's still-falling diastolic pressure is a result of health care, as required by Donabedian's definition, or lifestyle?

The processes of health care are indeed complex and conflicting, and they have many outcomes. There are few or no final results of health care as long as the person remains alive. It is much easier to define the output of a specific process, especially for a specific patient, and more useful clinically. Output is an engineering term denoting the immediate result of a process acting on an input. **Figure 9.1** shows a diagram of a generic process in which inputs go through a process and are converted to an output.

For example, consider a patient receiving treatment for a UTI. Three significant inputs to drug therapy are (a) the patient with the symptoms of a UTI, (b) an order for a therapeutic regimen, and (c) a drug product (in this case, nor-floxacin tablets). The output is a patient receiving therapy with norfloxacin. The output of continued therapy is symptom resolution and disappearance of bacteriuria, and the outcome (cure) results from many such outputs and uncontrollable environmental circumstances.

The process view is consistent with an older view of health care as consisting of discrete episodes, e.g., office visits or hospitalizations. **Figure 9.2** is a diagram of a continuous sequence in which each output forms a part of the input to the next set of processes. For simplicity, the diagram shows only one generic process to represent a large variety of specific processes that a patient might go through during care. To continue the UTI example, the output from one visit—a person beginning treatment with norfloxacin—becomes part of the input to the next. The first process might have been diagnostic services by a physician. The second process may be dispensing and advising by a pharmacist. The third process might be a follow-up visit or phone call or a prescription refill.

The outcome of these continuous processes of care would be (a) the patient's health status when care was terminated, e.g., when the UTI was cured or the patient was discharged, or (b) when health status had stabilized. We could speak meaningfully of the outcome of continuing chronic disease management if the outputs of each episode were relatively constant. Otherwise, we should think of them as outputs that can change in response to changes in the processes of care.

Figure 9.3 is a diagram of a pharmaceutical care system as it would illustrate the care of a single patient. This system is a continuous sequence where each output forms part of the input to

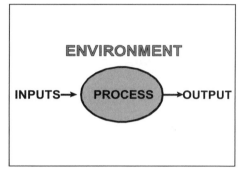

Figure 9.1. Diagram of a Simple Process.

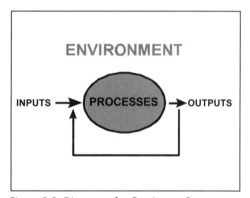

Figure 9.2. Diagram of a Continuous Process.

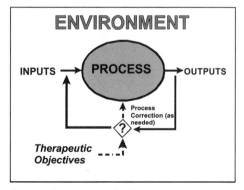

Figure 9.3. Diagram of a System.

the next process. In a system, outputs are evaluated against some standard or expectation, as shown by the diamond-shaped box with a question mark in it. If an output appears satisfactory, no action is taken. If a problem is recognized, action is taken to correct it.

The professional evaluates subjective and objective information—clinical indicators—by comparing them to an independent standard, shown in Figure 9.3 as the therapeutic objective.[a] If the clinical indicators are consistent with desired progress, no action may be taken and another follow-up visit may be scheduled. If therapy has not progressed satisfactorily toward the therapeutic objective, the professional should try (a) to identify the basic reason and (b) to change (correct) the process of care appropriately. For example, the therapeutic regimen (drugs, doses, frequencies, routes, durations) may be changed.

A clinical pharmaceutical care indicator may be defined as a therapeutic result that can be used to monitor and evaluate patient progress toward defined outcomes of drug therapy. A pharmaceutical care indicator is not a complete measure of therapeutic results (patient progress). Rather, it is a tool that can be used to assess progress and that can address attention to issues within the drug therapy of the patient that may require more intensive evaluation.[b]

Appropriate clinical indicators depend on the patient, the disease, and the therapy. Examples include a blood or serum drug level, a coagulation test, a patient's report of symptom status, and even the use of other drugs, especially drugs that reflect symptom status.

A therapeutic objective is an intended, proximate result of therapy (an output). A pharmacist or physician often should be able to specify a therapeutic objective even if unable to state definitely what outcome of drug therapy should occur or when it should occur. For example months of negative urine cultures may be necessary before one can announce the cure of some recurrent urinary tract infections (an outcome). However, an obvious therapeutic objective of antibiotic therapy is remission of symptoms and disappearance of bacteriuria. This distinction between symptom remission and cure is important, and different terms would help keep the difference clear. Reaching the therapeutic objective is not the same as reaching the outcome, merely a step toward it. Not reaching this therapeutic objective in a few days, however, may suggest that the patient is unlikely to be cured with that regimen.

An outcome, such as a cure, is usually more valued than an output, but outcomes are harder for professionals to define and control and often require more time. Outputs, although less significant, are more achievable—that is, they are easier to define and to control and usually occur sooner. The term output is rarely used in health care to mean an achieved therapeutic objective. It sounds too cold and objective. However, it is important that neither patients nor professionals confuse output and outcome (as in confusing symptom remission with cure). A term for an achieved therapeutic objective should distinguish it from both a desired objective and an achieved goal. The closest term in common usage for an output is progress, as in "the patient continues to make progress."[c] The terms therapeutic result, intermediate outcome, process-outcome, or therapeutic outcome also express the precise outputs of a defined therapeutic process. These therapeutic results must be definite in order for drug therapy to satisfy the definition of pharmaceutical care given above.

A major element in the management of drug therapy, therefore, is to identify, in advance, possible or likely therapeutic results and to specify approximately when they should be expected to appear. For example, in a particular patient first-dose dizziness from hypotension from ACE inhibitors may be expected (if it is going to occur) between 1–4 hours after administration. Symptom remission from antibiotic therapy of a UTI should appear within 24–48 hours. If symptoms persist beyond this time, a prompt change in therapy is indicated. Also, if the patient is not able to correctly interpret results, their significance should be specified in advance. This is common practice in inpatient care when a physician writes a chart note to the effect of "Call me if . . . ."

Monitoring

Monitoring is the process of obtaining and evaluating clinical indicators and other relevant information. In order for a pharmaceutical care system to work correctly, monitoring must be planned, intelligent, active, coordinated, and responsive.

1. A monitoring plan should be written in a patient's care record after the pharmacist understands the therapeutic objectives and before the prescription is dispensed. This can be as simple as a note to telephone the patient in 48 hours to inquire about symptom resolution, early appearance of side effects, etc.

2. Intelligent monitoring is individualized. It emphasizes therapeutic results known to be significant in this patient's past therapy (e.g., an idiosyncratic sensitivity to CNS side effects) or with this regimen (e.g., frequency of beta-agonist MDI inhaler use by an asthmatic patient).

3. Active monitoring means that the pharmacist would seek necessary data in contrast to waiting for the patient to mention it. Active monitoring also includes active listening: asking the patient how he is getting along, expecting a real answer, and then asking follow-up questions.

4. Coordinated monitoring allows the pharmacist to efficiently obtain information from the patient, caregivers, and professional colleagues. Each person involved in care may be better suited to obtain certain monitoring data than others. Regardless of who collects the information, it should be documented and communicated to others who may need it.

5. The professional should appropriately interpret and follow up on the information obtained.

Corrective Response

A corrective response should follow if a problem is found in monitoring. For example, if a pharmacist learns that an asthmatic patient is waking up more at night, coughing more, and having trouble getting up stairs that were usually not a problem, she might interpret this information to suggest that a serious exacerbation might be coming.

Referral without recommendation. A pharmacist's response to learning about therapeutic results can involve a referral, notifying another responsible person (e.g., the patient, a family caregiver, the patient's physician) of the possible significance of the results. This is the basic monitoring level—collection of data and recognition of a potential or actual problem.

Intervention and referral with recommendation. In other cases, the pharmacist may choose to respond to such data by defining the problem, choosing a solution, and either implementing the solution or recommending the solution to another. This is participation in managing therapy. For example, suppose pharmacist Spencer has learned that a patient with asthma is using his rescue inhaler (adrenergic metered dose inhaler) too frequently, coughing more, and waking up at night because of asthma. Depending on how severe these results seem to be, she might (a) recommend a visit to the physician without delay, (b) telephone the physician's office herself to recommend an appointment for that day for the patient, (c) telephone the physician with advice about starting a short-term course of corticosteroids, or (d) arrange for transporting the patient to an emergency room.

Points of View: Perception of Therapeutic Results and Outcomes

Monitoring and managing drug therapy in ambulatory care often requires information available only from the patient or caregiver and actions that can be taken only by the patient or caregiver. Patients may have different therapeutic objectives than professionals and certainly may experience therapeutic results and outcomes differently. Furthermore, humane practice requires that caregivers respect patient values and preferences. For these reasons, professionals should recognize the different points of view involved in the management of therapy, in particular the patient's point of view, and negotiate common goals if possible. The following example is intended to illustrate one possible combination of a patient's preferences and understanding of therapy.

Euripedes Pence is a 50 year-old tailor. He is a weekend fisherman and bowler. He was diagnosed with hypertension last year. His physician, Dr. Neil Perry, initially tried a low-salt diet and aerobic exercise, but when Mr. Pence's blood pressure did not fall, he moved on to diuretics and then to nadolol, a nonspecific beta blocker. Mr. Pence visited Dr. Perry yesterday. When the nurse took his blood pressure, it was 150/110. Dr. Perry told him that, if the hypertension was not lower in 4 weeks, he would increase the dose of medication.

Mr. Pence has telephoned to request a refill of his blood pressure prescription. The prescription is for nadolol, 40 mg. #60, sig: 1 q.d. for blood pressure. The last refill was a little more than 10 weeks ago.

The pharmacist, Ms. Dee Spenser, makes it a point to speak with Mr. Pence when he comes in, and after a little discussion about boats, she takes his blood pressure. It is 140/90, standing. Mr. Pence told her that it's usually about 130/90, sometimes a little higher, when he takes it himself at home.

Mr. Pence confides that he is reluctant to take any medication. He says that friends have taken medicine for their hypertension and, "never get off the stuff, like they get hooked or something." He is especially reluctant to increase the dose. On the contrary, he is thinking of stopping the medicine altogether. When Ms. Spenser asked why, he explained, in effect, that he never really agreed with Dr. Perry's decision to initiate therapy or to increase the dosage of the medicine.

He comments that he has no symptoms of hypertension and had been surprised when Dr. Perry told him he had it, because he's "not the nervous type." He admits that he has not been taking the medicine as prescribed but adds that "he has sufficient reason not to." He took the medicine as prescribed "for a while," and feels much better when he is not taking the prescribed dosage. While he was taking it he felt tired, dizzy, and depressed and he experienced occasional impotence; he thinks the nadolol is the cause.

He did not tell this to Dr. Perry. Dr. Perry has explained that hypertension is a serious disease, and Mr. Pence has not told him that he is skipping doses, especially on weekends. Mr. Pence says, "You gotta live while you're alive. You can't keep hoping to live forever."

Whose Therapeutic Objectives?

To have a patient as a partner, the professional should accept that the patient's primary reality is his illness experience. A patient may experience illness differently from what the health professional expects. People with diseases do not always feel ill or act sick. Sometimes, health professionals may be expecting the patient to follow instructions that have no basis in the patient's perception of reality. This raises an important question, which can be only be touched upon here: whose outcomes are important?

Perhaps what the patient wants most from therapy is less interference by his disease in his ability to enjoy certain activities of life. Some patients may be willing to cooperate in therapy only as long as it does not interfere with such activities. This may not imply recklessness or foolishness. Difficult compromise is sometimes preferable to the theoretically ideal therapeutic plan. Suppose that a patient's blood pressure is not quite as good on thiazides as it had been on beta blockers, but the patient has better quality of life. For whose outcomes is the team supposed to work?

From a clinical perspective, the pharmacist should be actively monitoring medicine use and clinical results and keeping the team informed. However, the pharmacist also has an opportunity to know how the therapy is affecting the patient's life and to keep the team informed about it.

Disease and Illness

A fundamental and essential distinction is made in the sociology of medicine between the personal experience of disease and its vicarious professional experience. This distinction is involved in the case of Mr. Pence, described above.

Illness, Wellness, and Quality of Life

The terms illness and wellness refer to a person's subjective experience, e.g., feelings, perceived ability to function. For example, Mr. Pence knew that he occasionally felt tired, dizzy, and depressed. Furthermore, the person may or may not act sick, i.e., change his activities as a result of illness. Illness experience and sickness behavior are the primary realities of health care. That is, patients experience them directly. They often comprise the motivation for, and basis of, health care and they may powerfully influence a person's other life experiences.

Although there is no generally accepted definition for quality of life, the concept refers to a person's satisfaction with life, sense of well-being (subjectively experienced), and ability to perform certain activities.[6] These activities include recreational activities and those necessary to take care of oneself (activities of daily living) and to meet social role expectations (e.g., as worker, spouse, parent, friend).

Quality of life represents the functional effects of an illness and its consequent therapy upon a patient, as perceived by the patient. Four broad domains contribute to the overall effect: physical and occupational function, psychological state, social interaction, and somatic sensation.[7]

Diseases and Diagnoses

The term disease is reserved for the professional interpretation of a person's account of illness experience, physical examination, and laboratory tests. As an interpretation or inference, disease is a professional's secondary perception of the primary illness experience. Disease is an interpretation of reality, the theoretical reality of diagnosis, pathophysiology, and therapeutics.

For example, a person experiencing chest pain and shortness of breath may visit a doctor for tests. After examination and testing, the physician may diagnose his condition as a recognized disease, perhaps angina pectoris or hiatal hernia, or as "essentially normal." Recognizing a patient's symptoms as a disease provides access to general knowledge that may be essential in managing the patient. In this example, although the doctor may actually know very little about this specific patient's angina, she may know a lot about angina from scientific studies and clinical experience. Nonetheless, it is necessary to remember that such general knowledge, no matter how scientifically based, is abstract knowledge about people other than the patient. It is obviously an academic complement, not a valid substitute, for the patient's primary experience.

Illness and Health-Related Quality of Life

Quality of life may be significantly influenced by non-health-related issues, such as socioeconomic status. Furthermore, some people's health-related quality of life may be influenced more by their feelings of illness or wellness than by objective disease status. Therefore, it is possible for the treatment of disease to increase feelings of illness or reduce quality of life more than the disease itself. For example, Jachuck et al.[8] reported on the outcome of the treatment of hypertension from the perspectives of physicians, patients, and family members. Physicians reported that 90% of the patients were doing better. Fifty percent of patients reported that they were feeling better, while the family members reported that 95% of the patients were doing worse. This raises an interesting contrast among the "outcomes" upon which the practitioner may focus. It also suggests that the distinction may be blurry between health-related and non-health-related quality of life.

Pharmacists should consider that therapy may influence a patient's illness and wellness experience and quality of life through simple or complex mechanisms, for example a patient may feel, as does Mr. Pence, that drug therapy is reducing quality of life because of side effects; therapy may affect the lives of family and friends; and family and friends may affect a patient's quality of life. Mr. Pence may be attributing symptoms to his therapy that are actually caused in part by his disease.

Also, pharmacists and other health professionals should be careful not to ignore a patient's illness just because the patient appears not to have a disease known to have a symptom or to be taking a drug known to have a particular side effect. A professional would only rarely overtly deny a patient's illness experience; however, ignoring it, depreciating it, or stating that nothing can be done for it is not uncommon. Chronic pain and some presentations of mental depression are common examples.

When the professional wants an outcome and the patient does not cooperate, such patients are called noncompliant. What should we call a professional who does not respond to symptoms (illness) in the apparent absence of disease? There is no equivalent term for a noncompliant professional, but "professional arrogance" might come to mind. That may not be entirely accurate, however. Sometimes the cause is excessive preoccupation with scientific models of disease and inadequate attention to what the patient is experiencing and trying to describe. Sometimes the cause is a difference in knowledge, values, and time horizon.

The case of Mr. Pence illustrates some important issues in the management of drug therapy. Psychological issues and clinical issues often interact. Mr. Pence has a reasonable, short-term, commonsense view that happens to include a number of mistakes. He felt worse when he took nadolol than when he did not. He concluded that his medicine was the problem, rather than his asymptomatic disease. He seems willing to trade present quality of life for future undesirable consequences of untreated hypertension. He confuses chronic therapy with drug addiction. For some reason he is unwilling to describe his concerns and the facts of his medications use with Dr. Perry. He may have some misunderstandings about his disease and its treatment. His secretive noncompliance could actually start a downward spiral, because Dr. Perry seems to believe that his present nadolol dosage is too low. Pence might be able to tolerate other regimens more easily. However, his beliefs about hypertension, assumptions about therapy, and secretive relationship with Dr. Perry might interfere with new therapies just as they did with the nadolol. Pence's behavior might change if his understanding changed. Recognizing Mr. Pence's perceptions, causal attributions, and goals might facilitate changing his misunderstandings.

In summary, understanding outcomes is essential for safe and effective clinical practice. The care of most patients consists of a series of observable results, which we have termed outputs or therapeutic outcomes. These results should be compared to definite expectations and therapeutic objectives so that the progress of therapy can be followed toward the intended outcome and deviations from the path can be corrected. Patients and professionals may have different views of both the reasons for and the objectives of drug therapy. Since patient cooperation in care is often necessary, especially in ambulatory care, professionals, patients, and family caregivers need to agree as much as possible about therapeutic objectives.

Systematic Improvement of Outcomes

The second major topic of this chapter is the improvement of systems and outcomes in groups or populations of patients. The philosophy of systematic improvement of outcomes originated in industrial production management. It has been known under various names, but we will refer to it as quality improvement. Quality improvement is

> *The combination of principles and methods that create both a quality and customer focused environment and the capability to identify, assess and constantly enhance the efficiency and effectiveness of those processes that determine important organizational results.*[9]

Even though the origins of pharmaceutical care are in clinical practice, not industrial management, both quality improvement and pharmaceutical care are continuous, systematic approaches to achieving defined outcomes. The philosophies of pharmaceutical care and quality improvement are analogous, especially as quality improvement is applied to health care. Pharmaceutical care is, in some respects, the application of quality improvement principles to patient outcomes, one patient at a time.

The components of a quality improvement system are guidelines, performance indicators, a database, and standards. **Figure 9.**4 shows the relationship of indicators, guidelines performance database, and standards in a generic quality improvement system. The diagram shows a pharmaceutical care system (one patient at a time) nested within the quality improvement system (many patient encounters or episodes).

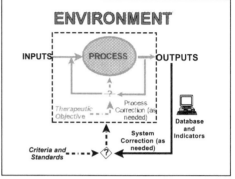

In a quality improvement system, outputs are evaluated against a standard or expectation, as shown by the diamond-shaped box with a question mark in it. Compliance with a therapeutic guideline (e.g., management of heart failure) can be measured through a pro-

Figure 9.4. Diagram of a Continuous Improvement System.

cess indicator (e.g., patients with heart failure receiving ACE inhibitors) and outcome indicators (e.g., patients with preventable cardiac decompensation). If outputs appear to be satisfactory, no action is taken. If a problem is recognized, it is defined, root causes are sought, and a solution is implemented as soon as possible. Also, a follow up might be scheduled in a shorter interval. The results may document an opportunity for improvement through changes in the guidelines and raise the expected performance standards.

Guidelines

A guideline is a description of a desired process, a standardized specification for care of a patient in the typical situation. Guidelines should be based on evidence as interpreted by experts. This should be done, whenever possible, through a formal, consultative process. Related terms and synonyms include clinical criteria, practice parameter, protocol, algorithm, review criteria, and preferred practice pattern. Guidelines codify the care process to achieve some degree of uniformity and predictability in the patient care process. Deviation from guidelines may be necessary for individual patients. To provide a specific example, a consensus may exist, based on clinical research, that the treatment of heart failure should include ACE inhibitors.

Indicators

Both a pharmaceutical care system and a quality improvement system may use indicators of performance or status. A performance indicator for use in a quality improvement system is defined as "a statistical value that provides an indication of the condition or direction over time of an organization's performance of a specified process, or an organization's achievement of a specified outcome."[10] According to an earlier definition, *an indicator is a quantitative measure that can be used to monitor and evaluate the quality of important . . . clinical and support functions that affect patient outcomes. . . . An indicator is not a direct measure of quality. Rather it is a tool that can be used to assess performance and that can direct attention to . . . issues that may require more intense review within an organization.* [9]

Two types of indicators for pharmaceutical care refer to process and therapeutic outcomes. Process indicators measure adherence to general or specific guidelines. Outcome indicators measure the achievement of defined outcomes. Process indicators measure definite activities that are a part of care, e.g., conformity to a prescribing guideline. Process indicators may be especially appropriate in quality improvement systems where

1. no valid and reliable therapeutic result is available,

2. some causes of the therapeutic result are not humanly controllable,

3. a process has a very strong, demonstrable link to outcome, or

4. a process is interesting in itself.

Rate-based indicators are corrected for the volume of events. For example, given a guideline recommending ACE inhibitors for patients with congestive heart failure, a rate-based indicator would be expressed as rate = N/D, where N equals number of patients each month with congestive heart failure who received a new or refill prescription for an ACE inhibitor and D equals total number of patients with congestive heart failure during the same month.

Sentinel indicators have no denominator. They are so closely related to quality of care that they are always followed up, and their rate of occurrence is expected to be zero.

Indicator Selection

An ideal quality improvement system indicator would be technologically feasible, practical to use reliably by various personnel, and validly related to quality of care issues important to stakeholders (e.g., patients, practitioners, payers). More specifically, an indicator should be

1. Valid,

   a. clearly related to quality of care

   b. specific and sensitive

   c. interpretable

2. Reliable for intended purpose,

3. Feasible and practical from the perspective of data collection,

4. Quantitative, i.e., measurable or countable,

5. Related to results that can be significantly influenced by practitioners within the organization,

6. Relevant to the organization's strategic plan, and

7. Independent from political or economic obstructions.

Efforts to improve drug therapy have tended to focus primarily on a few criteria, such as drug product and effectiveness. The challenge for a drug therapy quality improvement system is to evaluate and improve all six performance dimensions.

Performance Database

A database is an organized collection of specific information related to performance. Indicators should be selected based, in part, on available data and vice versa. A performance database should allow the ready calculation and reporting of indicators. Computerized pharmacy dispensing records may compose a performance database if the information can be sorted as needed. Process indicators would be more accessible from a typical prescription database, but outcome indicators would be less so. For example, a pharmacy database might easily yield indicator data for therapeutic duplication, length of therapy, and refill intervals.

Standards

A standard is a statement of an expectation that defines the organization's governance, management, and clinical and support services' capacity to provide quality care. A guideline specifies what is expected without exception. Standards describe how often guideline adherence is expected. They should be ideally based on benchmarks (empirical evidence from comparable processes or published results) but be open to continual improvement. That is, standards should not become upper limits for quality.

The Continuous Improvement of Pharmaceutical Care

One could explain pharmaceutical care as the application of quality improvement principles to individual patients and a quality improvement system as the application of pharmaceutical care to groups of patients. Both pharmaceutical care and continuous improvement are obligations of practitioners, not a departmental or organizational function to be delegated to a select few. A necessary part of a quality improvement system is the creation of a measurement system to improve patient care related processes that have a favorable impact on therapeutic results or outcomes. Figure 9.4 illustrates the use of multiple patient experiences to create a database that provides information about the process and results of treatment. This approach may aggregate data from multiple practice settings, a single hospital, a patient care unit, or even an individual practitioner.

Root Causes

Searching for root cause is an essential element of both patient care and quality improvement systems. This idea is very familiar to health professionals as the basis of rational therapeutics. For example, precordial chest pain can be relieved with analgesics; however, no competent health professional would choose this treatment until certain causes had been eliminated, especially angina pectoris and gastroesophageal disease. This is based on an educated understanding of cardiac and gastroesophageal pathophysiology. Analgesic treatment would be inappropriate because it would treat symptoms but neglect the underlying disease. If the pain is caused by coronary ischemia, coronary vasodilators (which are not analgesics) may provide temporary relief of chest pain, because they increase myocardial perfusion. The ischemia is caused by underlying coronary artery disease, caused by elevated serum cholesterol, which in turn is caused by a patient's metabolism, diet, and exercise. Treating symptoms without correcting causes may be dangerous. Correcting causes is often more effective, efficient, and permanent than treating symptoms, but it requires more understanding. This principle is as true for managing quality in a medication-use system as it is for managing patients.

Changes in a quality indicator within a patient population may be explained superficially, for example, as attributable to a few physicians who do not follow prescribing guidelines or a few noncompliant patients. Or, root cause analysis may show that the change in the indicator results from fundamental changes in the system, such as third-party formularies or payment policies.

A quality improvement system[d] and a pharmaceutical care system may trigger corrective action according to different criteria. A pharmaceutical care system addresses one patient at a time. It may not initiate corrective action unless a problem (defined as an obstacle to a desired outcome) can be found. A quality improvement system considers large aggregations (samples) of outputs and assumes that the processes leading to those outcomes can be improved. The issue is not so much whether to take action but which action to take.

A quality improvement system in operation is based on the following quality improvement principles:

1. understand patients' needs,
2. understand root causes of quality variations,
3. focus on root causes and prevention of problems, e.g., the system rather than the individuals or departments involved,
4. make decisions based on data,
5. follow up results of interventions and, when possible, use statistical process control tools

Using these principles, the characteristics of the ideal pharmaceutical care quality improvement system are to

1. measure and monitor performance of teams and individuals,
2. stimulate and facilitate continual improvement,
3. be cost effective,
4. meet accreditation and third-party performance requirements, and
5. be an integral part of providing pharmaceutical care.

Drug Use Evaluation Programs versus Quality Improvement System

Most pharmacists are familiar with drug use evaluation or drug use review programs. Drug use evaluation has been defined as "a structured, ongoing, organizationally authorized, quality assurance process designed to ensure that drugs are used appropriately, safely, and effectively."[11] The concepts of drug use evaluation apply to all practice settings.

Drug use evaluation evolved from the Joint Commission on Accreditation of Healthcare Organizations accreditation requirements that focused on the usage patterns of high-cost antibiotics in the early 1980's. The emphasis was on appropriate use, narrowly defined, as the old saying went, as the right drug for the right bug. This concept of appropriate use gradually evolved to include dose, regimen, monitoring, and even cost effectiveness, but still had a primary focus on the prescribing of high-cost drug products.

Drug use evaluation was based on the older philosophy of quality assurance, not quality improvement. Drug use evaluation, as typically practiced, emphasized process (prescribing). It held individuals (usually physicians) responsible for prescribing while the pharmacy department collected data and often carried out interventions. Although useful, it had several shortcomings. It sometimes created an adversarial relationship between physicians and pharmacists and did not reflect the realities of patient care from multidisciplinary teams. It compartmentalized responsibility for improvement processes that included many departments.

In contrast, where drug use evaluation emphasizes the prescribing process, quality improvement is consistent with the philosophical emphasis of pharmaceutical care on outcomes. Where drug use evaluation emphasizes physicians, quality improvement is consistent with the philosophical emphasis of pharmaceutical care on cooperation and shared responsibility. Where drug use evaluation emphasizes individual action, quality improvement emphasizes system performance. The transition from drug use evaluation to quality improvement system can be accomplished by (a) adopting quality indicators that go beyond drug, dose, and duration into the overall processes and outcomes of medication use by physicians and patients and (b) application of quality improvement principles. This is a profound change. Imagine for a moment that pharmaceutical care had never been described. Then consider what kinds of systems improvements would naturally result from the consistent application of quality improvement principles and methods to the medications use process. Logically, the application of quality improvement to medications use would eventually arrive at a pharmaceutical care system. Who knows how far quality improvement can take drug therapy beyond pharmaceutical care?

Summary

Pharmaceutical care is intended to achieve definite outcomes that improve a patient's health-related quality of life. This discussion has emphasized outcomes that can be accepted as important and valuable to all parties in a health care system and serve as the focus of measurement and improvement efforts. Various definitions of outcome and quality of life may produce considerable confusion among health care providers and patients. This confusion can be resolved somewhat if the patient's primary illness perspective is harmonized with the practitioner's disease orientation—for example, by considering professional and patient responses to "What do you want to achieve from this therapy?" and "How can we improve it?"

Pharmaceutical care is about measuring, monitoring, and improving a patient's quality of life. The quality improvement system uses the pharmaceutical care data and associated processes from many patients to improve the care of future patients. Both pharmaceutical care and quality improvement system are customer focused, require teamwork, use a feedback system, and are based on shared responsibility. They are indivisible and cannot be successfully practiced separately.

References

1. Kohn LT, Corrigan JM, Donaldson MS. To err is human: building a safer health system. Washington DC: National Academy Press; 2000.

2. Angaran DM. Quality assurance to quality improvement: measuring and monitoring pharmaceutical care. *Am J Hosp Pharm.* 1991; 48:1901–7.

3. Hepler CD, Strand LM. Opportunities and responsibilities in pharmaceutical care. *Am J Hosp Pharm.* 1990; 47:533–43.

4. Webster's Seventh New Collegiate Dictionary. Springfield, MA: G&C Merriam Company; 1971:264, s.v. effect (syn.).

5. Donabedian A. The role of outcomes in quality assessment and assurance. *QRB.* 1992; 18:356–60.

6. MacKeigan LD, Pathak DS . Overview of health-related quality-of-life measures. *Am J Hosp Pharm.* 42:2236–45.

7. Schipper H, Clinch J, Powell V. Definitions and conceptual issues. In: Spilker B., ed. Quality of life assessments in clinical trials. New York: Raven Press; 1990.

8. Jachuck SJ, Brierley H, Jachuck S et al. The effect of hypotensive drugs on the quality of life. *J R Coll Gen Pract.* 1982; 32:103–5.

9. Primer on indicator development and application: measuring quality in health care. Chicago: Joint Commission on Accreditation of Healthcare Organizations; 1992.

10. The measurement mandate: on the road to performance improvement in health care. Oakbrook, IL: Joint Commission on Accreditation of Healthcare Organizations; 1993.

11. American Society of Hospital Pharmacists. The ASHP guidelines on the pharmacist role in drug use evaluation. Practice Standards of ASHP 1992–93. Bethesda MD: ASHP.

Footnotes

[a] In systems language, this information is called feedback.

[b] Adapted from the definition of a performance indicator on page 10.

[c] Outside of psychiatry or rehabilitation, this is strange usage, as it seems to imply that progress is something the patient makes. Patients who do not make progress are often described as having failed therapy. In fact, the therapy makes progress or fails the patient.

[d] Quality improvement systems are also known as Performance Based Evaluation Systems (PBES).

Appendix 9.1. Outcome Definition, Classification, and Listing of Some Outcomes of Health Care

Adapted from reference 4.

A. Clinical

   1. Reported systems that have clinical significance
   2. Diagnostic categorization as an indication of morbidity
   3. Disease staging relevant to functional encroachment and prognosis
   4. Diagnostic performance—the frequency of false positives and false negatives as indicators of diagnostic or case-finding performance

B. Physiologic–biochemical

   1. Abnormalities
   2. Functions

      a. Loss of function

      b. Functional reserve—includes performance in test situations under various degrees of stress

C. Physical

   1. Loss or impairment of structural form or integrity—includes abnormalities, defects, and disfigurement
   2. Functional performance of physical activities and tasks

      a. Under the circumstances of daily living

      b. Under test conditions that involve various degrees of stress

D. Psychologic, mental

   1. Feelings—includes discomfort, pain, fear, anxiety (or their opposites, including satisfaction)
   2. Beliefs that are relevant to health and health care
   3. Knowledge that is relevant to healthful living, health care, and coping with illness
   4. Impairments of discrete psychologic or mental functions

      a. Under the circumstances of daily living

      b. Under test conditions that involve various degrees of stress

E. Social and psychosocial

   1. Behaviors relevant to coping with current illness or affecting future health, including adherence to health care regimens and changes in health-related habits
   2. Role performance

      a. Marital

      b. Familial

    c. Occupational

    d. Other interpersonal

  3. Performance under test conditions involving varying degrees of stress

F. Integrative outcomes

  1. Mortality

  2. Longevity

  3. Longevity, with adjustments made to take account of impairments of physical, psychologic, and psychosocial function—"full-function equivalents"

  4. Monetary value of the above

G. Evaluative outcomes

  1. Client opinions about, and satisfaction with, various aspects of care, including accessibility, continuity, thoroughness, humaneness, informativeness, effectiveness, cost

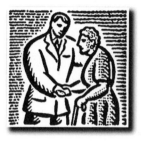

Part 2: Implementation of Pharmaceutical Care

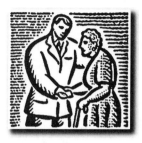

Chapter 10:
Pharmaceutical Care:
The Scope of Practice

Daniel Albrant, Pharm.D.

Lucinda L. Maine, Ph.D.

Richard P. Penna, R.Ph., Pharm.D.

Introduction

The primary purpose of this chapter is to describe the scope of practice encompassed in the term pharmaceutical care as it has been implemented in a variety of different practice environments. In addition, the progress that has been made in implementing this patient-focused pharmacy practice will be described in the context of a model of transformational change.

To achieve these objectives, the chapter will review the evidence that pharmacy has identified a major public health need and has made a commitment to fill that need. Key issues associated with the increased recognition that medication use is central to quality health care and that traditional methods of medication-use management are falling short in terms of patient safety and effectiveness of therapy will also be addressed.

The implications of these forces and the profession's attempts to address them will be studied in detail. This chapter will close with a review of the scope of pharmaceutical care practice, both today and in the future, in four distinct environments of pharmacy practice.

Transformational Change in Pharmacy Practice

A Framework for Transformational Change

Evidence mounts that the delivery of health care services, and the management of medication use specifically, is ripe for major, transformational change. Tinkering around the boundaries of inpatient and outpatient care delivery, financing, and accountability systems will not provide patients the safer, more effective, and caring health services model they desire and need. Nor will it rebalance the financial value equation. Those who study the escalation in health care costs say society cannot sustain continued increases in health spending in the face of so much evidence of waste and rework resulting from poorly executed and poorly coordinated health care services.

177

Former House Speaker Newt Gingrich outlined a model of transformational change that can be applied to medical care. The model begins with a clear and compelling vision of what the change will yield. Clearly no change of any magnitude will occur overnight. The model acknowledges that, for a substantial period of time, encompassing the movement from the current reality (health care as delivered today) to a midpoint where progress toward change is more evident, those attempting to lead the transformation will likely spend more effort on defensive strategies than on offensive measures designed to promote the necessary changes. From the midpoint on, defense will still be required to protect both important elements of the former systems and elements of change; however, more of the time and energies of change agents can be directed toward activities leading to the transforming change model. Ultimately, for the transformation to occur, the leaders must be able to articulate to the public why the change is beneficial to the individual. There must be a sustained and effective public communication process to create the groundswell of support for the proposed transforming change to occur.

Applying the Framework to Pharmaceutical Care

There are direct parallels between the change model and how the pharmacy profession is moving toward a transformed vision of practice. As will be noted in subsequent sections of this chapter and elsewhere in this book, the profession of pharmacy has been populated by leaders with a clear and compelling vision for transformational change. Brodie, Millis, Hepler, Strand, Manasse, Gans, and others have, over a period of decades, described the need for a new approach to medication use and for opportunities for pharmacists, as medication experts, to apply their body of knowledge and skills to improve patient health.

Opposition to change is part of human nature and the reason why change leaders must mount defensive strategies. Certainly organized medicine has been one source of opposition to introducing pharmaceutical care into mainstream health care. Corporate health care and some pharmacy organizations have long ignored the profession's attempts to introduce change. The inclination is to defend the known; individual practitioners and employers of pharmacists have often felt threatened by the suggestion that the roles of pharmacists in all settings must expand from overseeing the distribution of drugs to caring for patients who use medications. Policymakers have too often defended the status quo rather than enabled change through the passage of laws that expand pharmacists' scope of practice and that create public financing systems for medication use.

It has been difficult for the profession to find its voice and deliver a compelling message for the need for change. Medications throughout most of the twentieth century were not costly and were widely believed to be very safe. Oversight of medication use was generally assumed to be the primary responsibility of prescribing physicians. Limited evidence had accumulated about the potential and actual harm to patients that drug-related problems caused. At the turn of the twenty-first century, however, that began to change as the cost of medications and the untoward effects of mismanaged medication use took a center stage in health care and health policy. Without question, a process of transformation has been unfolding, with pharmacy's progressive leaders working hard against the opposing forces. Has the profession reached the midpoint? Possibly so, but there is still a significant amount of progress to be made before the delivery of pharmaceutical care is the standard of care and pharmacy practice.

What Encompasses Pharmaceutical Care?

Throughout the 1990's much of the profession's attention turned to developing and studying the practice model of pharmaceutical care. Even this process had its controversies. Was pharmaceutical care best delivered as a comprehensive approach to patients' medication use or could a disease-specific approach qualify as the new patient-centered practice model? Were only pharmacists capable of delivering care and where was the best site for the delivery of such services? Would any payers, including consumers, be willing to pay for pharmaceutical care services and, if so, exactly what services would they be buying?

Although there are no quick and simple answers to these questions, there is a touchstone resource that was produced to enable the profession to clarify what activities pharmacists do in delivering a wide range of services, including pharmaceutical care. The *Pharmacy Practice Activity Classification (PPAC)* outlines taxonomy of pharmacy practice activities in four domains.[1] Domain A, Ensuring Appropriate Pharmacotherapy, essentially delineates the nature of services pharmacists would render in providing pharmaceutical care. To a great extent, the activities are not influenced by where the services are delivered (i.e., in-patient versus outpatient services) or by the type of patient receiving them.

The work of the profession over decades now positions pharmacy to realize the vision of those leaders who have long seen the need for transformational change. The next section will revisit that history before launching more deeply into the scope and context of the practice of pharmaceutical care.

Roots of Pharmaceutical Care

Pharmacy: A Profession Familiar with Change

Pharmacy, like all professions, must evolve continuously to meet the needs of society and is therefore no stranger to change. As with most professions, pockets of resistance within the profession challenge the innovators and slacken the pace of change, which is nonetheless inevitable. Rufus A. Lyman,[2] founding editor of the *American Journal of Pharmaceutical Education,* noted the following with respect to change in pharmacy education:

> *Some were violently opposed, the majority was indifferent. Support did come from a few farseeing laymen who recognized the importance of the pharmacist and the drugstore in the public health service. It also came from a handful of practicing druggists who were readers of pharmacy's history and who had learned the part the pharmacist has played in the past in science, in industry, in research, in education, and in the art of living, and who had a vision of greater things for the future.*

Change through History

As detailed in chapter 2, in the pharmacy profession's earliest days, its practitioners were primarily involved with the gathering, identification, testing, and purification of natural drug products and with research on those products. Compounding those products into dosage forms that were safe, stable, and palatable was the predominant role of pharmacists in the pre-industrial era.

These traditional roles changed with the establishment of the pharmaceutical industry. Pharmaceutical companies, which were often founded by pharmacists, took the key scientific knowledge of the pharmacy profession and developed large, efficient systems for producing a dizzying array of pharmaceutical dosage forms. Increasingly, pharmacists accepted the responsibility to ensure that already-manufactured drug products were readily available to the public by maintaining systems of efficient, safe, and accurate drug distribution.

Change of major proportions is once again confronting the profession. The major expansion in the fundamental professional responsibilities of pharmacists—that of caring for people and for the outcomes of their medication use—represents a paradigm shift for practitioners, educators, and regulators. In short, all elements of the pharmacy profession are affected by this change.

The Concept of Role Expansion

Although profound change has been and is occurring in the profession, pharmacy is not abandoning the responsibilities the public has historically conferred upon it. Indeed, pharmacy continues to promote the pharmaceutical sciences, which support research and development in pharmaceutical industry. Increasingly, the clinical and biomedical sciences are directly applied to patient care. A growing area of scientific inquiry, that of outcome assessment, will provide the foundation upon which much of contemporary clinical practice, including pharmaceutical care, will be built.

The profession has accepted new responsibilities in practice as well, without completely abandoning the old ones. Many pharmacists continue to compound finished dosage forms, although in some cases the types of products are vastly different from those compounded in the past. Radioactive pharmaceuticals for diagnostic and therapeutic use, intravenous admixtures, and nutritional support products are examples of modern-day compounded products most often prepared by pharmacists. For two of the examples cited above (nuclear pharmacy and nutritional support pharmacy), the Board of Pharmaceutical Specialties (the specialty-recognizing body in the profession) certifies that practitioners involved in such practices possess specialized knowledge and skill.

Safe and effective systems of drug distribution remain very much within the scope of responsibility of many of today's pharmacists. However, as will be noted in more detail later in this text, automation and technical personnel will play increasing roles in executing the drug distribution function, making it possible for more pharmacists to apply their skills to the caregiving functions essential to pharmaceutical care.

The continuing expansion of pharmacists' professional roles and responsibilities into clinical specialties, long-term care, home health care, and a myriad of other areas reflects the consistent response of the profession to the changing needs of society. It also underscores the unique knowledge and services that pharmacists can bring to the health care system.

Signposts on Pharmacy's Road of Change

In a century filled with change of the magnitude and pace of that which pharmacy has experienced, it is not surprising to note that the profession's leaders have dedicated considerable effort to studies and reports that chronicle the status of the profession and how practitioners have met the needs of society. In the first half of this century, such reports were primarily concerned with the nature of the services pharmacists were providing and how those services were perceived, received, and appreciated by the public. In the middle of the twentieth century, it was clear that changes in the practices of pharmacy and drug manufacturing had called into question what the societally sanctioned role of the pharmacist truly was. Toward the mid-1980's, pharmacy turned its attention to strategic planning by inquiring about the future and by asking what the public's existing needs were and how the unique knowledge and skills of pharmacists could be useful in addressing those needs.

A brief summary of these chronicles, which were originally published as survey findings, key speeches, or study commission reports, provides a roadmap of the philosophical journey of the pharmacy profession toward pharmaceutical care. The summary will show that the leaders of the profession have made a transition from documenting practice to strategically envisioning how practice must be transformed to secure a professionally viable role for pharmacists.

The earliest report in this chronology, *Basic Material for a Pharmaceutical Curriculum,* is a report of the Commonwealth Fund Study and Survey of Pharmacy.[3] Dr. W. W. Charters and his team visited hundreds of pharmacies throughout the United States to investigate and tabulate the duties and functions of the pharmacist. Thousands of prescriptions were checked for ingredients and frequency of ingredients. Colleges of pharmacy and state boards were encouraged to use the report as a foundation for both curricula and state board examinations to ensure that individuals entering practice were equipped with relevant and adequate knowledge and skill to perform their socially sanctioned duties.

In reporting on the survey to the American Pharmaceutical Association (APhA), National Association of Boards of Pharmacy (NABP) Secretary H. C. Christensen noted that the profession should not depend on the results of this survey indefinitely and alluded to a concern that the profession was not evolving as rapidly or consistently as necessary. He called for continued surveying of the activities of pharmacists as a mechanism for continuously moving the boundaries of pharmacy practice forward and remaining in step with societal needs.

The Great Depression and World War II stalled subsequent analyses of the status or functions of pharmacists until 1948, when the American Council of Education published The Pharmaceutical Survey, also known as the Elliott Report.[4] The purpose of the survey was to ensure that pharmacy continued to occupy its proper place among the health professions in a post-war era marked by expanding opportunities for greater service to the public.

The survey covered all phases of the practice of pharmacy, with particular emphasis on professional education. Unlike the Charters study, which addressed the need to document the practice of pharmacy itself, the Elliott Report contained recommendations directed toward increasing the pharmacist's prestige and standing both in the community and among his fellow heath care professionals. This difference in study goals reflects a profound change in pharmacy practice. This change was brought on by the explosion of prefabricated medications and increased sophistication and profitability in the pharmaceutical industry. These developments altered the day-to-day functions of pharmacists markedly, and, called upon much less frequently to prepare or compound dosage forms, pharmacists began to struggle with a clear definition of their new role.

The Elliott Report devoted a considerable amount of attention to the supply and preparation of manpower for the pharmacy profession's emerging roles and to the quality of faculty and curricula at colleges and schools of pharmacy. The report recommended that the four-year program of education and training be fortified with a stronger base in both the pharmaceutical sciences and economics. Curricular emphases noted in the study spanned the entire spectrum from drug procurement and preparation to preparing students to provide "professional services to the public appropriate to the basic functions of pharmacy in its role as a health profession." The report also recommended that the American Association of Colleges of Pharmacy (AACP) and the American Council on Pharmaceutical Education (ACPE) take steps to develop an educational program leading to the professional doctor of pharmacy degree.[4] Significantly, the concept of "clinical pharmacy" was not yet recommended as the focus for the doctor of pharmacy degree program since the development of clinical pharmacy was still 15 years off.

Donald Brodie[5] articulated a key concept, which can be credited with shifting the inquiry of pharmacy's leaders from "What do pharmacists do?" to "What is the mainstream of pharmaceutical service?" Brodie conceptualized "drug-use control" as the keystone of pharmaceutical service, the mainstream of pharmacy. He noted that, although many felt that dispensing pharmaceuticals was the main activity of pharmacy professionals, this was not necessarily true. He quoted from the *Mirror to Hospital Pharmacy* to point out the frailty of this belief: "The dispensing function of the pharmacist, while important and even vital for patient care, is essentially a superficial practice of the profession which, by itself, does not utilize knowledge or skills sufficiently basic to merit professional recognition to the depth that lies within the grasp of hospital pharmacists."[6] This argument applies to all pharmacists, regardless of where they practice.

Brodie defined drug-use control as that system of knowledge, understanding, judgments, procedures, skills, controls, and ethics that ensures optimal safety in the distribution and use of medication. It is patient oriented and applies to the practices of all pharmacists, educators, journalists, and regulators. It extends from the point of drug discovery on the scientist's bench, to the pharmacy, and, ultimately, to the point of drug administration. Through his writings, Brodie brought the vision of the profession markedly closer to and more in line with the modern vision of pharmaceutical care.

Did Brodie's vision reflect the perception of the American public regarding the role their pharmacists played? Another key study, this one of the perceptions of consumers, revealed, troublingly, that people did not view the average pharmacist of the 1970's as the same kind of professional as the physician or dentist. Respondents more closely aligned a businessman with primarily commercial motivations with pharmaceutical manufacturers than patients and other professionals.[7] These beliefs were fortified by the environment in which most community pharmacists practiced. The study did not examine the public's perception of hospital pharmacists.

A lack of public awareness of the services pharmacists could and often did offer was noted as a compelling reason for the public's lack of trust in pharmacists. The public took for granted that pharmacists packaged and labeled medications properly and maintained the appropriate quality of products in inventory. Failure to provide personal attention and to establish a personal relationship with patients decreased customer confidence that pharmacists could provide professional services warranting professional status in the community. The research did reveal, however, a strong public desire for such a relationship, while noting that the rebuilding effort would not be an easy one for the profession.

A 1975 report entitled Pharmacists for the Future, commissioned by AACP, signals more change both within the profession of pharmacy and outside of it. The report begins by noting the tremendous concern among all elements of society regarding drug purity, efficacy, and safety, as well as the misuse and the cost and benefits of drugs. Commission chairman John Millis notes further that, although pharmacists are naturally concerned about these issues, they are also concerned about their role in society. Impressions of the role the pharmacist might fill in efforts to improve the drug-use process spanned from no role for an obsolete profession to a key role in filling the gaps in health services involving drugs.

The Millis Commission report noted a discontinuity regarding the generation of new knowledge about pharmaceuticals and the application of that knowledge in clinical use. Much drug research is done within the proprietary boundaries of the pharmaceutical industry, and findings are disseminated to busy therapy prescribers via vehicles of the industry's making. This process leaves a true gap in a system of optimal drug use. The commission proposed that "pharmacy should be conceived as a knowledge system which renders a health service by concerning itself with understanding drugs and their effects upon people and animals." As they make up an integral subsystem of the larger national health service delivery system, pharmacists, armed with essential information about drugs and their use, should be fully engaged in applying their professional judgment to weighing the expected benefits against possible risks of drug therapy.[8] This commission's wide-ranging recommendations for pharmacy education and practice are still being studied and implemented today.

In keeping with the profession's desire to examine periodically what pharmacists do in the course of their practices, APhA and AACP conducted a pharmacists' task analysis in 1977 and 1978. (A subsequent Scope of Practice study was conducted in 1992.) The Standards of Practice for the Profession of Pharmacy provided a comprehensive definition of pharmacy practice.[9] The standards were used by the NABP as the basis of its NABPLEX licensing examination and by schools and colleges of pharmacy as the basis for building a pharmacy curriculum.

Perhaps motivated by the stark realization, articulated by the study commission, that the future of the profession was insecure unless aggressive steps were taken to redefine the role of pharmacists, the profession turned its attention in the 1980's to first defining and then strategically charting the future course of pharmacy practice and education. Brodie again stated the need to capture the essence of pharmacy in the form of "a theory of practice" in his Harvey A. K. Whitney Award Lecture in 1980.[10]

He called for an articulation of the theoretical base of pharmacy and, in doing so, underscored the evolution that had been occurring in the profession for decades.[11] The theories that make up this base reflect the evolution from drug product focus to patient focus and ultimately state that the pharmacist is responsible for the outcomes of drug therapy used by patients and other professionals in the health care system. The four theories noted by these authors are

- theory of pharmacy as a drug-use control system,
- theory of pharmacy as a knowledge system,
- theory of pharmacy as a clinical profession, and
- theory of pharmacy as the interface between mankind and drugs.

The profession embraced the concept of clinical pharmacy in the 1970's and 1980's. Although this term can be defined in many ways, it is often used to distinguish those functions that are primarily informative and advisory from the more standardized, distributive functions of drug-use control. Hepler[12] challenged participants at a 1985 conference, entitled Directions for Clinical Practice and hosted by the American Society of Hospital Pharmacists (ASHP), to understand that limiting the scope of clinical pharmacy to just informative and advisory functions does not allow for conveyance of the maximum value of pharmacy's professional services to the public. Defining pharmacy in terms of responsibilities to the public for the appropriate use of drugs in patients more clearly suggests the societal value of pharmaceutical services.

The pharmacy profession was concerned that clinical pharmacy, often cited as the future of the profession, might fail to secure pharmacists' place beside physicians and other recognized professionals. A series of strategic planning efforts, actually beginning as early as 1984, unfolded over the next decade. Some were professionwide and others focused on a single area of practice but all shared the commitment to clearly articulate a vision for pharmacy and to set forth strategies to enable pharmacists to achieve that vision.

Schwartz[13] reviewed the considerable effort invested in the late 1980's by the profession's leaders in shaping the future of the profession. While noting that developing a strategic plan is a difficult undertaking for a large and diverse profession, the author suggested several mechanisms for strategically moving the profession forward.

The first of a series of professionwide strategic planning efforts began in 1984 with a conference entitled Pharmacy in the 21st Century, Planning for an Uncertain Future.[14] Five years later, a second Pharmacy in the 21st Century Conference was sponsored by 17 major national professional pharmaceutical organizations. The purpose of this conference was to identify and prioritize the major issues that would confront the profession during the next 15 to 20 years.[15] At this conference, the keynote speaker, C. Douglas Hepler, challenged participants to identify pharmaceutical care as the profession's major societal purpose and to establish standards and models of such care.

Participants clearly embraced this challenge, as evidenced by the strength of the consensus on key statements generated by work groups. Key statements receiving a score of greater than 4.5 on a 1 to 5 scale included (1) the need to develop a mission statement for pharmacy, (2) the need to develop standards for pharmaceutical care, and (3) the need for pharmacy to demonstrate and communicate its value in health care.

The American Society of Consultant Pharmacists (ASCP) also convened a strategic planning conference in 1989. This conference resulted in the articulation of a mission statement for consultant pharmacy and five strategies to guide the society and provide leadership to consultant pharmacists. The outcome statements from this conference reflected a strong desire to assist consultant pharmacists in realizing their role in optimizing pharmaceutical and related care and to help develop broad recognition for the value of pharmaceutical care.

These national conferences spawned several state and regional strategic planning efforts, and pharmacy's leaders increased their efforts to help practitioners and educators understand the importance of enunciating a new mission for the profession. These subsequent planning efforts encouraged participants to identify obstacles to pharmacy's advancement and set forth strategies that would allow the practice of pharmacy to meet contemporary societal needs.

Recognizing the importance of keeping pharmacy education positioned to produce graduates whose knowledge and skills meet society's needs now and in the future, AACP initiated its own planning process. The Commission to Implement Change in Pharmaceutical Education began its work in 1989 and a year later issued the first of five background papers. The first articulated a mission for the profession and a mission for pharmaceutical education, which, in general, was consistent with the concept of pharmaceutical care. Additional papers examined the core competencies needed to prepare pharmacists for contemporary practice, the structure of the degree program, and postgraduate training and education needs of the profession in light of the profession's chosen mission.[16]

APhA also charged a task force with examining the needs of society, ways the profession should prepare to meet those needs, and obstacles to pharmaceutical care. The report, entitled An APhA White Paper: The Role of the Pharmacist in Comprehensive Medication Use Management, describes the drug-use problems in today's society and defines pharmaceutical care as the services provided by pharmacists that can address those problems. Three broad areas preventing pharmacy from delivering these services were identified along with a series of 20 principles or areas for action.[17]

In 1993, ASHP and the ASHP Research and Education Foundation conducted a conference entitled Implementing Pharmaceutical Care. The objectives of the conference included identifying the implications of pharmacists' assumption of the responsibility for the outcome of drug therapy, the barriers to and opportunities for implementing this practice, and practice-level processes for pharmaceutical care implementation in organized health care settings. The national conference was to establish the basis for regional, state, and department-level planning efforts and catalyze the widespread adoption of the pharmaceutical care practice model.

Another professionwide conference carrying the Pharmacy in the 21st Century title was convened in October 1994 to continue the effort of identifying obstacles to the delivery of pharmaceutical care and designing strategies to overcome them. This conference addressed obstacles in all venues of practice and took advantage of the emergence of models of pharmaceutical care practice in ambulatory, managed care, acute, and long-term institutional settings.

Two additional conferences, in 1999 and 2001, took additional steps to examine how pharmacy could make the transformation from product-centric to patient-centered practice. Again in 1999, the Joint Commission of Pharmacy Practitioners (JCPP) took the lead in convening a professionwide strategic planning conference. This conference attempted to broaden the input on how best to manage medication use in the U.S. health care system by inviting the disciplines of medicine and nursing, as well as representatives of the pharmaceutical industry, to join with pharmacy's leaders in these discussions. Conferees agreed that appropriate medication use requires a multidisciplinary model of care that keeps the patient at the center. Vastly improved information technology and redefined scopes of practice were other priorities defined by the twentieth century's last strategic planning conference related to pharmacy.

In late 2001, the Pharmacy Manpower Project convened a strategic conference with a very different purpose than the earlier ones. Identifying the professionally-determined need for pharmacists in the year 2020 was the goal of this October 2001 meeting. Using best-practice analysis, experts attempted to estimate how many pharmacists might be needed in each of four dimensions of contemporary practice: order processing, primary care (ambulatory), secondary and tertiary care (institutional), and nondirect patient care roles. Regardless of the absolute number of pharmacists projected, it became clear in the discussions that pharmacists in the future must assume additional responsibility for direct patient care and the management of medication use. Of interest in these discussions was the belief that, as the profession has evolved in education and practice, no other profession has proven itself as capable of serving as society's medication use specialist as the twenty-first century pharmacist.

A New Model of Medication-Use Management in an Information Age

Role of Professions

As Buerki and Vottero discussed in substantial detail in chapter 1, professions are sanctioned by a society to provide a service that members of the society can not provide for themselves. Supporting the profession's status are a specialized body of knowledge, recognition by licensure, an ethical code, internal controls, a professional culture, and a system of organization.

The clear articulation of exactly what contemporary problems the profession of pharmacy is sanctioned to address is therefore critical to its transformation. Also, it is insufficient for the pharmacy profession alone to identify these problems. The lay public, other professionals, and society itself must agree on pharmacy's societal purpose.

Until recently, the public had been led to believe that pharmaceuticals were highly safe and universally effective. Consumers believed that their physicians and the government were their allies, and advertisers lent credence to both these allies. Patients did not believe that the prescriptions physicians so readily wrote to cure diseases and ameliorate symptoms could cause any harm, and physicians believed that their patients were equipped with the knowledge needed to ensure proper drug use. The public thought that because of federal regulations demanding a long and expensive approval process that only safe and effective drugs reached the market. Advertising for the nonprescription drugs, which were available in almost a half-million retail establishments, lulled consumers into the belief that an arsenal of highly safe and very effective products was available to treat every ailment. The late 1990's flood of direct-to-consumer advertisements for prescription drugs added to this belief system. What need could society see for the druggist beyond conveniently, accurately, and efficiently packaging what the physician or another prescriber had directed?

Manasse[18] characterized that need in his examination of drug misadventuring, which is profiled in this book in chapter 6. Adverse drug reactions, suboptimal response to therapy, and unnecessary institutionalization are all examples of societal problems that compound our nation's health care emergency.

In 1995, in response to national efforts to reform the health care system by the Clinton administration, a variety of national organizations (AACP, American College of Clinical Pharmacy, Academy of Managed Care Pharmacy, ASHP, APhA, ASCP, National Pharmaceutical Association, and the Consumers League) established the Consumer Coalition for Access to Pharmaceutical Care. One outcome of that coalition was the support of a study by Johnson and Bootman[19] that put the cost of drug-related morbidity and mortality in the United States at $76 billion per year.

Yet public perception regarding the potential for adverse consequences to accompany the use of medications did not begin to change until two reports on the quality and safety of the U.S. health care system were released by the Institute of Medicine in 1999 and 2001. Entitled *To Err is Human: Building a Safer Health System* and *Crossing the Quality Chasm: A New Health System for the 21st Century*, these landmark reports branded in the public psyche the fact that consumers of health care should not take for granted the safety and quality of care.[20,21] Pharmacy benefitted from the prominence medication-use problems assumed, especially in the study of medical errors. The 1999 report gained unprecedented attention in the consumer press, because the committee generating the report expressed the potential for fatalities attributable to improper delivery and management of patient care services.

The inescapable conclusion from the Institute of Medicine, coupled with the growing cost of medications and the recognition that the cost of adverse medication events exceed $1 to 2 billion annually, positions pharmacy to answer the question of what society needs from pharmacists. However, is there evidence that the profession can deliver what society needs?

Pharmacists' Efforts to Intervene in the Drug-Use Process

As noted by Strand, Cipolle, and Morley,[22] much of the drug-use problem is not in the drugs themselves but rather in the way the drugs are prescribed, dispensed, and used. Strand et al. identified the major reasons why drug therapy goes awry.

- *An error is made in the drug therapy decision-making process.* A drug is prescribed when none is indicated; no drug is prescribed when one is indicated; or the wrong drug is prescribed.

- *The implementation of the therapeutic process is faulty.* The patient is not administered the drug because the drug isn't delivered to the patient care area; the patient doesn't pick up the drug at the pharmacy because the patient cannot afford the medication; or the pharmacist makes an error in the dispensing process.

- *Patient behavior is faulty.* The patient does not comply with therapy.

- *Monitoring fails.* Monitoring for compliance, therapeutic effect, or for adverse effects does not occur or is lax.

Several studies specifically examine the application of pharmaceutical care practice models in ambulatory care.[23] An examination of these studies reveals a diversity in approach and expected outcomes that is not surprising given the fact that pharmaceutical care as a concept is still relatively new to most practitioners and researchers. Outcomes research examining the scope of drug-related problems and the impact of interventions is needed in three key dimensions: clinical, economic, and humanistic outcomes.

Appendices 10.1 and 10.2 provide a brief description of how pharmacists in different settings have evolved patient-focused practices that indeed appear to improve patient outcomes, yield economic savings to patients and payers, and provide a more satisfying practice for pharmacists.

Is Pharmaceutical Care a Philosophy or a Practice?

As has been noted previously, Brodie[5] first called upon the profession to articulate a theory of practice in the mid-1960's and finally proposed a multiple-theory concept of pharmacy 25 years later. His theories recognize the need for a drug-use control system using the "knowledge, understanding, judgements, procedures, skills, controls, and ethics that assures optimal safety in the distribution and the use of medicines." They also encompass the interface between mankind and drugs and argue that pharmacy should be responsible for the outcomes of care, the promotion of health, and the prevention of disease.[11]

The remainder of this book examines in depth many aspects of pharmaceutical care delivery both in the United States and other countries. The inescapable conclusion is that redirecting the pharmacist's focus from drugs to patients and drawing the pharmacist's attention to the outcomes that drug therapy achieves in individuals are fundamental to the new practice of pharmacy. Failure to accept responsibility for helping patients to achieve optimal outcomes will limit the professional role of pharmacists in the future and perhaps even threaten the existence of this profession.

Is this shift, now broadly referred to as pharmaceutical care, a philosophy of practice or is it a new process for practicing an age-old profession? Clearly, it is both. It represents a fundamental change in perspective for practitioners, educators, and regulators, who must stop defining what pharmacists do in terms of drug products and begin associating it with the needs of the individual patient.

In order to make this change, however, a complete restructuring of the manner in which pharmacists practice is needed. Relinquishing direct control for drug distribution and entrusting this task to adequately trained technical personnel and automation (and perhaps another pharmacy) is an essential first part of the process of change. The caregiving portion of the pharmaceutical care process has been defined as "the pharmacist's workup of drug therapy (PWUDT)."[21] For this to be successful, pharmacists must establish a direct, caregiving relationship with the patients who trust them with the responsibility of managing medication use.

Redefining both the philosophy and practice models of a profession is a Herculean task, and leaders in the profession of pharmacy do not underestimate that fact. Evidence of this understanding can be found in their commitment to pharmaceutical care. This commitment is reflected in mission statements, study commission reports, conferences, and research materials that have been released during the last five years or so and universally supported by pharmacy practice organizations. An examination of this evidence and a review of work yet to be completed forms the remainder of this chapter.

The Response of the Profession

Mission Statements of Professional Organizations

In strategic planning, the mission statement defines the core business of an organization. Considering the challenge by Hepler to adopt pharmaceutical care as the new mission of pharmacy, it is not surprising that an outcome statement of the Pharmacy in the 21st Century Conference in 1989 was the call for the profession to articulate a new mission. Before that conference had even adjourned, one of the work groups presented a draft mission statement to the conferees.

Subsequently, a subgroup of JCPP began the process of drafting a mission statement for pharmacy. Finding common language acceptable to the leaders of such diverse groups of pharmacists as those represented at the JCPP table proved difficult, but ultimately consensus was reached on a relatively simple statement of pharmacy's mission which read, "The mission of pharmacy is to help patients make the best use of medications."

The boards and deliberative bodies of numerous national associations have adopted the JCPP mission statement and several have gone on to articulate, within their own organizations' strategic plans, missions that reflect their commitment to pharmaceutical care. Likewise, the results of state and regional strategic planning activities have universally demonstrated the broad commitment to this paradigm shift within the profession.

NABP Model State Pharmacy Practice Act

Licensure is one mechanism to distinguish a group of professionals from society at large. Pharmacy in this country has been licensed for more than a century through state boards of pharmacy. At the national level the boards are represented by NABP, which provides a uniform licensing exam used by almost all states, assists with reciprocity, and provides leadership on emerging issues confronted by the states as they strive to protect the public interest by regulating the practice of pharmacy.

A major effort was undertaken in the late 1980's and early 1990's to prepare an updated model state pharmacy act. NABP, with significant input from state boards and state and national practitioner organizations, released the model act in 1992 with model rules for many specific aspects of practice (e.g., nuclear/radiologic pharmacy, sterile practice, and continuing education).

The NABP model act included model rules for pharmaceutical care that establish minimum requirements for facilities, personnel, and practice. The inclusion in state law of language that at least acknowledges the pharmacist's responsibility to provide pharmaceutical care is one step toward establishing a new standard of practice.

Pharmacy Education and AACP Policy on Entry Degree in Pharmacy

A lack of emphasis on the patient in pharmacy curricula was previously noted as one of the impediments to improving the drug-use process and reducing patients' drug-related problems. Reference has also been made to the AACP Commission to Implement Change in Pharmaceutical Education, which issued five background papers. Pharmacy education's commitment to making the changes in education needed to support pharmaceutical care is clear.

A significant step towards making changes in education came in 1992 when the AACP House of Delegates adopted the recommendation of the Commission and supported curricular changes that include the institution of the doctor of pharmacy degree as the single, entry-level degree for the practice of pharmacy. As outlined in other background papers from the Commission, this degree would provide the patient focus, communication skills, and problem-solving ability so critical to pharmacists' ability to deliver pharmaceutical care. United in philosophy over the appropriate entry-level training model, pharmacy education leaders defined specific competencies for graduates and current practitioners; made curricular changes in both undergraduate and postgraduate training and education programs; and identified the human, fiscal, and clinical resources that will be needed to change pharmacy education.

ACPE Revised Standards and Guidelines

ACPE is charged with establishing standards and guidelines for pharmaceutical education and surveying schools and colleges of pharmacy to certify adherence to these standards. Periodically, ACPE undertakes a revision of its standards to ensure that they continue to produce graduates equipped to meet contemporary and future societal needs.

A revision of ACPE standards and guidelines began in 1989 with a declaration of intent to undertake such an action. Reflected in the declaration was the belief of the council that the new standards should recognize the doctor of pharmacy degree as the single entry-level degree for the practice of pharmacy. The initial draft of the standards and guidelines, which was subject to numerous open hearings at national meetings, also stated that schools and colleges of pharmacy should adopt the philosophy of pharmaceutical care as the framework for curricular design.

APhA White Paper on the Pharmacist's Role

The previously cited APhA white paper was commissioned by the APhA Board of Trustees and was directed to all pharmacists in the United States in an attempt to define pharmacy's mission in the twenty-first century and determine what the profession must do to achieve its goals. It was intended to both stimulate pharmacists' thinking and challenge their professional beliefs and practice behavior. It is considered a blueprint for action aimed at moving the profession toward new roles.

ASHP Statement on Pharmaceutical Care

ASHP issued a statement on pharmaceutical care, which was adopted by its House of Delegates in June 1993, with the purpose of assisting pharmacists in understanding pharmaceutical care, as such understanding must precede efforts to implement the concept.[24] The ASHP statement defined pharmaceutical care, articulated its principal elements, and examined its implications for pharmacists, patients, other providers, information systems, educators, and researchers.

Scope of Pharmacy Practice Project

Fundamental to defining the emerging roles for pharmacists as pharmaceutical care providers and to charting the course for achieving those roles is the question of what pharmacists and pharmacy technicians do today in their daily practices. A major study exploring the contemporary practice of pharmacy in all settings, the Scope of Pharmacy Practice Project, was completed in early 1994. The intent of the four national sponsoring organizations (AACP, APhA, ASHP, and NABP) is to use the outcomes of the study for a variety of credentialing activities, to understand better how pharmacists apply their knowledge and skills in the care of patients, and to see how technical personnel support those efforts.

Environments for Pharmaceutical Care

The nature of pharmaceutical care will vary according to the environment in which it is rendered. **Appendices 10.1, 10.2,** and **10.3** provide short analyses of pharmaceutical care in the community pharmacy, hospital pharmacy, and long-term care environments.

References

1. Maine LL. Pharmacy practice activity classification. *J Am Pharm Assoc.* 1998; 38:139–48.
2. Kremers L, Urdang J. History of pharmacy, 4th ed. Philadelphia, PA: Lippincott; 1976.
3. Christensen HC. Dr. Charters' commonwealth survey report. *J Am Pharm Assoc.* 1927; 16:351–3.
4. Elliott EC. The pharmaceutical survey, a resume. *Am J Pharm Ed.* 1949; 13:230-44.
5. Brodie DC. Drug-use control: keystone to pharmaceutical service. *Drug Intell.* 1967; 1:63–5.
6. Francke DE, et al. *Mirror to hospital pharmacy.* Washington, DC: American Society of Hospital Pharmacists; 1964.
7. What is the Dichter Institute saying about you? *J Am Pharm Assoc.* 1973; NS13(il):638–41.
8. Millis JS, et al. Pharmacists for the future: the report of the study commission on pharmacy. Ann Arbor: Health Administration Press; 1975.
9. Kalman SH, Schlegal JF. Standards of practice for the profession of pharmacy. *Am Pharm.* 1979; NS19:21–35.
10. Brodie DC. Need for a theoretical base for pharmacy practice. In: Harvey A. K. Whitney Award Lectures: 1950–1992. Bethesda: American Society of Hospital Pharmacists; 1980.
11. Brodie DC, McGhan WF, Lindon J. The theoretical base of pharmacy. *Am J Hosp Pharm.* 1991; 48:536–40.
12. Hepler CD. Pharmacy as a clinical profession. *Am J Hosp Pharm.* 1985; 42:1298–306.
13. Schwartz MA. Envisioning pharmacy's future: a further commentary on strategic planning. *Am J Pharm Ed.* 1990; 54 (Summer):1–8.

14. Bezold et al. 1985.
15. Cocolas GH. Proceedings of the pharmacy in the 21st century conference: executive summary. *Am J Pharm Ed.* Winter 1989; 53:1 S–5S.
16. AACP 1993.
17. American Pharmaceutical Association. APhA white paper: the role of the pharmacist in comprehensive medication use management. Washington, DC: American Pharmaceutical Association; 1992.
18. Manasse Jr. HR. Medication use in an imperfect world. Baltimore, MD: ASHP Research and Education Foundation; 1989.
19. Johnson JA, Bootman JL. Drug-related morbidity and mortality: a cost-of-illness model. *Arch Intern Med.* 1995; 155:1949–56.
20. Institute of Medicine. To err is human: building a safer health system. Washington, DC: National Academy Press; 1999.
21. Institute of Medicine. Crossing the quality chasm: a new health system for the 21st century. Washington, DC: National Academy Press; 2001.
22. Strand LM, Cipolle RJ, Morley PC. Pharmaceutical care: an introduction. Current Concepts. Kalamazoo: The Upjohn Company; 1992.
23. Michel NE. Projects study pharmaceutical care outcomes in ambulatory patients. *Am J Hosp Pharm.* 1993; 50:1524–7.
24. American Society of Hospital Pharmacists. ASHP statement on pharmaceutical care. *Am J Hosp Pharm.* 1993; 50:1720–3.

Appendix 10.1. Community and Ambulatory Care

Community Practice

Long heralded as the most accessible point for patients to meet a health care provider, the nation's 50,000 plus community pharmacies truly represent a paradox in the evolution of pharmaceutical care practice. Few people are more than a few miles from a pharmacy, whether free-standing, part of a mass merchandiser, in a grocery store, or in a medical office park. During each hour the pharmacy is open, each facility has some of the most highly trained health professionals and society's true medication specialist. Chronically ill patients may interact with pharmacy personnel on a monthly basis, if not more frequently than that.

To suggest that pharmaceutical care is the standard of care in this or virtually any other ambulatory care setting, however, would be wrong. Most pharmacists practicing in this setting spend the majority of their time involved with order fulfillment, third-party program management, and administration of the pharmacy department. However, the promise that they can do more, as suggested by the success of several research and demonstration projects, is encouraging.

What limits progress? Historically it is two primary factors: the fact that the community pharmacist is relatively isolated from other health care providers and the limitation in financial transactions for the delivery of services in community practice. More recently the increasing volume of prescriptions in a tight labor market for pharmacists has also limited practice change.

Throughout the decade of the 1990's, several important demonstration projects were undertaken that yielded evidence that when the practice of patient-focused care was cultivated in community settings great improvements in health status and cost of care were measured. In addition, in separate projects in Minnesota and Florida, Drs. Strand and Hepler made great contributions in establishing community-based pharmaceutical care practices.

What did these projects teach the profession about delivery of pharmaceutical care in community settings? First, the practice must support a coordinated relationship among the patient, the pharmacist, and the referring physician. Second, the ability of pharmacists to collect, assess, and use patient-specific monitoring information (e.g., blood sugar, cholesterol, A1C level) is essential for their monitoring and patient management. Third, the pharmacist must become the patient's coach and help the patient assume increasing responsibility for managing his or her own care. Finally, it is virtually impossible for the same pharmacist to deliver patient care and be directly involved in the order fulfillment process. They can certainly be provided in the same environment but they must be separated in terms of personnel.

Ambulatory Care

There are other exciting ambulatory care practice models, including those at fully integrated health systems (e.g., Kaiser Permanente, Veterans Administration), and more and more pharmacists are finding practice opportunities in physicians' practices. Fully utilizing the knowledge, skills, and abilities of clinical pharmacists in primary care is essential for quality medication use now and in the future.

Appendix 10.2. Pharmaceutical Care Practice in Hospitals: Present and Future

Hospital pharmacists have long been leaders in providing services to patients and colleagues. This began with the implementation of unit-dose medication distribution and continues to evolve into a highly patient-centered, team care approach to improve a patient's health. Milestones along the way have been clinical pharmacy initiatives (e.g., therapeutic drug monitoring), pharmaceutical care initiatives (e.g., identification of drug therapy problems), and the newest practice that combines the best of both models and expands the profession into a holistic and integrated model of patient care.

Many pharmacist-led patient centered programs have been initiated in response to regulations promulgated by such entities as NCQA and JCAHO. The latter has been a major force in demanding change in the practice of hospital pharmacy, and indeed to the inpatient health care system as a whole. Although not all of the regulations have paid direct patient care dividends, the overall system is safer and of a more predictable quality since the review standard changes that were made in the late 1980's.

The problem that has plagued hospital pharmacist patient care is the episodic nature of the interaction with the patient; most prominently the inpatient. With inpatient hospital stays averaging around four days, there is little time to adequately assess and implement a care plan with a patient. It is quite likely that the patient will leave the hospital to the care of a primary physician or physicians and not be seen again by the hospital pharmacist. No followup is obtained from the practitioner(s), nor does the pharmacist typically initiate any followup.

The future of hospital pharmacy practice is truly one of integration. Hospitals continue to buy physician practices and link them through a common computer system that is more complete than the billing systems that have characterized hospitals in the past. Computer systems now can link clinical care (e.g., lab and radiology test results online) with physician office records and scheduling and billing data. Although pharmacy modules are still not fully integrated into many platforms, some progress is being made. Before too long, all patient information will be accessible by hand-held, wireless technology from anywhere within a health system. This will allow pharmacists to promote appropriate therapeutic choices, monitor and revise therapy in "real" time, develop innovative strategies to improve persistence and compliance with medications, and have all of this data available across the health care system. Interactions with community-based pharmacists will lead to a seamless system of care that will protect the patient and provide optimal outcomes. Outcomes will then be measured and reported, and a true assessment of quality practice (and possibly comparisons of system quality) can be performed.

Appendix 10.3. Pharmaceutical Care for the Elderly in Long-Term Care

One of the developed world's most striking trends is the aging of its population. In the United States this phenomenon is widely recognized as the aging of the baby boomer cohort; the group of post-World War II children whose travel through each age of development redefined the way sociologists, policymakers, and others characterized society. It is widely believed that the impact of this group on aging, retirement, and health care for the elderly will be no different. From the perspective of health care services and medication use, the aging of the baby boomers should have an extraordinary impact on the need for pharmaceutical care services.

The vulnerability to medication-use problems of those 65 and older is a widely appreciated aspect of both health care and aging. The federal government recognized this in regulation over 30 years ago when writing quality assurance guidelines for the nation's nursing home population. Regular retrospective drug regimen reviews provided by pharmacists, monthly for those needing the highest level of skilled nursing care and less frequently for others, became a requirement for payment from such federal programs as Medicaid. A new cadre of pharmacists known as consultant pharmacists emerged to meet this defined need for medication control in nursing homes.

During the 1990's, consultant pharmacists began to critically examine the delivery of patient care services in nursing homes and other long-term care environments. The leaders in the area were not convinced that monthly retrospective reviews that were too frequently ignored by the patient's physician or other health care providers was the most effective model of medication management. An ambitious effort known as the Fleetwood Projects was undertaken by the American Society of Consultant Pharmacists Foundation to redefine individualized pharmaceutical care for elderly patients taking multiple chronic medications.

The Fleetwood Project had three phases. Phase I served to quantify the cost of medication-related problems in the nursing home population. Significant opportunities for quality improvement and cost savings were identified. Phase II identified which subgroups of nursing home patients were most at risk of medication-related problems and hence the target for a different model of pharmacist intervention. The project further articulated what the shift from a retrospective to a prospective model of pharmacist service would entail and tested the delivery of such service in a limited population of at-risk patients.

Prospective pharmaceutical care in the long-term care setting finds pharmacists increasingly involved in patient assessment, designing pharmaceutical care plans, identifying the need for and making clinical interventions to improve medication use, having direct interaction with nursing home residents and their family members, and experiencing increased collaboration with the interdisciplinary patient care team. Initial results from testing this model yield evidence of improvements in patient status and overall increases in satisfaction with pharmacy services from other participants in the patient care process.

Phase III of the Fleetwood Project was funded by the Commonwealth Fund in 2001 and is designed to implement and evaluate the prospective pharmaceutical services model in an intervention and control group design during 2002. The results will add another significant piece of evidence of how pharmaceutical care improves overall health quality and decreases avoidable medication-related problems.

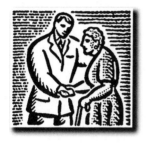

Chapter 11: Marketing Pharmaceutical Care

Orsula Voltis Thomas, Pharm.D., M.B.A.

Calvin H. Knowlton, R.Ph., M.Div., Ph.D.

Introduction

Consumers know little about the concept of pharmaceutical care. Patients rarely consider the extent to which a pharmacist's assessment, evaluation, medication management care planning, and monitoring can optimize their pharmacotherapy outcomes. Patients are usually unaware of the benefits of pharmaceutical care. Pharmaceutical care is of little concern to health insurance payers and is largely unknown by patients' primary care providers. The lack of universal provision and standards for pharmaceutical care has posed barriers to the diffusion of these services and to its widespread acceptance in the United States.

As pharmacogenomics replaces the "one-medicine-fits-all" approach with an "appropriate medication for this particular patient, first time" approach, pharmacists will have more opportunities to incorporate the features and benefits of pharmacogenomics into pharmaceutical care.[1]

Upon completion of this chapter, the reader will have an understanding of the following concepts:

- The concept of marketing,
- The traditional military language of marketing,
- The difference between marketing and sales,
- The usefulness of market research,
- The importance of communicating product features and benefits,
- The notion of branding,
- The opportunity that pharmacogenomics presents for pharmacists, and
- The importance of marketing for the future of pharmaceutical care.

What Is Marketing?

There are many ways to define marketing. Phil Kotler,[2] a lead authority on marketing,

197

characterizes it as, "A social and managerial process by which individuals and groups obtain what they need and want through creating, offering, and exchanging products of value with others." Marketing is the action taken to elicit a desired response from a particular group or audience.

Defining Needs, Wants, and Demands

Human needs are the essentials of life, such as food and clothing. Wants are specific items that will meet an expressed need, such as a particular brand (e.g., Campbell's or Banana Republic). A demand, however, requires both a desire for a specific product or service and a willingness to pay. Marketers can influence demands by satisfying people's wants and needs.[2]

In pharmacy, one may consider access to medication a basic societal need. Accurately dispensed prescriptions may meet society's desire to receive the expected prescribed medication. Pharmaceutical care can meet the desire for safe, effective, and appropriate medication use. The job of marketing is to induce the demand for pharmaceutical care, and to assess the societal value for cost-effective pharmacotherapy care that ensures optimized pharmacotherapy endpoints (clinical markers) and outcomes (effects on quality of life) in the health care system.

Value and Satisfaction

Differentiating amongst various service and product offerings is based upon the ability of the offering to provide value and satisfaction to customers. Value is the ability of the product to meet the need at a favorable price. Satisfaction is the pleasure, fulfillment, and contentment a customer feels as a result of the purchase.

An example of this is the willingness of patients not only to pay for diabetes management services of pharmacists but also to find pleasure in the knowledge gained and positive health outcomes as a result of the service provided.

Exchange

An exchange occurs when at least two parties provide each other with something of value. This is commonly considered a value creation process because the exchange usually provides greater value to each party as a result. A medication care plan, created and monitored by a pharmacist, can save thousands of dollars in direct and indirect medication costs to payers, and can allow patients to have improved functionality and quality of life. If the patient paid $50, and the entire process took the pharmacist 10 minutes, then the monetary value was greater than the actual monetary exchange for both parties.

Relationships and Networks

Relationships and networks are created as a result of working to continually meet the needs of clients. Networks are partnerships of stakeholders in a defined market. Network presence usually results from being in a market for long periods of time, building trust with clients, learning the synergy amongst stakeholders, and creating strategic alliances. One can achieve network presence by, for instance, serving on the boards of local and national organizations of a specific disease market. Relationship building and networking can be the basis for company growth strategies. These concepts are the foundation for relationship marketing.

Markets, Marketing, and Prospects

A market exists when various potential customers have the same particular need or want and are willing to pay for a solution that will satisfy that need or want.[2] The size of the market is the number of potential clients that have a willingness to pay for goods or services. Marketing is the activity within a market geared toward actualizing an exchange.[2]

Attributes of Market-Oriented Businesses

Organizations that are market oriented, or market driven, understand the factors that influence market behavior and the buying influences of market decision-makers.[3] Understanding the market is the responsibility of not only the marketing and sales departments but also the departments of finance, quality, operations, human resources, and administration. Employees of a market-oriented company should be knowledgeable about the market they are in, regardless of their positions within the organization.

A successful organization's product offering is determined by the needs of the market. When needs assessment or market research is disseminated throughout the organization, opportunities can be identified using the various perspectives of the people in the organization who do not work in marketing and new business development.

Equally important is the ability of the operations department and others to participate in the decision-making process of the type of customer with whom the organization would like to do business.[3] When customer selection does not incorporate the influence of operations, operational teams may be reactive to the needs and desires of customers instead of proactive by focusing on the desired product mix offering.

Removing barriers amidst departments facilitates incorporation of the expertise of specialists within an organization. Departments that are unable to work together often cannot meet the expectations set by marketing or sales. The ability of a department to influence strategic decisions also provides the opportunity to get the "buy-in" needed for successful implementation.

Departmental cooperation on implementing a marketing program is important for successful execution. Including those responsible for implementing the plan in the planning process fosters mutual collaboration and enhanced communication. An execution plan crafted by a single department can cause coworkers in other functional units to regard themselves as unimportant and to feel negatively toward new ideas or processes.

Successful organizations attempt to embrace shared communication. The marketing teams that respect the needs of other departments find it easier to successfully focus on and meet the changing needs of competitive markets.[3]

Traditional Steps in the Marketing Process

According to Kotler, there are five basic steps in the marketing process: (1) researching a market opportunity, (2) targeting segments of that market in a superior way, (3) creating the 'marketing mix' that will differentiate the product and position it for success, (4) implementing the marketing strategy, and (5) evaluating feedback and results, and adjust the plan as part of the strategic process.

Although pharmaceutical care has been formally defined as a method of pharmacy and adopted as a practice, no one has yet taken the steps to market it. Using the steps listed above, one can determine how pharmaceutical care is doing in regards to marketing.

- *Researching a marketing opportunity.* Many articles point to the fact that a significant number of people suffer and die as a result of drug-related problems.

- *Targeting segments of the market in a superior way.* Many segments have been targeted, such as the elderly, those with chronic disease, preventative medicine, insurance payers at risk, etc.

- *Creating a marketing mix.* A consistent message touting the benefits of pharmaceutical care is not being relayed to the target market segments—an inconsistent message can be more detrimental than no message at all.

- *Implementing the marketing strategy.* Planning a marketing strategy and implementing the tactical plan to targeted markets includes defining the strategy, outlining the tactics and timeline, and estimating a budget. A tactical plan may include syndicated newspaper articles in specific target market publications or the sampling of pharmaceutical care services at designated locations.

- *Evaluating feedback and results.* Although it is difficult to assess when and how often to measure the outcome of marketing strategies and tactics, it is important to do this to ensure that the marketing team's efforts are effective and that budgeted dollars are being well spent. It also provides a means to update or change marketing and tactics based on results.

Whether pharmacists are perceived as having the professional expertise that allows them to be the sole providers of this service is questionable. Payers often feel that they are already paying for these services through physicians and nurses. They may even have the expectation that pharmaceutical care should be provided as part of the dispensing fee for the product. The profession could benefit from writing, executing, implementing, and evaluating a marketing program for pharmaceutical care.

The Marketing Mix: The Four Ps and Cs of Marketing Pharmaceutical Care Services

The four Ps are the basic components of the marketing process. Simply stated, when designing a marketing strategy, the following factors need to be considered in implementation and budget planning: product, price, promotion, and place.[4]

Some argue that the four Ps represent the seller's point of view and not the client's or buyer's perspective. When considering the buyer's perspective, each marketing tool must be designed to deliver a customer benefit. These are referred to as the four Cs.[5]

As with the four Ps, the four Cs must also be consistent when designing a marketing plan. The four Cs consist of the following: customer needs and wants, cost, convenience, and communication. **Table 11.1** shows how a marketing plan for pharmaceutical care might take into account the four Ps and four Cs.

Table 11.1. The Four Ps and Four Cs in Relation to Pharmaceutical Care

Four Ps	Example	Four Cs
Product	Pharmaceutical care	Customer needs and wants
Price	$100/hour	Cost
Place	In pharmacies throughout the country or telephonically	Convenience
Promotion	Through alliances with medication safety programs	Communication

Adapted from reference 2.

The Marketing Planning Process

Typically, company leadership develops the strategic mission and vision. Each department within the organization (marketing, sales, performance, human resources, finance) then creates its own strategic plan to carry out the vision and mission of the corporation.

In marketing, the strategic business unit for each product or service must have a strategic tactical plan to meet the business plan goals of the organization. These plans are used to create a roadmap for the marketing team, direction for the sales team, and a framework for the marketing budget.

Marketing plans are typically written annually, but they are generally outdated soon after being printed. This occurs when the outcomes of marketing programs cause a change in the strategy.

A comprehensive marketing plan includes a definition of the market, identification of competitors in the market, risks to the organization based on changes that may take place in the future (e.g., political unrest, change in Medicare reimbursement, vendor influences), identification of the product offering including a "SWOT" analysis (evaluation of offering Strengths, Weaknesses, Opportunities, and Threats), distribution channels, marketing strategies and tactics, timelines, and evaluation tools. User-friendly software programs are available to assist organizations in creating marketing plans.

Marketing Strategy: Using Military Warfare Concepts in Business

Many military warfare strategies can effectively be applied to business strategy. One could argue that business/marketing strategies are dissimilar from strategies used in warfare since human lives are not at stake; however, people who do not receive pharmaceutical care are at risk, and our profession should indeed "take arms" to promote pharmaceutical care.

The pharmaceutical battles that pharmacists face daily are caused by rapid change, disruptive events, small windows of opportunity, lack of available data, and the overall sense of urgency to "fix" the health care system. Pharmacists' enemies include opinion-based medicine (as opposed to evidence based) and medication misadventures.

Military commanders can teach pharmaceutical care providers that outmaneuvering the enemy can overcome the challenge of the rapidly changing combat environment.[6] The focus is not on overpowering rivals but on targeting their weaknesses.

How does one apply warfare strategies and tactics to marketing pharmaceutical care? The argument against pharmaceutical care is that no one will pay for it and, therefore, it has no value. Thus, to market pharmaceutical care the value created as a result of the product or service must be clearly presented.

Pharmaceutical Care Warfare Marching Orders: Identify the Enemies' "Achilles Heels"

- Exploit the reality—Medication costs have consistently increased by 15–20% over the last few years, but prescription benefits managers market the "savings" that result from the use of prescription card formulary systems.

- Target critical vulnerabilities of competitors—Other health care providers lack the education and experience of a clinical pharmacist.

- Take risks and use the element of surprise to achieve sizable results—Participate in research or studies showing the value of pharmaceutical care.

- Focus resources at critical points in the process. Identify and take advantage of available opportunities while allowing individual "troops" to make real-time decisions in the field.

- Deploy and implement plans quickly.

- Partner with others to combine arms when synergistic returns are greater than those realized individually—Align with other health care providers with access to patients or information not available otherwise.

Carefully calculated business strategies can outflank pharmaceutical care competitors in the marketplace and allow pharmacists to overcome barriers to the provision of pharmaceutical care and enemies of the practice. Understanding key concepts of marketing strategies and tactics is one way to overcome these challenges. The use of military jargon seems to get the emotive juices flowing.

Marketing versus Sales

Marketing is the process of listening to, researching, and responding to the wants and needs of clients whose ideas can provide greater efficiency, cost savings, and satisfaction for a company's product and service offerings. Marketing begins prior to product conception and continues through the life of the product, assessing performance and finding new product applications.[7]

Marketing is not selling, although it is part of any successful sales process.[8] The focus of marketing is to identify a client's wants and needs. Marketing teams must discover precisely what people (potential consumers) are thinking. Marketing cannot be confined to just one department—the job of everyone in the organization is to meet and exceed customer expectations.

Selling is the process of inducing the demand for products or services. Selling begins when the product comes off the manufacturing line. Whereas marketing is getting into the minds of current and potential clients, selling is getting into their wallets (**Table 11.2**).

Table 11.2. The Marketing-Focused versus Sales-Focused Organization

Marketing Focus	Selling Focus
Customer's wants and needs emphasis	Product/service emphasis
Wants and needs considered in the creation of new products and services	Make the product first and figure out how to sell it
Management is profit-oriented	Management is sales volume-oriented
Planning is long-term	Planning is short-term
Business stresses wants of buyers	Business stresses needs of sellers

Adapted from Stanton WJ, Futrell C. Fundamentals of marketing, 8th ed. McGraw-Hill; 1987:11–2.

The Importance of Market Research

The reality of business is that many entrepreneurs follow their gut instincts, even in the midst of data that is unfavorable to the product or service. However, conducting market research is an essential step in the new product development process for marketing and sales success. First, it is important to assess for which unmet needs or problems the product or service can be positioned as a solution. Simply communicating the features and benefits of the firm's products or service offerings without first finding out the value of such for the client will prevent an organization from fully understanding and achieving its own potential.

Market research can be outlined as a five-step process[2]:

1. defining the problem and research objectives,
2. developing the research plan,
3. collecting the information,
4. analyzing the information, and
5. presenting the findings.

Focus groups are the most popular tool in marketing research.[9] Over 5,000 research organizations conduct focus groups. Focus groups are particularly useful during the exploration process, where little is known about the topic of interest.[10] In the market research process, focus groups are considered to be a starting point from which to assess the perception of the product or service offerings by various stakeholders (**Table 11.3**). Though, like any research tool, the data from focus groups has limitations. These include the semblance of qualitative data, as well as the inaccurate representation of the general population.

**Table 11.3. Common Goals of a Focus Group Meeting—
a Quantitative Market Research Tool[10]**

- Obtaining general background information about a topic of interest;
- Generating research hypotheses that can be subjected to further research and testing using more quantitative approaches;
- Stimulating new ideas and creative concepts;
- Diagnosing the potential problems with a new program, service, or product;
- Generating impressions of products, programs, services, institutions, or other objects of interest;
- Learning how respondents talk about the phenomenon of interest—this can be useful in designing materials like survey questionnaires, etc.; and
- Interpreting, confirming previously obtained quantitative results.

Focus groups can also be used to confirm or discount beliefs held within an organization regarding their product, service, or the success/failure of a marketing campaign. Unlike clinical research, market research is usually limited in size.

Market research may result in the creation of tools to assist in the marketing and selling of products and services. It may also show that it is too early or too late to enter a market. Although costly, market research can save an organization a significant amount of money by ensuring that the product or service will be positioned appropriately for the market in which it is intended. The research may also provide evidence of applications for products in different market segments.

Features and Benefits

It is important to promote product and service features and benefits. An example of a product feature is the patient information leaflet that is included with a newly dispensed medication. This feature is a benefit to the patient because it includes access to information about the medication, gives the patient the ability to review and plan for potential medication problems (and thus precludes the need to stop a medication—e.g., constipation with opioid pain medications), and serves as a reference should the patient think he or she is experiencing an untoward side effect. **Appendix 11.1** contains more examples of benefits delivered by pharmaceutical care.

The Importance of Product Branding

Managing a brand successfully is the key to attracting and keeping customers. Brands are not just logos, slogans, or trademarks. A brand is a distinctive identity that differentiates a relevant, enduring, and credible promise of value associated with a product, service, or organization—and indicates the source of that promise.[11] Successful brand identities can command premium pricing and profitability. Consumers are not only buying a product or service when they choose a brand; they are counting on the added value that only that specific brand can bring.

The Opportunity Presented by Pharmacogenomics in the Pharmaceutical Care Process

Many wonder why a particular medication can be used in one patient effectively while being ineffective or the proximal cause of an adverse effect in another. Most likely, it has less to do with environmental factors than with genes that modulate the effect of medications in the body. Marketing pharmaceutical care will assuredly embrace the emerging tool of pharmacogenomics.

The discipline known as pharmacogenomics is defined as the understanding of the relationship between variances in DNA resulting in changes in the response to medication therapies. Variances from a reference DNA are known as polymorphisms. These polymorphisms are what change the way most drugs work for us.[12] Pharmacogenomics is a growing field aimed at assessing the genetic basis for differences in drug efficacy and toxicity, and it uses genome-wide approaches to identify the network of genes that govern an individual's response to drug therapy.

The Human Genome Project has mapped all 30,000 genes, made up of 3 billion base pairs. Humans are 99.9% the same. The variations occur in 1 of each 300 base pairs (or, 1 in every 2,000 genes), which result in differences in proteins and their functions. These changes make some of us, for instance, poor metabolizers of certain medications.

So far, scientists know that there are more than 25 drug-metabolizing enzymes, more than 7 drug transporters, and more than 25 forms of drug receptors (i.e., about 60 different areas) where genetic differences can affect the action of medication differently per individual.[13,14]

The ultimate goal of pharmacogenomics is to "define the contributions of genetic differences in drug disposition or drug targets to drug response, thereby to improve the safety and efficacy of drug therapy through use of genetically guided, individualized treatment."[15] The vast amount of new data emerging from the human genome projects, including the genetic determinants of drug responses and effects, is rapidly being understood. This new data is being translated into more rational drug therapy.

The opinion-based, shotgun approach to medication management used today does not account for interindividual differences in human DNA. Adverse drug reactions could be preventable, with knowledge of a patient's genetic predisposition to such an event. Pharmacogenomics will bridge the gap in knowledge about which medication will be most appropriate in a particular person by identifying those people who should be treated; those who should not be treated because of their propensity for an adverse event or lack of response; and those who need a modified dose based on the severity of the polymorphism.[12] As a result, pharmacogenomics will bring a new level of safety and effectiveness to the medication-use process. It may well become the cardinal tool in pharmaceutical care.

Predisposition to toxicity can occur for a number of reasons, including an inherited deficiency in drug metabolism, or a receptor mutation in the target tissue. In theory and in practice, with individual genomic data, the subset of patients who are identified to be at risk for an adverse event or for no response at all would be treated with different dosages or alternative medications.

The study of pharmacogenomics started about 20 years ago with the cloning of the gene that metabolizes codeine to morphine, debrisoquin hydroxylase, also known as CYP2D6. In some patients, a lack of this enzyme prevents the conversion of codeine to morphine, rendering codeine therapy ineffective in this subset of patients. In the United States, it is estimated that 10% of the population do not have CYP2D6, which precludes the activation of morphine and results in zero analgesic response. In addition to this 10%, another 25-30% have one good copy of the gene and one bad copy, requiring a dosage adjustment for optimal effect (**Figure 11.1**).

Codeine is just one example. Others medications are shown in **Table 11.4**.[12]

Table 11.4. Examples of Medication-Related Clinical Consequences as a Result of Polymorphism in Genes

Medication Class	Clinical Consequences of Polymorphism in Genes
ACE inhibitors	Cough
ß2-Blockers	Desensitization, CV effects
ß2-blockers	Antihypertensive effect
Heparin	Thrombocytopenia
Aspirin	Antiplatelet effect
Sulfonylurea	Insulin release
Thioridazine, Haloperidol	Tardive dyskinisa, akathisia, and response to therapy
Levodopa and DPA	Hallucinations
Antidepressants*	Response to therapy

*(e.g., clomipramine, fluoxetine, paroxetine, fluvoxamine)

There is a way to prevent adverse patient outcomes due to medication therapy: knowing which patients should not use a medication or which patients are genetically predisposed to requiring a higher or lower dose for the desired effect. Incorporating pharmacogenomic information into the pharmaceutical care process would ensure the safe and appropriate use of medications in the majority of patients. Pharmacogenomics will improve the pharmaceutical care process.

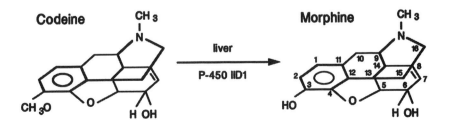

Figure 11.1. Metabolism of Codeine to Morphine.

The Importance of Marketing Pharmaceutical Care

There is a growing body of knowledge regarding the need for pharmaceutical care as a part of the health care delivery process (see, especially, chapter 6). There are three conditions that can be considered market opportunities: (1) a product or service is in short supply, (2) an existing product or service that is superior to that which exists can be supplied, and (3) a new product or service can be supplied.

All three conditions are applicable to society today regarding pharmaceutical care services. Using the ECHO model,[16] which focuses on Economic, Clinical, and Humanistic Outcomes, pharmaceutical care can be marketed and positioned as a superior product to the medication management systems that exist today.

Identifying the market opportunity for pharmaceutical care means finding the consumer in need of pharmaceutical care services and creating a way to meet the need. Wherever a need exists, an opportunity exists. Marketers of pharmaceutical care must first identify a group whose pharmacotherapy outcome needs have not yet been met or are less than desirable. As with many professional services, consumers may not realize just how unsatisfied they are with current medication management. Educating consumers about the risks or problems with prescription medications, without providing additional pharmaceutical care services, can force unmet needs to surface as unmet wants or desires, inducing a demand for pharmaceutical care.

Even so, one of the greatest challenges faced by companies that market pharmaceutical care is the absence of a standard model for compensation of pharmaceutical care services. Although pharmaceutical care has been recognized as having monetary value, a standard and widely accepted model for reimbursement (such as the fee-for-service model for physicians) does not exist. Thus, there is an opportunity to align payment for pharmaceutical care with that of other stakeholders, i.e., those who are paying for it.

Two options for compensation of pharmaceutical care exist: (1) the capitated shared-risk model for a mix of patients with diverse needs and (2) the per-diem model in a group of patients at equal risk. A model incorporating both of these options can combine the cost of medications with pharmaceutical care services or can bill medications under the traditional Average Wholesale Price model plus capitation or per diem for pharmaceutical care services. The former is more effective at lowering overall pharmaceutical care costs, since the pharmaceutical care provider is "at risk" for the cost of medications. Data are emerging to show that pharmaceutical care services reduce the cost of medication while enhancing the quality of care.

It is easy to see the difference between incentives in the fee-for-service and incentives in the per-diem model in a patient using multiple inhalers and oral medications for the treatment and symptom management of asthma. In a fee-for-service model, the pharmacy is only paid for the product, and not for the outcome of the patient. The pharmacist's economic incentive is to dispense medication. Considering that the poor management of asthma and misuse of medications (e.g., ineffective inhaler administration) benefits the pharmacist who is paid for product dispensing, this incentive structure is illogical.

In the per-diem model, payment to the pharmacist is a fixed dollar amount that is independent of product use. Thus, the pharmacist has an incentive to ensure successful achievement of patient endpoints (adherence to medication, symptom control) and outcomes (patient functionality), and not merely to dispense more medication. The pharmacist may choose to invest in activities that ensure positive outcomes, such as patient education and monitoring.

The Value Proposition of Pharmaceutical Care for Society

In order to position pharmaceutical care as a strong brand, one must identify a strong position in the minds of buyers. This position is termed a value proposition—a compelling reason for the buyer to purchase the offering.

To create a value proposition, a broad position must be established, followed by a specific focused position.[7] For example, pharmaceutical care has a broad position of being "essential for one's health"; its specific position could be that, when provided by competent pharmacists, patients have the best health performance outcomes. Once these positions have been established, the value positioning or price can be set. There are five value positions to consider[7]:

- More for more—higher price to cover higher costs
- More for the same—higher quality for the same price
- Same for less—consistent quality for lower price
- Less for much less—downscaled version of the offering at a lower price
- More for less—what everyone wants and typically is offered by those with the greatest buying power: largest selection, lowest price

A buyer will only decide to make the purchase if the total value proposition considers all of the features and benefits of the service.

Average pharmaceutical spending from 1994–1999 was 12.8% of health care expenditures, which is only slightly higher than 1987–1994 of 11.9%. During the former dates, drug expenditures were due in equal parts to the direct effects of increased prices and utilization growth. Yet, during the latter years, 80% of the growth was due to increase in utilization. Berndt[17] explains that the reasons for this change in type of growth are that

- Pharmaceuticals are a modest share of health care spending and have registered as a high ticket market sector for cost-containment strategies;
- The dramatic growth of third-party prescription coverage. Since 1997, 46% of spending on average is from growth in new drug product innovations;
- Successful new product innovations produced by the pharmaceutical industry;
- Pharmaceutical firms' success in technology transfer and marketing efforts. The amount of dollars spent on marketing compared to sales is 12.3% in contract to Intel, 5.8% and Revlon, 24%. Direct-to-consumer advertising for pharmaceuticals was $1.8 billion in 1999, up 40% from 1998.

IMS Health estimates that pharmaceutical companies spent $13.9 billion on marketing.[18] The pharmaceutical industry will likely continue to increase marketing efforts as consumer demand for information increases and marketing rivalries among products become fierce as they try to differentiate themselves.

Pharmaceutical care brings the value proposition of bridging the gap between medication cost-effectiveness and pharmacotherapy outcomes. The ensuing result would be the needed balance between the pharmaceutical industry's marketing prowess and appropriate, rational, cost-effective use of medications.

The value proposition of pharmaceutical care is more for much less. Direct medication costs can be lowered and costly adverse outcomes can be avoided, while the quality of life for stakeholders including payers, patients, and providers of pharmaceutical care is enhanced.

Conclusion

Inducing consumer demand is crucial for pharmaceutical care to be considered an essential part of the health care delivery system in the United States. The need for pharmaceutical care to ensure safe and appropriate medication use has been established. The benefits of pharmaceutical care are clear. Inducing the demand for it is the next step in the marketing process.

Organizations that effectively market pharmaceutical care can be successful. Pharmaceutical care models exist that align payment incentives to ensure optimal and appropriate medication use. Stakeholders in models where payment incentives are aligned are highly satisfied. The role of marketing in pharmaceutical care is to differentiate the value that these services can bring. By showing the economic, clinical, and humanistic outcomes created for patients, payers, and other health care providers, marketers can induce the demand for pharmaceutical care.

As Dick Penna[19] described in his acceptance speech of the Remington Honor Medal, stakeholders, including pharmacy associations, have not made the investment needed in marketing to change attitude and behaviors that would induce the demand for pharmaceutical care in our society. Until patients recognize the benefits for pharmaceutical care and a system for payment that ensures appropriate compensation is in place, our profession is at risk for losing the battle against medication misadventures and poor health outcomes.

Acknowledgement

The authors wish to acknowledge Jena Salon of excelleRx, Inc. for her editorial expertise and comments.

References

1. Robertson JA, Brody B, Buchanan A et al. Pharmacogenetic challenges for the healthcare system. *Health Affairs.* 2002; 21(4):155–67.
2. Kotler P. Marketing management: analysis, planning, implementation and control, 9th ed. Prentice Hall, NJ: Simon & Schuster; 1997.
3. Shapiro B. What the hell is 'market oriented'? *Harvard Business Review.* 1988; 66:199–25.
4. McCarthy E. Basic marketing: a managerial tool, 12 ed. Homewood, IL: Irwin; 1996.
5. Lautenborn R. "New marketing litany: 4P's passe; C words take over." *Advertising Age.* October 1, 1990:26.

6. Clemons EK, Santamaria JA. Maneuver warfare: can modern military strategy lead you to victory? *Harvard Business Review.* April 2002:57–65.

7. Kotler P. Kotler on marketing: how to create, win, and dominate markets. New York: The Free Press; 1999.

8. Allessandra T, Barrera R. Collaborative selling: how to gain competitive advantage in sales. New York: John Wiley & Sons; 1993.

9. Clancy K, Krieg P. Counter-intuitive marketing: achieving great results using uncommon sense. New York: The Free Press; 2000.

10. Stewart DW, Shamadasani PN. Focus group theory and practice. Applied social and research method series, vol. 20. Newbury Park: Sage Publications; 1990.

11. Ward S, Light L, Goldstine J. What high-tech managers need to know about brands. *Harvard Business Review.* 1999; 4:85–95.

12. Evans WE, Johnson JA. Pharmacogenomics: the inherited basis for interindividual differences in drug response. *Annu. Rev. Genomics Hum. Genet.* 2001; 2:9–39.

13. Evans WE, Relling MV. Pharmacogenomics: translating functional genomics into rational therapeutics. *Science.* 1999; 286:487–91.

14. Evans WE, Johnson JA. Pharmacogenomics: the inherited basis for interindividual differences in drug response. *Annu. Rev. Genomics Hum. Genet.* 2001; 2:9–39.

15. McLeod HL, Evans WE. Pharmacogenomics: unlocking the human genome for better drug therapy. *Annu. Rev. Pharmacol. Toxicol.* 2001; 41:101–21.

16. Kozma CM, Redder CE, Schultz RM. Economic, clinical and humanistic outcomes: a planning model for pharmacoeconomic research. *Clin Therapeu.* 1993; 15:1121–32.

17. Berndt ER. The U.S. pharmaceutical industry: why major growth in times of cost containment? *Health Affairs.* 2000; 20:100–14.

18. Data from IMS Health as reported in Pharmaceutical Industry Profile; 2000:figure 5–7.

19. Penna RP. Views from a woerk in pharmacy's vineyard. Remington lecture, American Pharmaceutical Association Annual Meeting. Philadelphia, PA: March 17, 2002.

Appendix 11.1. Features and Benefits of Pharmaceutical Care Exercise

Features	Benefits
Clinically Trained Pharmacists	Medication experts that understand the importance of your health care goals and desired outcomes
Consultation with Prescribers	When your doctor is unaware of a problem with a medication, our pharmacists take the time to ensure your safety when it comes to medications

Review of Medication Profile	Expert review of your profile reduces your risk of having drug–drug interactions, drug–food interactions that can cause medical problems, or even death
Customized Medication Care Plan	Even the best selling medications are not for everyone. By evaluating your medical history, we can customize your medication profile to ensure optimal pharmacotherapy outcomes (i.e., provide what is appropriate for you)
Personalized Follow-up Monitoring Plan	Lifestyle considerations are important in creating a monitoring plan that is easy to follow and ensures your safety. Monitoring your medication outcomes can reduce your risk of adverse drug effects and unplanned doctor and emergency room visits. In addition, you can be ensured that the goals of therapy are being met
Automated Medication Dispensing	Automated dispensing reduces the chance of an error that can cause pain and suffering
Refill Reminders	Increases adherence to the medication regimen ensuring positive pharmacotherapy outcomes
Direct Delivery	Saves time and money, ensures patient confidentiality
Ensure Optimized Pharmacotherapy Outcomes	Significant return on investment for payers increasing profitability and patient satisfaction
Web site access	Provides access to information and other support tools when you need them, thereby increasing the efficiency of the health care process

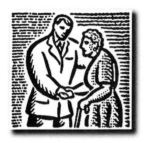

Chapter 12: Practice Changes Facilitated by Pharmaceutical Care

Brian J. Isetts, Ph.D., B.C.P.S., F.A.Ph.A.

Bernard J. McKone, Dip.Pharm, M.Pharm, F.N.Z.C.P., F.P.S.

"The best way to predict the future is to invent it."
Alan Kay (conceiver of the laptop computer)

Overview

The purpose of this chapter is to describe and discuss changes in the way pharmacists care for patients as a result of pharmaceutical care. Pharmaceutical care is a measured and predictable response to any drug-related need that a patient may have. This consistent and systematic process helps patients achieve desired therapeutic outcomes while avoiding or minimizing the adverse consequences of taking medications. Equipped with a standard process for helping a patient with any drug-related need, pharmacists can take comfort in knowing that when a patient needs help they will know exactly what process to use to help that patient. In this sense, pharmacists truly can predict the future because the future of pharmacy has been invented through the implementation of pharmaceutical care practices.

Introduction

In order to discuss practice changes attributable to the advent of pharmaceutical care, it is important to first define what constitutes a health care practice. Pharmacists have previously defined a practice on the basis of a set of daily professional activities. All other health care practices have time-honored rules in place describing the essential elements of those health care practices. A practice may be viewed as the application of knowledge, guided by a commonly held social purpose, to the resolution of specific problems, in a standard manner accepted and recognized by society. Reference textbooks and articles describing the details of caring for patients within a pharmaceutical care practice are available elsewhere.[1-4]

To present a discussion of pharmacy practice changes facilitated by pharmaceutical care, it will help to briefly review a few important aspects of a pharmaceutical care practice. Pharmacists have found that an understanding of the practice components and characteristics of a pharmaceutical care practice provides them with a clear target or goal for working towards advancing practice and improving the care delivered to patients.

Pharmacists have long been rated highly by the public in terms of honesty, integrity, and ethical standards.[5] Communities throughout America generally view pharmacists as a middle-class profession and have counted on pharmacists to be a reliable source of health care information. Although the importance of pharmacists to their respective communities is rarely disputed, a patient's description of what a pharmacist actually *does* can vary widely.

All other health professions fulfill a unique contribution to society and have a care process that is identifiable by patients. Dentists care for a patient's dental needs and conduct an oral examination using a standard process.[6] Physicians care for a patient's medical needs and engage in a standard differential diagnostic process to develop a patient's medical problem list.[7] Similarly, pharmaceutical care is helping pharmacists care for a patient's drug-related needs through the use of a consistent and systematic patient care process.

As discussed earlier in this book the profession of pharmacy is witnessing a paradigm shift toward caring for people and for the outcomes of their medication use. For the last 25 years the profession of pharmacy has sought to define a pharmacist's unique contributions to society. In his 1980 Harvey A.K. Whitney Lecture Award address, Brodie[8] called for establishing a theoretical base for pharmacy practice. Brodie predicted that as the theoretical base took form it would clarify the social purpose of pharmacy and provide the basis for new ideological concepts about the relationship between the profession and society.

Problems in the medication-use process became increasingly evident. Manasse developed the term "drug misadventuring" through an extensive literature search of the less than desirable consequences of medication use.[9] Johnson and Bootman[10] later described the alarmingly high magnitude of drug-related morbidity and mortality. Evidence continued to mount on the nature and extent of medication-use complications.[11-15] One prominent report compared and contrasted the current medication-use system to that of the air traffic control system.[16] The preeminent physician and author Lucian Leape has noted that if the air traffic control system were designed in a manner similar to our medication-use system results could be expected to be routinely catastrophic.

In 1988 Strand and colleagues[17] culminated 10 years of work by describing a systematic problem-solving process applied to the use of medications. Other health care professions use a systematic problem-solving process to meet a patient's health care needs, but there was no such process applied to the use of medications in place. The Pharmacist's Workup of Drug Therapy was developed as a way to describe the cognitive thought process for identifying, resolving, and preventing problems patients encounter in the medication-use process. In 1990 the landmark article, "Opportunities and Responsibilities in Pharmaceutical Care," described the theoretical constructs necessary for a pharmacist to assume responsibility for a patient's drug therapy outcomes. This article set the foundation for the development of a new professional practice, as there was no individual or profession responsible for ensuring that patients achieve desired, positive therapeutic goals while avoiding or minimizing the adverse consequences of medication use.[18]

Within the philosophy of pharmaceutical care, the unique social need that pharmacists fulfill is minimizing or avoiding drug-related morbidity and mortality. Clarifying this social purpose provides the basis for defining the scope and domain of a pharmaceutical care practice. The scope and domain of pharmaceutical care provide the context for defining how pharmacists can address a problem better and more systematically than other individuals or professions. The scope of pharmaceutical care is drug therapy problems, and the domain is the practice in which a practitioner assumes responsibility for all of a patient's drug-related needs and is held accountable for this commitment.

Brief Description of the Practice

Having a consistent problem-solving process to identify, resolve, and prevent drug therapy problems is important but can't be applied if there is not a system in place to support the delivery of this service. The three components of a pharmaceutical care practice are the philosophy, patient care process, and the practice management system. The philosophy of practice includes meeting a unique social need, having a patient-centered approach, caring for a patient through a therapeutic relationship, and having clearly defined patient care responsibilities.

As part of any redesigned medication use system there must be an individual or profession responsible for all of a patient's drug therapy outcomes. Acknowledging this patient care responsibility provides an opportunity for discussing the integration of generalists and specialists in pharmacy. In a redesigned medication-use system, there will need to be practitioners with a primary care focus who can account for all of a patient's drug-related needs and for specialist practitioners who can fulfill drug-related needs that are beyond the expertise of a primary care or generalist practitioner.

The patient care process describes what actually happens between the practitioner and the patient when pharmaceutical care is provided. First, the practitioner conducts an assessment for the purpose of ensuring that (1) all of the patient's drug therapy is indicated and that all conditions are appropriately treated and (2) the patient's drug therapies are effective, safe, and convenient and drug therapy problems are identified. A care plan is designed outlining the practitioner's and the patient's activities and responsibilities for achieving intended therapeutic goals and for resolving and preventing drug therapy problems. Then, a follow-up evaluation is scheduled to determine progress toward achieving desired therapeutic goals and to determine if the patient has any new drug-related needs. The purpose of defining a common patient care process is to accomplish patient care objectives, not to constrain decisions of individual practitioners. Within a given profession, practitioners may execute the standard patient care process slightly differently.

The practice management system is the underlying organizational framework to support a practice. This includes an organization's mission statement, description of resources needed to provide the service, system for evaluating progress toward meeting goals and objectives, and reward mechanism. The reward mechanism includes compensation systems necessary for financial stability.

The most important piece of the practice management system is the practice management plan. A practice management plan guides daily decisions and activities and holds the organization accountable. A practice management plan contains four key elements: a clear description of the service provided, a list of resources required to deliver the service, a practice evaluation process, and a revenue stream. A sample practice management plan is presented in **Table 12.1** so that the reader may obtain an appreciation of the steps in

Table 12.1. Sample Pharmaceutical Care Practice Management Plan[a]

(For an ambulatory pharmacy located in a primary care clinic)

PRACTICE PLAN/ MISSION	1 MONTH	3 MONTHS	6 MONTHS	12 MONTHS
Service Provided	1) Assess all the patient's drug-related needs in a systematic and comprehensive manner for the purpose of achieving all therapeutic goals and to identify drug therapy problems 2) Develop a care plan for the patient to achieve goals of therapy and resolve and prevent drug therapy problems 3) Evaluate the actual patient outcomes and status	Continue same service mission	Continue same service mission	Continue same service mission
Patients Receiving Care	Patients in the ACME Insurance Plan demonstration project	1) ACME Plan patients 2) Patients from Pediatric Asthma Clinic	1) ACME Plan patients 2) Pediatric Asthma Clinic patients 3) Senior living facility patient appointments	1) ACME Plan patients 2) Pediatric Asthma Clinic patients 3) Senior living facility patients 4) General clinic referrals
Number of Patients	One new patient per day (M–F)	Two new patients per day plus follow-up evaluations	Three new patients per day plus follow-up evaluations	Four new patients per day plus follow-up evaluations
Growth Schedule for Practice	15–20 total patients in active care plans	75 patients in care plans	200 patients in care plans	500 patients in active care plans

PRACTICE PLAN/ RESOURCES	1 MONTH	3 MONTHS	6 MONTHS	12 MONTHS
Personnel/Time	1) One pharmaceutical care practitioner at 0.5 FTE 2) One support technician at 0.2 FTE	1) One practitioner at 0.75 FTE 2) One support technician at 0.25 FTE	1) Two practitioners at 0.75 FTE 2) One support technician at 0.5 FTE	1) Two practitioners at 1.0 FTE 2) One support technician at 0.5 FTE	1) Two practitioners at 1.5 FTE 2) One support technician at 0.75 FTE
Physical Plant	1) Modify patient consultation area in pharmacy 2) Assist clinic in preparing the old cast room for pharmaceutical care appointments	1) Add pictures and posters to consult area 2) Install data port to clinic exam room 3) Install file cabinets	1) Install interactive web-based kiosk 2) Schedule patient appt's in clinic room	Continue minor improvements on both patient interaction areas
Educational Resources	Update reference textbooks	Add medical library Internet access	Obtain CD-ROM reference materials	Attend international pharmaceutical care retreat in Auckland, NZ
Documentation	Use paper charts for first 10 patients	Utilize Microsoft Access to construct a patient database	Purchase pharmaceutical care software program	Link interactive kiosk to documentation system and patient home internet
Financial Goals				
Costs	$1,500 per month	$2,000 per month	$3,000 per month	$4,000 per month
Revenues	$250 per month	$500 per month	$2,000 per month	Start five-year business plan
Savings	Individual patient savings documented on paper	Prepare drug therapy problem database	Submit info to Univ for start of econ study	Start pharmacoeconomic study in ACME University analysis

Table 12.1. Sample Pharmaceutical Care Practice Management Plan[a] (cont.)

(For an ambulatory pharmacy located in a primary care clinic)

PRACTICE PLAN/ EVALUATION	1 MONTH	3 MONTHS	6 MONTHS	12 MONTHS
Patient Care	1) Review total number of drug therapy problems identified 2) Establish a patient advisory panel to discuss program impressions 3) Keep track of number of patients achieving desired therapeutic goals	1) Monthly practitioner case presentations focusing on common drug therapy problems 2) Develop patient satisfaction survey items with advisory panel 3) Compare number of goals achieved at initial and follow-up appts	1) Utilize monthly case presentations by practitioners to determine level of congruence with selected clinical practice guidelines 2) Administer patient satisfaction survey	1) Conduct independent, blinded practitioner reviews of cases to obtain feedback on patient feedback in relation to the care that has been documented 2) Utilize evening dinner meeting sponsored by local pharmaceutical company to launch post-marketing surveillance initiative
Practice	1) Review the number of patients receiving pharmaceutical care 2) Keep track of the most commonly encountered medical conditions in patients receiving pharmaceutical care 3) Implement an accounts receivable system for introductory program payments	1) Compare patient enrollment goals to actual number of patients in care plans 2) Collect practitioner productivity statistics 3) Reconcile accounts receivable	1) Analyze process flow between clinic and pharmacy 2) Determine expansion opportunities for third-party reimbursement demonstration projects	1) Compare actual numbers of patients in care plans to program goals 2) Discuss patient satisfaction survey results 3) Compare actual revenues to initial program revenue goals 4) Commence five-year business plan based on revised program revenue goals

[a]Reprinted, with permission, from the American College of Clinical Pharmacy. Issetts B. Pharmaceutical Care. In: Mueller BA, Bertch KE, Dunsworth, TS et al., eds. Pharmacotherapy Self-Assessment Program, 4th ed. The Science and Practice of Pharmacotherapy 1 Module. Kansas City, MO: AACP; 2002:166–7.

building a practice.[19] This appreciation will provide insight into how innovative pharmacists have used the principles of pharmaceutical care to advance practice.

Specific Practice Changes and New Opportunities

From a consumer perspective, pharmaceutical care is a new and emerging concept. The general public is witnessing dramatic change in the way pharmacists are functioning in society within a relatively short period of time. However, discussions with elders about experiences they have had with their family apothecary often lead to the recollection of a care component strikingly similar to the philosophical underpinning of pharmaceutical care as a covenantal relationship between a patient and a pharmacist. The industrial era gave rise to a significant number of pharmacists fulfilling dual roles as "druggists" and retail merchants. Up until the mid-1960's pharmacists were precluded by the American Pharmaceutical Association–Code of Ethics from informing the patient of the name of the medication, much less the intended actions and side effects. Then, the consumerism movement prompted patients to begin questioning authority relative to the medications that they were putting into their bodies.

The lack of a theoretical base clarifying the social purpose of pharmacy and a profession sometimes fragmented into differentiated academic degrees with practices defined by the location, commercial enterprise, or by a drug and disease focus of interest are also factors affecting public recognition of pharmacists' unique social contributions. This may explain why it has been difficult for some patients to identify a standard care process used by pharmacists for the application of drug therapy knowledge to the resolution of drug therapy problems. Public recognition of a defined social purpose for the profession of pharmacy may be as important to the implementation of pharmaceutical care, and to the rate of practice change, as are realigned payment incentives.

In order to characterize the development of pharmaceutical care practices, it is important to analyze the interrelated conditions, or environment, in which pharmaceutical care exists. Systems must be in place in the medication-use process that account for both acts of commission (i.e., prescribing, dispensing, and medication administration errors) and acts of omission (i.e., the absence of any individual or profession responsible for patient medication outcomes). When a system is analyzed for both what is and what is not being done to help patients achieve desired therapeutic outcomes and avoid undesirable consequences, the context of pharmaceutical care can then be described as a systematic failure related to the use of medications. A central focus of this chapter is the effect that a new medication-use system, which includes an individual (i.e., a pharmaceutical care practitioner) responsible for medication outcomes, can have on a patient.

The following sections highlight practice changes that occur when pharmacists apply the principles of pharmaceutical care by focusing on the care patients receive in the most common settings. With little variation, practitioners who practice pharmaceutical care daily are those individuals who have accepted responsibility for what happens to patients when they take medications, who have assimilated the consistent and systematic patient care process into daily professional activities, and who have secured compensation for the delivery of these services. This transformation is an evolutionary process that takes time. It is sometimes helpful for pharmacists to view the journey toward providing complete and comprehensive pharmaceutical care services as moving up a pharmacy practice ladder. Viewed in this manner, the practice management plan presented in Table 12.1 contains discrete steps in the ladder so that pharmacists can know exactly where they are in practice transition.

Impact on Patients in the Hospital Setting

Experiences of clinical pharmacists have been important to the development of pharmaceutical care by helping the profession of pharmacy move one step closer to providing patient-specific care and addressing all of a patient's drug-related needs. There is a notable difference in role delineation between early clinical pharmacy pioneers and current pharmaceutical care practitioners. The role of early clinical pharmacists was to serve the physician, typically for a pharmacokinetic consult or some other one-time, limited focus consultation, as opposed to establishing their own practice. Although the services provided to patients through these limited focus consultations had a significant impact on those patients, only a very small percentage of patients received assistance from these services. Nevertheless, the services delivered by clinical pharmacists helped to develop new practice opportunities because these services began sensitizing patients, physicians, and other health care providers to the value of having pharmacists work toward improving a patient's drug therapy outcomes.

Similar to other segments of the profession, hospital pharmacists are striving to shift the focus of frontline practice from one practice model to another. As discussed in an earlier chapter, this means shifting from the old model of dispensing a drug product accurately to a patient to the new model of helping a patient make the best use of medicines. Although this new professional direction has been embraced throughout pharmacy, there was some initial variability in the way pharmacists provided pharmaceutical care. To help reduce this variability, the pharmacy organization that represents the largest number of hospital pharmacists developed guidelines on a standard method for providing pharmaceutical care.[20]

Although justifying the implementation of, and compensation for, pharmaceutical care services in hospitals might require rigorous economic analysis it may actually be patient safety that compels society to demand these services. A study published in 1998 estimated that 106,000 hospitalized U.S. patients experience fatal adverse drug reactions each year.[15] This figure ranks as the fifth leading cause of death in the United States.

As increasing numbers of patients experience medication-use complications and realize that this is not an inevitable or acceptable consequence of health care, the public clamor for answers and solutions can be expected to intensify. Patient medication safety has been the driving force for many significant health care advances, such as the 1937 elixir sulfanilamide tragedy (safety requirements of the FD&C Act), the European thalidomide experience (safety and effectiveness requirements of the1962 Kefhauver Drug Amendments), and the incidence of adverse drug events in nursing homes (1972 consultant pharmacists' law).[21]

Evidence continues to mount regarding pharmacists' contributions to improving drug therapy outcomes and reducing drug-related morbidity and mortality. A few noteworthy findings include pharmacist review of medication orders in the intensive care unit prevents errors, and pharmacist consultation reduces drug costs[22]; hospitals with pharmacists stationed on the medical wards (i.e., decentralized pharmacists) have a 45% decrease in medication errors and a 94% decrease in medication errors that adversely affect patient care outcomes[23]; and for every $1 invested in clinical services provided by pharmacists, approximately $17 is returned in the form of health care system cost savings.[24]

There have also been efforts to study and coordinate patient care responsibilities of pharmacists working in hospitals and other institutions and to develop continuity of care initiatives between the institutional and ambulatory sectors. One study evaluating systems for exchanging patient information among hospital, long-term care (LTC), and ambulatory pharmacies was conducted in a small mid-western city. It was reported in this study that hospital and ambulatory care pharmacists documented more interventions when information was supplied to the pharmacist (experimental group) compared with a group of patients for whom no information had been supplied.[25] The amount of time that a patient spends in a hospital is relatively short and the coordination of patient care responsibilities among pharmaceutical care practitioners across practice settings is of great importance.

Hospital pharmacists are in a unique position to utilize the standard patient care process by virtue of access to a patient's hospital records and proximity to other health care professionals providing care to the patient in the hospital. Pharmacists functioning in acute care settings have developed the skill of using the observations of family members, nursing staff, and other health care providers to determine a patient's drug-related needs. The implications for patients in the hospital setting related to the provision of pharmaceutical care include decreased medication errors, improved effectiveness of administered medications, better continuity of care between care settings, and the creation of "fail-safe" systems that place responsibility for what happens to patients in the medication-use process squarely on the shoulders of a pharmacist functioning at the patient's bedside.

Impact on Patients in the Long-Term-Care Setting

Experiences of consultant pharmacists functioning in long-term-care facilities (e.g., nursing homes) have been important to the development of pharmaceutical care practices. Consultant pharmacists have provided solutions to medication-use problems occurring in the LTC setting. Noteworthy is recognition by federal legislators that pharmacists are required for the appropriate use of medications in these settings.

Consultant pharmacists are in a unique position to provide pharmaceutical care by virtue of access to the patient and the patient's medical records and because of repeated follow-up visits that provide the opportunity for evaluation of actual patient outcomes. When patients present with significant physical disabilities or cognitive impairment, consultant pharmacists utilize the observations of family members, nursing staff, and other health care providers to determine a patient's drug-related needs—a skill developed through necessity by acute care pharmacists in the hospital setting. It is interesting to note that, in the study regarding exchange of information between pharmacists in different patient care settings, there were no differences observed in the rate of documentation of interventions when information was supplied to the LTC pharmacist following patient discharge from the hospital (experimental group) compared with a group of patients for whom no information had been supplied to the LTC pharmacist.[25] This observation can be explained by the fact that LTC pharmacists routinely receive information about patients discharged from the hospital so the information supplied to them in this study was already available to the LTC pharmacist.

It has been found that for every dollar spent on drugs in nursing facilities at least an additional $1.33 is consumed in the treatment of drug-related morbidity and mortality.[26] The American Society of Consultant Pharmacists has been a leading proponent in helping consultant pharmacists fulfill the social purpose of identifying, resolving, and preventing drug therapy problems in nursing home patients. A significant aspect of a consultant pharmacist's responsibility in the nursing home is to conduct drug regimen reviews for the purpose of ensuring that all drug therapies are appropriately indicated, effective, safe, and conveniently administered. When actual or potential drug therapy problems are identified, consultant pharmacists work in collaboration with physicians and nursing home staff to resolve and prevent these problems. Physicians and nursing home staff accept more than two-thirds of consultant pharmacists' recommendations regarding solutions for resolving and preventing drug therapy problems.[27]

Demonstrating improved therapeutic outcomes attributable to the care delivered by consultant pharmacists represents the third phase of the three-phase Fleetwood project. The Fleetwood project has used a comprehensive approach to examine patient outcomes and the cost of drug therapy problems. Researchers conducting this project believe that consultant pharmacists can improve outcomes significantly and save billions of dollars annually by avoiding many drug therapy problems for elderly patients.

Knowing the actual outcomes in patients receiving medications represents the accountability of pharmaceutical care. This focus on ascertaining the actual outcomes of drug therapy has profound implications on the care patients receive and on the future of the profession. The anticipated benefits of knowing the actual outcomes of drug therapy will be discussed at greater length in the section of this chapter on new patient care opportunities facilitated by pharmaceutical care.

Impact on Patients in the Ambulatory Care Environment

Pharmacists who see patients in a clinic examination room benefit from having access to the patient and the patient's medical record; community pharmacists benefit from exposure to large numbers of patients who frequent the pharmacy to obtain new and refill prescriptions. It is common for patients with pharmaceutical care plans to have a chart that complements their medical records.

One of the first attempts to translate the theory of pharmaceutical care into practice occurred in 1992. Practitioners working in 20 community pharmacies throughout Minnesota participated, as co-investigators, in a demonstration project to help determine what pharmaceutical care would look like in practice. The work of all types of pharmacists providing care to patients in a myriad of clinical settings was used to help Minnesota Project pharmacists formulate these practices. A key ingredient missing from previous experiences of pharmacists functioning in clinical pharmacy positions was the description of a consistent and systematic process of care to guide pharmacists in the delivery of pharmaceutical care.

There were numerous locations where pharmacists embarked upon efforts to translate the theory of pharmaceutical care into practice. A few other noteworthy projects that have helped shape the practice of pharmaceutical care today have been conducted in locations such as Iowa, Virginia, Washington, Florida, Mississippi, Wisconsin, Canada, New Zealand, and the Indian Health Service and Veteran's Affairs health care facilities, just to name a few. The value of these pharmaceutical care initiatives resides in developing a mounting body of evidence supporting pharmacists' contributions to improving patient clinical, humanistic, and economic outcomes of drug therapy and in reducing drug-related morbidity and mortality.

The need for integration of services and collaboration with a patient's primary care team is an important challenge being overcome by pharmacists functioning in the ambulatory care setting. An unpublished finding of the Minnesota Project was that patients with pharmaceutical care plans had more physician office visits during the study than they had before the project, according to third-party payer claims data. In retrospect, it was noted that few of the pharmaceutical care sites were integrated with patients' primary care clinics. Therefore, when drug therapy problems were identified, patients commonly returned to their primary care clinic to resolve these problems because the mechanisms for collaboration between the physician and pharmacist were not in place. Collaboration among patients, pharmacists, and physicians has been demonstrated to be an effective means of helping patients achieve desired therapeutic goals.[28,29] Today, laws enabling collaborative drug therapy management agreements have been enacted in approximately two-thirds of the United States (see **Figure 12.1**).

Innovative community pharmacy practitioners have found it helpful to redesign their patient care areas and professional policies and procedures in order to create a care environment similar to that experienced when patients visit other health care professionals. When patients see that pharmacists provide care in a manner consistent with social norms and that pharmacists are working in collaboration with other primary care providers, patient payment and demand for these services increases.[a]

Pharmacists working in clinics have access to patient medical records and to other primary health care providers. One of their biggest challenges has been the constraint of a billing system based on the provision of discrete physician procedures, rather than on the achievement of desirable patient outcomes. It is anticipated that this billing constraint may be alleviated as health care payment incentives focus on achieving actual patient outcomes. Some clinic practitioners have started building complete and comprehensive pharmaceutical care practices using limited funding available through programs designed to improve outcomes in patients who have specific medical conditions such as diabetes, atrial fibrillation, or dyslipidemia. Results from one such practice show that patients and providers have saved more than $172,000 in preventable hospital stays, emergency room visits, and office appointments.[b]

Impact on Patients Receiving Home Health Care and Hospice Care Services

Patients increasingly select health care treatment options that defer or avoid institutionalization. As larger numbers of patients seek to avoid institutional health care encounters, there is a subsequent increase in the number of patients who are taking complex medication regimens at home. Pharmacists who care for patients in these settings benefit from using a common care process designed to ensure that all therapies are appropriately indicated, effective, safe, and convenient for the patient to take. The opportunity to receive as many health care services as possible in the comfort of the home is desirable for many patients.

COLLABORATIVE PRACTICE AGREEMENT FOR THE PROVISION OF PHARMACEUTICAL CARE

This collaborative practice agreement is established for pharmaceutical care provided to patients in Fairview Clinics and Pharmacies. This agreement has been facilitated by the 1999 revisions in the Pharmacy Practice Act, Minnesota State Statutes 151.21 related to the establishment of Collaborative Practice Agreements in the State of Minnesota.

Specially trained pharmacists holding the distinction of "Certified Pharmaceutical Care Practitioners" are authorized to provide pharmaceutical care to patients in Fairview Clinics and Pharmacies. Evidence of this distinction includes successful completion of a 120-hour, 8-week, 50-patient certificate preparation program administered by the Peters Institute of Pharmaceutical Care at the University of Minnesota.

Pharmaceutical care is defined as, "a practice in which the practitioner takes responsibility for all of a patient's drug-related needs and is held accountable for this commitment." Pharmaceutical care practitioners meet with patients to systematically review all of the patient's drug-related needs for the purpose of ensuring that all therapies in use by the patient have an appropriate medical indication, are as effective as possible, are as safe as possible, and are convenient to use. A care plan is then established to meet mutually agreed upon goals of therapy, and to resolve or prevent any drug therapy problems that may interfere with a desired, positive patient (therapeutic) outcome. Periodic, scheduled follow-up evaluations are then established between the patient and the pharmaceutical care practitioner for the purpose of documenting actual therapeutic outcomes.

This agreement is established on this ＿＿ day of ＿＿＿＿＿＿＿＿＿ in the year ＿＿＿＿ between the physician and pharmacist listed below.

＿＿＿＿＿＿＿＿＿＿＿＿＿＿＿＿

A. Physician, M.D.,

Fairview Oxboro Clinic

＿＿＿＿＿＿＿＿＿＿＿＿＿＿＿＿

A. Pharmacist, R.Ph., B.C.P.S., C.P.C.

Fairview Dept. of Pharmaceutical Care

Figure 12.1. Pharmaceutical Care Collaborative Practice Agreement.

Impact on Patients in Other Countries

Pharmaceutical care has universal appeal because drug-related morbidity and mortality knows no boundaries. The consistent and systematic process of providing pharmaceutical care holds true without regard to the language spoken. Similar to the process dentists throughout the world use to start their oral examination, pharmaceutical care practitioners in other countries use the same process to commence the assessment of a patient's drug-related needs. Pharmacists in at least 24 countries are prepared to deliver pharmaceutical care.[c] The implementation of pharmaceutical care in New Zealand is an example.

A group of pharmacists in New Zealand, working in conjunction with the Pharmaceutical Society of New Zealand (PSNZ), expressed a keen interest in pharmaceutical care shortly after the landmark paper published by Hepler and Strand[18] in 1990. The PSNZ invited individuals such as Strand, Hepler, Knowlton, Isetts, and others to make presentations and conduct workshops at national conferences held throughout New Zealand. In 1994 the PSNZ adopted quality standards for the practice of comprehensive pharmaceutical care (CPC) and appointed a national training manager. A group of New Zealand pharmacists also toured the United States extensively during this time to meet with practitioners, educators, and payers. The implementation of pharmaceutical care in New Zealand was guided by the lessons learned from lively international exchange of ideas and concepts, combined with a number of unique innovations developed through the work of the PSNZ.

During one of the visits to New Zealand, a study was conducted to determine if pharmaceutical care implementation rates could be accelerated with an on-site, collegial visit from an established pharmaceutical care practitioner shortly after pharmacists completed formal CPC training. Isetts and McKone made extended visits to 10 New Zealand pharmacies whose staff had received pharmaceutical care training. Collegial visits included guidance on executing the site's management plan and conducting collaborative patient work-ups. Sites were selected for collegial visits based on travel convenience from a pool of approximately 50 sites. Ten other sites, whose staff had received pharmaceutical care training but did not have a post-training collegial visit, were selected for comparison. The group of 10 sites without a collegial visit had similar demographic characteristics, such as location, size, and prescription volume, as the 10 collegial visit sites. One month after collegial visits, the total number of completed patient work-ups and total number of drug therapy problems identified were compared. Pharmacists at the 10 collegial visit sites completed six times as many patient workups (137 versus 22) and identified six times as many drug therapy problems (233 versus 36) as their counterparts who did not receive a collegial visit.[30] This study highlighted the need for the profession to undertake more work at the local pharmacy level to support and nurture this developing practice.

Another significant practitioner training innovation occurred in 1999 with a memorandum of understanding between the New Zealand College of Pharmacists and the PSNZ creating a mechanism for the college to train all postgraduate pharmacists in CPC. As of January 2002, 10% of pharmacists on the professional register (574 of 3831 pharmacists) had been trained. This includes fourth year pharmacy students undertaking the CPC component of their training, thereby exempting them from that part of the CPC training offered to pharmacists. This initiative means that all graduates have been introduced to CPC training, and they can continue to seek accreditation once they are registered.

An important compensation development relates to a possible relationship between the numbers (or critical mass) of pharmacists actually practicing pharmaceutical care and compensation. In tandem with training offered by the pharmaceutical society and the college, the Pharmacy Guild of New Zealand successfully negotiated government remuneration for prescription review services undertaken by pharmacists. Approximately 5% of New Zealand's community pharmacist workforce are actively practicing CPC. The number of pharmacists actually providing pharmaceutical care has been cited as a reason that the government in that country was encouraged to fund the process.[31] This funding was achieved by separating funding from a previously profitable dispensing remuneration into a fund for cognitive services.

As further pressure has come on remuneration for dispensing, this move has protected pharmacists' ability to seek remuneration for prescription reviews, which forms an initial stage of the CPC process. The opportunity then exists for pharmacists to continue CPC with those patients, following through on drug-related needs exposed during the initial review. In addition, the New Zealand government's Clinical Training Agency recognized CPC as vital for pharmacists and provided a one-time grant of $250,000 to the New Zealand College of Pharmacists to further the CPC training of pharmacists.

Web-Based Phamacy and Cyber Space Implications

Establishment of a therapeutic relationship between the practitioner and the patient stands as a central tenet of pharmaceutical care. But does this mean that all pharmaceutical care encounters need to be conducted face-to-face with the patient and the practitioner sitting in close physical proximity to one another? The answer to this rhetorical question is no. Each patient will seek a certain comfort level or balance between conveniences offered through technological advances (high-tech) and the need for personal human interaction (high-touch). It is envisioned that high speed internet connections, visual telephones, tele-medicine/tele-pharmacy, and the use of home laboratory monitoring devices may allow the patient to use his or her own den or kitchen table as a setting for receiving virtual health care services.

Future Directions and
New Patient Care Opportunites

Pharmacists who will be caring for patients over the next 15–20 years may be wondering what to expect as pharmaceutical care practices continue to grow and expand. Pharmaceutical care practices can be expected to continue growing by contributing to the social purpose of achieving desired therapeutic outcomes while minimizing or avoiding drug-related morbidity and mortality. A prominent national Institute of Medicine report pointed out the need for fundamental changes in the American health care delivery system.[32] There is a gap, or chasm, between the health care that we have and the care we *could* have. Pharmaceutical care would help to fulfill at least nine of the 13 recommendations advanced by the high-profile expert panel charged with developing the evidence to support recommendations for fundamental change in health care delivery.

Pharmacists will have job descriptions with a decreasing emphasis on the physical aspects of dispensing medications, although a pharmacist will most likely remain responsible for making sure that dispensing systems are functioning correctly and that the patient receives the correct medications. New dispensing systems will incorporate the use of robotics, machines, certified pharmacy technicians, and the decentralized or off-site dispensing of medications. The development of new, targeted medication delivery systems may further decrease the emphasis on pharmacists dispensing medication.

Pharmacy manpower issues can be expected to change over time as well. Historically, the profession of pharmacy has witnessed the ebb and flow from manpower shortage to surplus. Economic forces may come into play as employers, patients, and payers realize that greater accuracy and productivity in the distribution of medications will occur if a one-half million dollar machine is used to dispense medications rather than paying five pharmacists $100,000 each in annual salaries and benefits. It's possible that the pharmacist shortage noted in 2002 may actually accelerate society's demand for redesigning medication-use systems that both improve medication dispensing accuracy and efficiency and help patients achieve drug therapy treatment goals that minimize or avoid drug therapy problems.

Consumer demand for pharmaceutical care can be expected to increase as more patients encounter, and benefit from, this service—but this will take time. For the last 50 years a large segment of the profession has relied upon the business of dispensing medications to support pharmacists' livelihood. The last two generations of society have an indelible image of pharmacists as "pill counters," rather than the caring apothecary of previous generations. The future of pharmacy depends on pharmacists making an investment in providing pharmaceutical care. For society to recognize that there is a solution to the health care crisis of drug-related morbidity and mortality, there must be an ample number of pharmaceutical care practices in existence. Witness the New Zealand government's willingness to pay for medication reviews when a critical mass (i.e., 5%) of pharmaceutical care practitioners was reached. Consumer demand for, and public recognition of, pharmaceutical care must be present before pharmacists will be routinely compensated for pharmaceutical care services.

Future health care payment systems may also include patient incentives to actively collaborate with pharmaceutical care practitioners and other providers to achieve desirable drug therapy treatment goals. Results from the Asheville, North Carolina project and from Project ImPACT: Hyperlipidemia demonstrate that when consumers actively collaborate with pharmacists and other health care providers to attain mutually-desirable treatment goals there are substantial effects on clinical, economic, and humanistic outcomes.[29,30] It is foreseeable that a consumer health care credentialing system will emerge. Such a credentialing system would be based on a patient's active participation in meeting treatment goals with financial incentives provided to patients and providers by managed care organizations for achieving these goals.

The pharmaceutical manufacturing industry also will have an impact on the provision of pharmaceutical care services in the future. In the early 1990's some industry executives viewed pharmaceutical care skeptically as there were fears that this would introduce another layer of decision-making, potentially doubling promotion and marketing expenses. The manufacturing industry has repeatedly stated that drugs are the most cost-effective therapy available to patients. This is true if the medication therapy is appropriately indicated, effective, safe, and convenient for the patient to use. It is recognized that the most expensive medication is not the one with the highest acquisition cost but rather the one that has no intended use in the patient, is ineffective, unsafe, or not used appropriately. Future realigned health care payment incentives may include pharmaceutical industry contributions toward compensation for the achievement of actual patient outcomes.

After providing care to patients, pharmaceutical care practitioners will want to know how well they are doing. Practitioners can self-evaluate their performance by analyzing how well they care for a patient in comparison with established patient care process criteria.[1,3] Efforts to establish national pharmaceutical care benchmarking measurements have been ongoing since 1997. Practitioners working in conjunction with the Minnesota Pharmacists Association originally developed a four-part Pharmaceutical Care Competency Assessment Instrument. A Benchmarking Steering Committee, convened within the Quality Center of the American Pharmaceutical Association Foundation, is developing benchmarks based on the consensus driven Library of Medicine—Pharmacy Practice Activity Classification presented previously in this book. It is expected that these benchmarking measurements will be used, and adapted, in the future by employers, patients, consumer groups, and third-party payers as a way to evaluate practitioners and ensure the delivery of consistent services.

The advent of pharmaceutical care may also be accelerating recognition of pharmacists as health care providers at the federal level. A frequently cited reason for pharmacists' inability to be compensated for the care delivered is that pharmacists have not been included or recognized as health care practitioners or as providers of health care services in laws, rules, and regulations governing the financing of state and federal health care programs. Recall that the rules governing the conduct of other professional practices include acceptance and recognition by society of a standard process used to apply knowledge for the resolution of specific problems that fulfill a unique social purpose. It can be reasoned that, as legislators and their constituents continue to receive pharmaceutical care services, the unique social purpose of pharmacy will be further clarified through legislation.

Various Congressional bills and proposals have been advanced for a Medicare prescription drug benefit. Some of these legislative proposals have included budgetary allocations of approximately $50 million annually for a prescription drug benefit program with 10% of this money allocated for medication therapy management services. Initial descriptions and definitions of medication therapy management services contained in these bills have approached the tenets of pharmaceutical care. Much like the wording contained in the 1972 law calling for a consultant pharmacist to conduct monthly drug regimen reviews of nursing home patients, a Medicare prescription drug benefit law including medication therapy management services would have a significant impact on the profession of pharmacy.

Summary

There has been extensive professional discourse on the roles and responsibilities of pharmacists. Experiences of early clinical pharmacists paved the way for expanded professional responsibility. Pharmaceutical care emerged as a call for the responsible provision of drug therapy for the purpose of achieving definite outcomes that improve a patient's quality of life. The experiences of pharmacists seeking to incorporate this philosophy into everyday practice have led to the definition of a pharmaceutical care practice as one in which the practitioner takes responsibility for all of a patient's drug-related needs and is held accountable for this commitment.

The unique social need that is compelling society to demand pharmaceutical care is drug-related morbidity and mortality. The magnitude of drug-related morbidity and mortality continues to escalate and a national policy debate on this subject has generated interest in the causes of medical errors. Information and data related to the preventability of drug-related morbidity and mortality indicate that drug misadventuring need not be an inevitable consequence of the medication-use process.

Prior to the introduction of pharmaceutical care, a pharmacy practice was ill defined to society. Now pharmacists can describe their practices based not on the physical location or a disease state of interest but rather on the consistent and systematic means for achieving desired therapeutic goals and reducing drug-related morbidity and mortality. Pharmacists throughout the world are witnessing the rewards of having a theoretical base that clarifies the social purpose of pharmacy and provides an understanding of relationships between the profession and society. The rewards of pharmaceutical care apply to all health care stakeholders across all practice settings.

Pharmacists who practice pharmaceutical care have accepted responsibility for their patients' outcomes, have incorporated a consistent and systematic patient care process into daily professional activities, and have secured compensation for their services. In terms of public awareness, the pharmaceutical care movement may still be in its infancy, but the foundations for meaningful and enduring change in pharmacy and in the medication-use process affecting the health care of millions of patients for many years to come has been established.

References

1. Cipolle RJ, Strand LM, Morley PC. Pharmaceutical care practice. New York: McGraw-Hill; 1998.
2. Rovers JP, Currie JD, Hagel HP et.al. A practical guide to pharmaceutical care. Washington, DC: American Pharmaceutical Association; 1998.
3. Isetts BJ, Sorensen TD. Use of a student-driven, university-based pharmaceutical care clinic to define the highest standards of patient care. *AJPE*. 1999; 63:443–9.
4. Klein-Schwartz W, Isetts BJ. Patient assessment and consultation. In: Covington TR, ed. Handbook of nonprescription drugs, 12th ed. Washington, DC: American Pharmaceutical Association; 2000.
5. Carr JC. Gallup poll rates honesty and ethical standards. *Regul Toxicol Pharmacol.* 1999; 29:96.
6. Bricker SL, Langlais RP, Miller CS, eds. Oral diagnosis, oral medicine, and treatment planning. Philadelphia: Lea & Febinger; 1994.
7. Goroll AH, Mulley AG, eds. Primary care medicine: office evaluation and management of the adult patient. Philadelphia: Lippincott, Williams & Wilkins; 2000.
8. Brodie, DC. Need for a theoretical base for pharmacy practice. *Am J Hosp Pharm.* 1981; 38:49–54.

9. Manasse HR Jr. Medication use in an imperfect world: drug misadventuring as an issue of public policy. *Am J Hosp Pharm.* 1989; 46:924–44, 1141–52.

10. Johnson JA, Bootman JL. Drug-related morbidity and mortality. *Arch Intern Med.* 1995; 155:1949–56.

11. Johnson JA, Bootman JL. Drug-related morbidity and mortality and the economic impact of pharmaceutical care. *Am J Health Syst Pharm.* 1997; 54:554–8.

12. Bero LA, Lipton HL, Bird JA. Characterization of geriatric drug-related hospital readmission. *Med Care.* 1991; 29:989–1003.

13. Bates DW, Cullen DJ, Laird N et al. Incidence of adverse drug events and potential adverse drug events. Implications for prevention. ADE Prevention Study Group. *JAMA.* 1995; 274:29–34.

14. Leape LL, Bates DW, Cullen DJ et al. Systems analysis of adverse drug events. ADE Prevention Study Group. *JAMA.* 1995; 274:35–43.

15. Lazarou J, Pomeranz BH, Corey PN. Incidence of adverse drug reactions in hospitalized patients: A meta-analysis of prospective studies *JAMA.* 1998; 279:1200–5.

16. Kohn LT, Corrigan JM, Donaldson MD, eds. To err is human: building a safer health system. Washington, DC: National Academy Press; 2000.

17. Strand LM, Cipolle RJ, Morley PC. Documenting the clinical pharmacist's activities: back to basics. *Drug Intell Clin Pharm.* 1988; 22:63–7.

18. Hepler CD, Strand LM. Opportunities and responsibilities in pharmaceutical care. *Am J Hosp Pharm.* 1990; 47:533–43.

19. Isetts BJ. Pharmaceutical care. In: Mueller B, ed. Pharmacotherapy self-assessment program, fourth edition, book five. The science and practice of pharmacotherapy—I. Kansas City: American College of Clinical Pharmacy; 2002.

20. American Society of Health-System Pharmacists. ASHP guidelines on a standardized method for pharmaceutical care. *Am J Health-Syst Pharm.* 1996; 53:1713–6.

21. Sonnedecker G, ed. Kremers and Undang's history of pharmacy. Philadelphia: Lippincott, Williams & Wilkins; 1976.

22. Leape LL, Cullen DJ, Clapp MD et al. Pharmacist participation on physician rounds and adverse drug events in the intensive care unit. *JAMA.* 1999; 282:267–70.

23. Bond CA, Raehl CL, Franke T. Medication errors in United States hospitals. *Pharmacotherapy.* 2001; 21:1023–36.

24. Schumock GT, Meek PD, Ploetz PA et.al. Economic evaluation of clinical pharmacy service—1988–1995. *Pharmacotherapy.* 1996; 16:1188–1208.

25. Kuehl AK, Chrischilles EA, Sorofman BA. System for exchanging information among pharmacists in different practice environments. *Am J Health-Syst Pharm.* 1998; 55:1017–24.

26. Bootman LJ, Harrison DL, Cox E. The health care cost of drug-related morbidity and mortality in nursing facilities. *Arch Intern Med.* 1997; 157:2089–96.

27. Johnston AM, Doane K, Phipps S et al. Outcomes of pharmacists' cognitive services on the long-term care setting. *Consult Pharm.* 1996; 11:41–50.

28. Bluml BM, McKenney JM, Cziraky MJ. Pharmaceutical care services and results in Project ImPACT:Hyperlipidemia. *JAPhA.* 2000; 40:157–65.

29. Cranor CW. Outcomes of the Asheville diabetes care project. *Pharm Times.* 1998; Oct(suppl):S19–25.

30. Isetts BJ. Pharmaceutical care in New Zealand: customizing the blueprint. *JAPhA.* 1997; 37:301–4.
31. Dunlop JA. To link or not to link: pharmaceutical care and medication dispensing. *JAPhA.* 2001; 41:514–6.
32. Committee on Quality of Health Care in America. Crossing the quality chasm: A new health system for the 21st century. Washington, DC: Institute of Medicine— National Academy Press; 2001.

Footnotes

[a]Policies, procedures, and photographs on file from Family PharmaCare Pharmacy, proprietor Chad Shedron, West Lafayette, Indiana; Iverson Corner Drug, proprietor Paul Iverson, Bemidji, Minnesota; and Quinn's Gore Pharmacy, proprietor Bernard McKone, Gore, Southland, New Zealand.

[b]Wetzel S. Twin Cites health groups receive quality improvement awards: Fairview Health Services—Pharmaceutical Care Program receives silver prize. Buyers Health Care Action Group, Press Release, September 14, 2000.

[c]Data related to the numbers of pharmacists prepared to practice pharmaceutical care in other countries based on information from international pharmacists participating in formal preparation programs. Data on file in the Peters Institute of Pharmaceutical Care at the University of Minnesota College of Pharmacy.

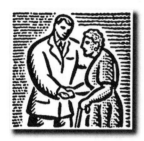

Chapter 13:
Compensation for
Pharmaceutical Care

Michael T. Rupp, Ph.D.

For pharmaceutical care to advance from philosophy to reality, a number of formidable obstacles must first be overcome. Some of these have been discussed in previous chapters. They include deficiencies in pharmacist education, barriers in the physical environment, and inadequate access to patient information. Overcoming these obstacles is an essential step toward ensuring that pharmaceutical care can become the standard of pharmacy practice. However, removing these barriers alone will not ensure that pharmaceutical care *will* become the standard of practice. For that to occur there is yet another critical condition that must be met: compensation.

This chapter presents an overview of compensation for pharmaceutical services, with particular emphasis on pharmacy's transition from a product-centered, task-oriented occupation to a patient-centered, outcome-oriented clinical health profession. Also, the meaning of the term "value" is explored within the context of pharmaceutical care. Developments in the definition and measurement of the value of physicians' services are described and their potential application to pharmacy is discussed.

The chapter continues with a comparison of alternative approaches for structuring payment for pharmacists' services. Components of an ideal compensation system are proposed and discussed. The chapter concludes with a discussion of recent events in the ongoing evolution of systematic payment systems for pharmaceutical care services.

Historical Perspective

The professional services that pharmacists historically performed were linked exclusively to the drug products they prepared and dispensed. Indeed, until the latter part of the twentieth century, the definition of pharmacy practice was virtually synonymous with the activities of drug dosage formulation and delivery. Although pharmacists have always recognized that proper use of medications is essential for achieving desired therapeutic outcomes, the pharmacy profession did not historically embrace this role as a professional responsibility of the pharmacist.

During the past several decades, a fundamental change has occurred in the definition of pharmacy practice and the recognized professional role of the pharmacist. Although it is impossible to say precisely when or where this transformation began, Brodie's assertion that drug-use control was the primary mission of pharmacy in 1967 represents a particularly noteworthy milestone.[1]

The continuing evolution of pharmacy practice was further reflected in the 1975 report of the Study Commission on Pharmacy, headed by Dr. John Millis, which concluded:

> *Pharmacy is a health service.* The only justification for inventing, manufacturing, distributing, prescribing, or dispensing drugs is that they can and do have a beneficial effect upon people who are ill and that drugs can cure disease, control disease, prevent disease, or ameliorate the sufferings of the victims of disease.[2]

The Millis Commission stated unequivocally that delivering pharmaceutical products to patients is not—or at least, it should not be—an end in and of itself. Rather, drug distribution is but a means to an end, and the end is the enhanced health and well-being of the patient. Clearly, the distributive activities that are involved in delivering drug products to patients remain important elements of pharmacy practice. However, as the profession has evolved, these activities no longer define the practice of pharmacy. That is, the drug product is no longer the social object around which the profession is organized. Rather, it is the patient, or perhaps more precisely, the interaction that occurs between the patient and the drug product, which represents the central focus of contemporary pharmacy practice.

In recent years, the concept of a patient-centered approach to pharmacy practice has been further advanced in a philosophy known as pharmaceutical care.[3] Although this emerging concept has not been fully operationalized, one aspect is clear: implementing pharmaceutical care requires the pharmacist to adopt a patient-centered approach to practice that focuses on ensuring the achievement of desired patient outcomes rather than only the performance of tasks.

The impact this concept has had on pharmacy practice is evidenced in the revised mission statement for the profession that was adopted by the American Pharmaceutical Association's (APhA) Board of Trustees in 1991. It states:

> *The mission of pharmacy is to serve society as the profession responsible for the appropriate use of medications, devices, and services to achieve optimal therapeutic outcomes.*[4]

However, as many professional organizations and educational institutions have rushed to embrace pharmaceutical care as the new mission of practice, it has become clear that practicing pharmacists face formidable barriers to consistently providing this level of care, particularly in the community setting.

In November 1990, the Office of Health and Human Services (HHS) Inspector General, Richard P. Kusserow, released a report titled *The Clinical Role of the Community Pharmacist.*[5] Several conclusions of the Inspector General's report are particularly relevant to this discussion. First, the report stated "there is strong evidence that clinical pharmacy services add value to patient care," and that the value created by these services "includes not only improvements in clinical outcomes and enhanced patient compliance, but also reductions in health care utilization costs associated with adverse drug reactions." Despite the recognized potential value of clinical services, the report concluded that these services "are not widely provided in community pharmacy settings. In the community pharmacy setting, significant barriers exist that limit the range of clinical services generally provided." One of the most formidable of these barriers is "a transaction-based reimbursement structure [which] links pharmacists' reimbursement to the sale of a product rather than provision of services."

The Inspector General's report recognizes that the relative absence of equitable compensation policies among payers represents one of the greatest barriers to the consistent provision of pharmaceutical care by pharmacists. For this reason, the development of compensation strategies that recognize the value of professional services and equitably reward pharmacists who competently and consistently provide these services represents a clear and urgent priority for the profession.

Professional Services: The Essence of Pharmaceutical Care

In recent years, there has been a surge of interest in professional services within the pharmacy profession. Pharmacists' growing acceptance of a new and expanded professional mission (i.e., pharmaceutical care) is partly responsible for this increased interest. However, there can be little doubt that this interest has also been fueled by a recognition that future reimbursement for the product component of pharmaceutical care will be increasingly restricted by third-party payers.

As interest in professional services has grown, a new vocabulary has emerged that seeks to better define and describe the contemporary professional role of the pharmacist. The pharmacy literature during the past decade is replete with references to pharmacists' "clinical," "professional," "cognitive," and "value-added" services. Despite this burgeoning jargon, a consensus has yet to be reached as to just what constitutes a professional pharmacy service. Since these are the very activities for which pharmacists are seeking compensation, it is important to clarify this term.

Many services are provided in pharmacies that may be legitimately argued to add value to the bundle of goods and services delivered to consumers. For example, the familiar distributive activities that are performed during the processing of a prescription order add value to the bulk drug product. Likewise, the various auxiliary services that many pharmacies offer, such as home delivery and mail service, also add value.

But many of these pharmacy services do not require the specialized knowledge, expertise, or professional judgment of a pharmacist. Many of these services can be—and are now—performed quite adequately by mechanical devices or supportive personnel, albeit with some supervision. So, although these services do technically add value, they cannot be considered value-added services in the professional sense.

Instead, professional services refers to the nondistributive cognitive (i.e., judgmental) activities that pharmacists are able to perform by virtue of their specialized knowledge, training, and expertise. Indeed, it is this inseparability of the service from the individual who performs it that represents one of the hallmarks of any professional service.[6] In pharmacy, these services include such things as compounding (as distinguished from simple reconstitution), prescription screening and intervention, self-care consultation, therapeutic drug monitoring, pharmacokinetics dosing, drug utilization review/evaluation, and patient counseling and education. Although they differ in their immediate objectives, each of these services share a requirement for the specialized knowledge and skill of the pharmacist to gather and interpret patient-relevant information and to make decisions or take actions to positively influence patient health outcomes.

It must therefore be concluded that it is the degree of professional judgment involved in the performance of a particular activity that merits, for some, the label "professional service." Since it is the profession that defines what constitutes professional judgment, it is pharmacists who are best positioned to determine whether or not a particular activity requires the specialized knowledge and skill of a pharmacist to ensure consistently competent performance.

Value, however, is another matter entirely. The value of a professional service—and indeed of *any* good or service—is determined not by the producer, but by the consumer. Moreover, it is important to recognize that value is not intrinsic to a product or service. Products and services have no intrinsic value. Rather, they are assigned or imbued with value by the consumer, based on the extent to which the consumer believes the use of the product or service will achieve desired benefits.

Value, Exchange, and Compensation

The relationship between the concept of value and economic compensation can be found in any marketing text. Central to the definition of marketing is the notion of the "exchange relationship."[7] The ultimate goal of all marketing activities is to enhance the voluntary exchange of values between producers and consumers of goods or services. This exchange is typically in the form of money from the consumer in return for a product or service from the producer.

For this voluntary exchange of values to occur, certain conditions must first be satisfied. Perhaps the most important of these conditions is that both the producer and the consumer must recognize the value of what the other brings to the exchange. Moreover, both parties must believe that they will receive something of equal or greater value from the exchange than they are being asked to give up. Without this shared recognition of value given and value received, voluntary exchange simply will not take place.

At one time, economists debated about whether the concept of value really had two distinct meanings. The debate centered on the question of whether things could have high value in use, and yet have little or no value in exchange, and vice versa. A similar type of reasoning has been used by pharmacists for many years to explain their inability to secure compensation for their professional services. Pharmacists have long argued that their professional services have high value in use, but little value in exchange, as demonstrated by the relative absence of compensation.

While some theoretical economists may still be debating the definition of value, from a more pragmatic marketing perspective the answer to this question is clear: If there is not a willingness on the part of consumers to exchange value (i.e., to pay) for a product or service, then that product or service has no value, at least not in the economic sense of the term. So, from a marketing perspective, the fundamental barrier in securing compensation for professional services in pharmacy is simply that the value of pharmacists' professional services is still not widely recognized by the economic consumers (i.e., payers) of these services. At the very least, this value has not been sufficiently quantified to serve as the basis for paying for these services.

Although simple to state, the solution to this dilemma is much more difficult to achieve: Pharmacy providers must demonstrate to payers, in specific, measurable, and relevant terms, the valuable outcomes that are created by their professional services. For this reason, defining and measuring the value of pharmacists' professional services is arguably the single greatest challenge that the profession will face in the coming years. For it is only from this shared recognition of value created and value received that meaningful dialog can begin between pharmacists and payers toward creating standard payment systems for pharmacists' professional services.

What Is the Value of a Professional Service?

Simply stated, the goal of pharmaceutical care is to maximize the positive outcomes patients can achieve through appropriate medication use while minimizing the negative outcomes they may experience. In recent years, a number of excellent articles have reviewed the published studies on the value of professional pharmacy services.[8-13] In general, these studies support Inspector General Kusserow's conclusion that pharmaceutical services add value to patient care by enhancing the achievement of therapeutic and economic outcomes.

However, the usefulness of much of the available research for contributing to the development of compensation policies is limited by two factors. First, most of these studies were conducted in institutional settings. Studies of pharmacy services delivered to patients in a single hospital are particularly prominent in the literature. As a result, the applicability of many of these studies to community practice is often limited. A second limitation of much past research is that calculation of the value of professional services was often restricted to measuring the effect of services on the costs of care only, especially costs directly associated with the drug product. To date, relatively few studies have attempted to measure the impact of professional pharmacy services on a more comprehensive battery of relevant patient health and economic outcomes. Fewer still have done so in the community practice setting.

An example of a study that overcame some of these limitations involved the prospective drug utilization review activities of pharmacists in 89 independent and chain community pharmacists practicing in five states.[14] In this study, researchers found that pharmacists intervened to correct prescribing errors on 1.9% of all new prescription orders they screened during the routine dispensing process. When these interventions were evaluated by a panel of experts, it was concluded that over 28% of the errors that pharmacists identified and corrected could have harmed the patient.

In a subsequent analysis of data collected during this study, the value of the pharmacists' screening and intervention activities was estimated by calculating the direct cost of medical care that was avoided as a result of these activities.[15] Using this approach, the mean estimated value of pharmacists' interventions was found to be $123 per intervention (in 1990 dollars). When distributed across all new prescriptions that were screened and dispensed during the study, the mean value that pharmacists added to each new prescription by screening for prescribing problems was estimated to be $2.32. Thus, in this study an attempt was made to estimate the effect of a dispensing-related professional pharmacy service on the total cost of health care.

Increasingly, the professional services that pharmacists provide, and for which they wish to bill, are not directly related to drug distribution activities. In 1997, Rupp, McCallian, and Sheth[16] reported on a community pharmacy-based asthma management service that had been successfully implemented and marketed to an HMO. During the first year of this program, HMO patients experienced significant improvements in quality of life and decreases in the use of health care services, including a 77% decrease in hospitalization, a 78% decrease in emergency room visits, and a 25% decrease in urgent care visits. As of the publication date, a contract with the HMO that paid the pharmacy a flat fee for each patient admitted to the program had been renewed for the third consecutive year.

Despite the relative dearth of published research that fully characterizes and quantifies the impact of pharmaceutical care and its component services on relevant patient outcomes in the ambulatory practice setting, a number of promising initiatives are currently ongoing. As results from these projects are released, the case for compensating pharmacists for their professional services may be further strengthened.

The Ideal Compensation Model

What are the characteristics of an ideal compensation system for professional pharmacy services? Although it is beyond the scope of this chapter to describe such a system in detail, several desirable qualities can be identified.

First and foremost, the system must be fair; it must recognize that pharmacists and other providers of prescription drug products who perform at different levels of service deliver different levels of value to patients. The system should be capable of recognizing and equitably rewarding providers who competently and consistently perform professional services that create desired patient outcomes, and must also have the capacity to distinguish those providers who competently and consistently perform these services from those who do not. This suggests that the system should also be supported by a comprehensive quality assurance program.

A second characteristic of the ideal compensation system is that it should be simple; conditions and criteria for payment must be clearly defined and easily understood by both providers and payers. Additionally, the process for submitting claims and receiving payment should be consistent with current electronic claims processing systems and not add unduly to an already burdensome administrative process.

Third, the ideal payment system must be dynamic; it must accommodate frequent adjustments to reflect the contemporary realities of a rapidly changing health care environment.

Developing a compensation system with these qualities will require providers, payers, and policymakers to work together to answer a number of difficult questions. Some of the thorniest of these questions are addressed below.

What Will Be Compensated?

To facilitate equitable compensation to pharmacists for the value their professional services create, it is necessary to "unbundle" pharmaceutical care into its separate component parts. Separating payment for the pharmaceutical product (reimbursement) from that for the professional service (compensation) is an essential first step. Pharmacists' dispensing and nondispensing services must also be separated and classified according to various criteria.

Figure 13.1 illustrates the concept of unbundling prescription pharmaceutical care by separating the valuable components of an outpatient pharmacy services benefit. As illustrated in the figure, professional pharmaceutical services can be divided into two broad classes: administrative services and patient care services. Administrative services, such as generic substitution, therapeutic interchange, and formulary enforcement, are typically performed by pharmacists in compliance with the requirements of a pharmacy benefit program. It has been well documented that these tasks add significantly to the cost of dispensing and create major hard-dollar savings to third-party payers.[17,18] Thus, a system whose fee schedules recognize and reward providers for the provision of these administrative services is desirable.

The final class of services in a traditional pharmacy services benefit comprises true patient care services that are routinely performed by pharmacists pursuant to implementing the therapeutic plan of a prescriber, such as prospective drug utilization review, drug therapy monitoring, and patient counseling. To ensure their consistent performance, payment policies must recognize the incremental value contributed by the routine provision of these services. This implies the need for separate professional fees that are tied to the competent and consistent performance of these services.

However it is accomplished, the unbundling of pharmaceutical care is important for communicating to patients, employers, and third-party payers that an outpatient pharmacy services benefit is—or should be—much more than merely a prescription drug benefit. Clearly, the drug product has potential value. However, it is important that the economic consumers of pharmaceutical care recognize that drug products per se do not confer therapeutic benefits to patients. Rather, it is the appropriate *use* of drug products from

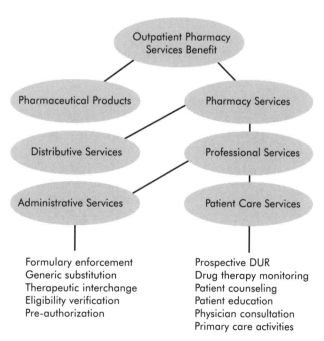

Figure 13.1. Components of an Outpatient Pharmacy Services Benefit.

which patient benefits accrue. The pharmaceutical product is merely a vehicle for the delivery of potential therapeutic benefits to patients. The degree to which these benefits are actually realized by patients depends on the nature of the delivery system through which patients gain access to these products. This is the pharmaceutical care role of the pharmacist, at least insofar as the prescription drug.

In addition to services that are routinely performed during prescription drug delivery, a true disaggregation of pharmaceutical care would include recognition of professional patient care activities that pharmacists perform outside of the traditional prescription dispensing role. For example, a comprehensive system would also be able to accommodate classes of services related to patient self-care consultation,[19] as well as a growing list of pharmacy-based services that target patients with special needs including screening and wellness,[20] disease state management,[16,21,22] home i.v. infusion therapy,[23] therapeutic drug monitoring,[24,25] and a host of others. As technology increases the ability of appropriately trained personnel to reliably perform many clinical laboratory analyses in the ambulatory setting, the number of specialized pharmacy-based services that employ this technology to screen for and monitor the progression of disease and the effects of therapy may be expected to increase.[26]

While still in its infancy in the United States, the concept of separating the professional components of care from the distributive aspects has been implemented in perhaps its broadest sense in l' opinion pharmaceutique, or "pharmaceutical opinion" program in the Quebec province of Canada. In this program, the pharmacist is paid a fee by the provincial government for rendering "a judgment concerning the therapeutic value of one drug or a drug regimen, as a result of the analysis of a patient profile."[27] In addition to the pharmaceutical opinion program, pharmacists in Quebec are currently paid the equivalent of twice the standard dispensing fee for refusing to dispense a prescription they believe to be erroneous or inappropriate.[28]

While the Quebec model may appear to represent an ideal approach to many American pharmacists, for many years it suffered from very low use by pharmacists in Quebec. In attempting to understand this low use, the Quebec Ministry of Health investigated and concluded there were three primary causes. First, although the level of payment that was available was not trivial, many pharmacists felt that it did not fully compensate them for the full costs of the time required to perform and document their opinions and interventions. Second, the administrative requirements for documentation and claims submission were thought by many pharmacists to be excessive given the level of compensation that was available. Finally, many pharmacists were concerned about harming their relationships with physicians by calling their prescribing decisions into question.

Responding to the first two concerns, in June of 1992 the provincial government of Quebec increased fees for both the pharmaceutical opinion and the refusal to dispense program. It also streamlined the administrative requirements for payment. As a result of these changes, pharmacist participation in both programs increased dramatically.[29]

The need to define and communicate services for which payment is being requested has been met in other medical professions by the creation of standard terminology systems for the efficient communication of professional services that are performed by its members. These systems facilitate precise and efficient communication between providers and payers regarding the service that was performed for which payment is being requested. An example is the Current Procedural Terminology (CPT) coding system employed by physicians.[30] The development of a similar coding and billing system in pharmacy represents an important priority for the profession as it seeks to structure standard compensation systems for pharmaceutical care services. Important recent initiatives in this area will be discussed later in the chapter.

As a final issue in determining what will be reimbursed, consideration must be given to selecting appropriate indicators of service performance upon which to base payment. For example, a seemingly logical basis for compensating pharmacists who consistently screen for prescribing errors would be to pay pharmacists on a per-intervention basis. That is, the more errors that pharmacists catch and correct, the more they would be paid.

However, further examination suggests that such a payment strategy, although intuitive and seemingly logical, may not reward pharmacists for the right thing. For example, if the pharmacist were practicing in a relatively closed system where the majority of prescriptions are routinely written by a relatively small and stable set of physicians, one would expect the pharmacists' interventions to produce a learning curve effect in which prescribers with whom the pharmacist has intervened could be expected to make progressively fewer errors over time. Thus, the overall quality of prescribing by physicians in the area would improve over time as a result of pharmacists' consistent monitoring and intervention activities. If, however, payment for pharmacists' prospective DUR activity were to be based entirely on the number of errors they catch and correct, pharmacists would essentially be penalized for having positively influenced the prescribing behavior of area physicians. So in this case, and perhaps many others, it may be more appropriate to base payment on some reliable measure of performance of the service itself (i.e., process), rather than on some narrowly defined output or outcome indicator in whose creation this service may, or appropriately may not, result. As pharmacist care services evolve beyond discrete medication-related services into the realm of disease management programs, the need to define appropriate processes and outcome indicators upon which to base payment will continue to grow.

Who Will Be Compensated?

Two related questions must be answered here: "What professional qualifications are necessary to ensure competent performance of professional pharmacy services?" and "How can patients and payers be assured that providers meet these qualifications?" Essentially, both of these questions relate to the broad issue of quality assurance.

It is generally assumed that any licensed pharmacist should be capable of ensuring the competent performance of the basic distributive activities required for routine prescription drug delivery, whether they personally perform these services or oversee their performance by others. Likewise, most licensed pharmacists should be capable of performing routine administrative services, such as drug product selection and structured formulary management activities. It is therefore unlikely that payers will require additional evidence of proficiency beyond professional licensure as a precondition for compensation for these types of services.

In contrast, the professional qualifications that are needed to ensure the proficient performance of some other professional services may not be as clear-cut in the minds of some payers. By definition, these services should not be performed by nonpharmacists.

However, whether professional licensure alone is a sufficient indicator of proficiency may depend on the nature of the service and the extent to which the knowledge and expertise that is required to perform it can be reasonably assumed to have been gained during a typical entry-level degree program.

It is not unrealistic to expect that for some professional services, additional evidence of proficiency, such as advanced training or experience, may be required as a condition of compensation. One mechanism by which these additional proficiencies might be gained is through advanced certificate programs that have been created by various professional associations, schools of pharmacy, and commercial providers to enhance practitioner competencies in such areas as long-term care, drug therapy monitoring, pharmacokinetics dosing, and a growing number of specific disease states.[31,32]

Of these providers of certificate training programs for pharmacists, perhaps the most active is the National Community Pharmacists Association (NCPA) through its National Institute for Pharmacist Care Outcomes (NIPCO) initiative. Currently, NIPCO offers certificate training programs in over a dozen therapeutic areas including respiratory care, arthritis and pain, immunization skills, cardiovascular care, osteoporosis, diabetes, and nutrition and weight management. Each program provides participants with a minimum of 15 hours of didactic and hands-on training.[33]

Upon completing one of these advanced training programs, pharmacists are typically awarded a certificate. These certificates, however, merely verify that the participant has successfully completed all requirements of the program. Importantly, they do not certify the pharmacist's competency in performing specialized care services related to the disease or therapeutic area of interest. Anticipating that third-party payers may eventually require the latter as a condition for payment led a consortium of four national pharmacy organizations (APhA, National Association of Boards of Pharmacy, National Association of Chain Drug Stores, and NCPA) to form the National Institute for Standards in Pharmacist Credentialing (NISPC) in 1998.

The purpose of NISPC is to credential pharmacists as competent to provide disease specific services that are, or could be, appropriately included in public and private health care plans. This credentialing is accomplished through a national examination process. At present, examinations exist in four areas: asthma, diabetes, dyslipidemia, and anticoagulation therapy monitoring. Additional examinations are currently in development.

Whereas some disagreement continues to exist about whether pharmacy should credential its practitioners in general pharmaceutical care or in specific areas of expertise, there appears to be growing consensus about the value of credentialing as a way to ensure some minimally acceptable level of quality.[34] A recently announced initiative by the National Committee for Quality Assurance (NCQA), the primary accrediting entity for health plans and managed care organizations, suggests that this credentialing concept will eventually be applied beyond providers to include the patient care and disease management programs they provide.[35]

In addition to personnel qualifications, a variety of structural, environmental, and organizational barriers to the consistent performance of professional services exist in many pharmacies. So, beyond the eligibility requirements associated with *who* may perform a compensatable professional service, it is not unlikely that certain conditions associated with *where* and *how* these services are performed may be required by some payers.

An example of one organizational barrier to the provision of professional pharmacy services was observed in the study by Rupp, DeYoung, and Schondelmeyer[14] of pharmacists' interventions to correct prescribing errors. When the researchers examined the data to explain the observed variance among participating pharmacies in their rate of error detection, they found that a marked negative relationship existed between pharmacists' intervention rate and the distributive workload (i.e., prescription volume) imposed on them by their employer. The authors concluded

> *The results of this study suggest that some pharmacists may be exceeding their personal dispensing threshold. In doing so, they are placing patients at an increased risk of harm from medication errors and related problems. Clearly, pharmacists themselves are responsible for taking sufficient time to fulfill their patient care role. However, correcting this situation will also require action by the payors of prescription care to recognize the value of pharmacists' extra-distributive professional services and to develop mechanisms to ensure that these services are routinely performed.[14]*

A final consideration regarding the issue of who will be paid is whether payment should be made to the pharmacy or to the pharmacist. This issue is particularly relevant in the majority of practice settings, where the pharmacist is a non-owner employee. Clearly, pharmacy organizations provide the resources necessary for the provision of care by their pharmacist employees. However, pharmacies do not provide pharmacist care, pharmacists do. If the reward system is directed exclusively toward the organization, employee practitioners may have no direct incentive to routinely perform professional services. Indeed, in busy community practices with high distributive workloads, the practicing pharmacist often faces significant barriers and even *dis*incentives to performing these time-consuming services.

It would probably be impractical for third-party payers to compensate employee pharmacists directly for their care services. However, the ideal compensation system would ensure that all billed services can be reliably traced to an individual pharmacist, and that the pharmacy organization maintains a practice environment and employee reward system that encourages and supports the delivery of pharmaceutical care.

How Will Services Be Compensated?

This question encompasses at least two separate questions: (1) How should fees be set? and (2) How will the operational mechanics of payment function?

Although various permutations exist, there are really only two approaches to establishing fees that are commonly used in health care: capitation and fee-for-service. Capitation is a pre-determined, fixed-fee that reimburses providers on a per-patient, per-time period basis. Capitation is intended to encourage providers to contain the costs of care by placing the net compensation they realize from their services at risk. As a result, the provider is theoretically given incentive to perform high-quality care at the lowest possible cost. However, some questions have been raised as to whether this effect is observed in actual practice. Some evidence exists in both pharmacy and medicine that capitation and other fixed fee arrangements may sometimes negatively affect the quantity and quality of services provided to patients[36,37] and the trust that patients place in their caregivers.[38]

Perhaps the most notable experiment with capitation in pharmacy was the ill-fated Iowa Medicaid capitation program of the late 1970's. Although not without early successes, this ambitious experiment revealed a variety of problems with implementing a capitation-based system in pharmacy. Among these were patient and provider resistance, lack of adequate risk-sharing by pharmacists, inadequate mechanisms for periodic readjustment of fees, and the failure to distinguish between the drug product and the pharmacist's services in the fee-setting process.[39,40]

Recognizing both the potential of capitation and the shortcomings of past experiences with it, former Health and Human Services Inspector General Kusserow has recommended that new demonstration projects using capitated payment be conducted.[5] These projects would include economic rewards and penalties tied to the achievement of defined patient outcomes.

The alternative approach to capitation for setting provider fees is broadly subsumed under the term "fee-for-service." Because physicians have the longest and most successful history of compensation for their professional services, it is instructive to examine the medical model for insight into alternative approaches to establishing fees for professional services that might be considered by pharmacy providers.

Historically, the professional fees that physicians charged resulted from free market transactions between individual physicians and their patients. Physicians would adjust their fees based, in part, on the willingness and ability of patients to pay these fees. With the advent of public and private health insurance, a third party was permanently and irrevocably inserted into the physician–patient relationship. But while the mechanics of payment changed, the underlying basis of fee setting did not, at least not immediately. Rather, physicians were initially able to successfully influence health policymakers to ensure that payment would continue to reflect the fees that physicians wished to charge for their services. Thus began the era of third-party payment based on the usual, customary, and reasonable (UCR) method of fee setting.[41]

By the early 1980's, the UCR method of compensation was widely considered to be a financially unsound approach that encouraged abuse by providers.[42] Simply stated, what physicians considered to be usual and customary was often not considered reasonable by payers. It was generally agreed among government payers that a new basis was need for determining fees for physicians' services. This opinion was particularly prevalent in the Medicare program, where it was concluded that a standard fee schedule was needed for physician services. The result of this decision was the Harvard Resource-Based Relative Value Scale (RBRVS) project.[43]

Funded in part by the Health Care Financing Administration (HCFA), now the Centers for Medicare and Medicaid Services (CMS), the RBRVS is an ongoing attempt to create a rational and systematic alternative to the prevailing methods of reimbursing physician services that is based on the estimated resource input costs to perform the services. The goal of this project is to create a system of resource-based formulas for establishing equitable physician fees for services rendered to patients.

Essentially, the RBRVS defines the resource inputs to physicians' services as consisting of three separate components: (1) work expended by the physician in terms of the time required before, during, and after the service and the intensity with which this time is spent; (2) the practice costs necessary to supply the service; and (3) the opportunity costs of training, including recognition of the income that physicians forego when they pursue additional education to qualify for specialty practice.[44] The RBRVS combines these resource inputs into a model that is intended to reflect the relative costs that efficient physicians would incur in providing a given medical service if a perfectly competitive market existed.

To create the RBRVS, researchers surveyed 3000 physicians in 18 specialties to determine the work necessary to perform over 400 medical services. Adjustments were made for between-specialty differences by having physicians in the 18 specialties identify pairs of services that required similar amounts of work. Since it was impossible to gather data on all 7000 Medicare procedure (i.e., billing) codes, the researchers instead grouped procedures into broad classes of services that were assumed to be relatively similar in terms of resource inputs. They then extrapolated results from the 400 surveyed services to procedures in their respective classes that were not surveyed. Perhaps not surprisingly, when they compared the resulting fee scale to actual physician charges, the researchers concluded that "current physician charges are not closely related to resource costs."[44]

The general approach used in the RBRVS received widespread support from policy makers, and even some physician organizations including the AMA. Moreover, similar input-based approaches to fee setting have been explored in other health professions, including dentistry.[45] In spite of the support that has been expressed for the RBRVS as a method of determining compensation for physician services, this approach has been criticized on a variety of conceptual and practical grounds.[46]

Even if payment schedules are regularly revised to account for changes in practice and technology, the RBRVS approach has a number of significant limitations as a measure of value, at least for purposes of serving as the basis for voluntary exchange. First, the RBRVS considers only the inputs of medical services, not the outputs, much less the outcomes. This is inconsistent with the realities of a free market. While the costs of inputs represents a rational basis for determining the price of a service from a producer's perspective, it is clearly not a reliable method of determining the value of a service from a consumer's perspective. In a competitive market, services whose prices exceeded consumers valuation of them would simply not be demanded, irrespective of the costs that producers incurred to produce these services.

A second, and related limitation of the RBRVS, is that it does not directly consider differences in the quality of services provided. Thus, providers of low quality services are paid at the same rate as those providing high quality services.

The Office of Technology Assessment has defined quality health care as "the degree to which the process of care increases the probability of outcomes desired by patients and reduces the probability of undesired outcomes given the current state of knowledge."[47] This definition of quality suggests that while the process of care (i.e., services of providers) is the primary object of quality assessment, the basis or rationale for this approach is what is known, or what is thought to be known, about the causal relationship between health care services and the outcomes desired by patients.

To many, one of the implications of this relationship is clear: if quality is to be assured in the provision of health care services, then it is necessary to somehow link the activities of providers to the achievement of desired patient outcomes. This would seem to present a compelling argument for including patient outcomes in the design of compensation systems for health care providers, including pharmacists. If so, a compensation model that considered both resource inputs as well as patient outcomes, i.e., a resource-*based*, outcomes-*adjusted* approach to valuing pharmaceutical care, may represent the ideal model.

As a final consideration on the subject of establishing rational and acceptable fee schedules for professional services, some have questioned whether it is realistic to expect that an entirely workable system can ever be created through a purely research-based approach. In this vein, arguments have been advanced for maintaining some element of negotiation in the development of future fee schedules, regardless of the systematic basis that is employed to assign value. As one critic has written,

> *Writing a fee schedule is the simplest part. The most urgent task is to design a decision-making system to allocate the money and resolve disputes. . . A standing negotiating system is indispensable for revising the fee schedules that are ultimately adopted, by reducing weights as work becomes simpler and by adding and pricing new procedures.*[42]

Operational Mechanics of Compensation

In addition to a rational basis for setting fees, a workable compensation system for professional pharmacy services must also be operationally efficient. Some of the issues discussed above, such as the creation of standardized service/billing codes and fees, the development of provider eligibility requirements, and the establishment of mechanisms to resolve disputes, will contribute to the creation of such a system. However, a workable model must also have an efficient means of processing claims and providing payment to providers.

In 1980, the National Council for Prescription Drug Programs (NCPDP) introduced the Universal Claim Form to facilitate the efficient submission, processing, and payment of pharmacy claims. In 1988, direct electronic submission and adjudication of claims in an online, real-time environment became possible. Since then, the Standardization Committee of NCPDP has assumed responsibility for developing and maintaining a standard format for the electronic submission of third-party drug claims. This standard defines data format, transmission protocol, and other telecommunication requirements, and is periodically revised by NCPDP to reflect changes in technology and the health care environment.

NCPDP recommends the use of their standardized format for electronic communication of claims among pharmacy providers, insurance carriers, third-party administrators, and others involved in the submission, processing, and payment of prescription claims.

In 1993, an ambitious new initiative was launched in the NCPDP. Spearheaded by the Professional Pharmacy Services work group, the objective of this initiative was to create "a standardized, practical framework that will allow the electronic documentation, storage, and transmission of clinical and billing data that describe the delivery of professional pharmacy services."[48] As part of this objective, a task group had been formed and charged with creating "a systematic listing of terms, definitions and identifying codes that describe the delivery of professional pharmacy services."[48]

As the primary pharmacy organization involved in the development of electronic prescription claims standards, this ongoing initiative at the NCPDP was considered to hold great promise for facilitating the routine billing of professional pharmacy services that are performed during the delivery of a prescription drug. However, the mere existence of such a standard does not necessarily ensure that pharmacists will be paid for their services. Rather, it merely enhances the speed and efficiency of claims submissions and processing where providers and payers can reach agreement on the value of these services. To date, the use of NCPDP's coding and billing system to pay pharmacists for their professional services has been disappointingly slow outside of a few pilot projects by selected prescription benefit managers (PBMs). Instead, where pharmacists are successfully billing and being paid for their services, they are doing so primarily through the patient's major medical carrier using the same HCFA-1500 universal claim form and CPT codes that physicians use.[49]

Recent Developments

In 1996, the 104th Congress passed Public Law 104-191 entitled "Health Insurance Portability and Accountability Act of 1996." Known informally as HIPAA ("hip-ah"), this law directed the Secretary of HHS to adopt national standards to enable health information—including claims transactions—to be exchanged electronically. The law also required the creation of regulations to ensure the privacy of patients' health information. The final rule for HIPAA was published in December 2000, and was originally set for implementation in October 2002. However, because of the complexity of standardizing the electronic exchange of health information, Congress passed legislation in late 2001 to extend the deadline for compliance of transactions and code sets until October 2003.

Although it is too early to know what the full impact of HIPAA will be, there is little question that it will have a profound affect on how the business of health care is transacted in the electronic environment. Within the context of professional pharmacy services, a particularly interesting development has occurred. As noted above, NCPDP is the standards development organization (SDO) that has historically maintained electronic data interchange standards in pharmacy. In recognition of this status, the HIPAA Final Rule on Standards for Electronic Transactions adopted the NCPDP Telecommunication Standard Format, Version 5.1, as the standard for pharmacy claims. However, another electronic standard, the ASC X12N 837 Health Care Claim, was adopted for professional health care claims that are billed to major medical carriers, including those of pharmacists. X12N is the insurance subcommittee of X12, a SDO that is involved in the development of electronic data interchange standards in a variety of industries.

As discussed earlier in this chapter, most pharmacists who are currently successfully billing third-party payers for their professional services are doing so through the major medical carrier using the HCFA-1500 universal claim form. Routine payment for professional pharmacy services has simply not made its way into prescription benefit plans in any meaningful way. Since, the X12N 837 claim represents the electronic equivalent of the HCFA-1500 form. The HIPAA ruling effectively eliminates NCPDP and its code sets from relevance in the future electronic billing for professional pharmacy services, except where the service was associated with the delivery of a prescription drug to a patient and the claim is being submitted to a PBM.

As this chapter was being completed, HHS was considering a petition by NCPDP to add their standard to that of ASC X12N 837 as a HIPAA-compliant standard for professional pharmacy services billings. Whether HHS will do so is unknown.

Another event of potentially profound significance to the future of compensation for pharmacist care services occurred on May 25, 2001, when Senator Tim Johnson (D-SD) introduced S. 974 entitled "Medicare Pharmacist Services Coverage Act" to the 107th Congress. If passed, this legislation would amend Title XVIII of the Social Security Act to provide beneficiaries with coverage for pharmacists' drug therapy management services under Part B of the Medicare program. By recognizing pharmacists as eligible health care providers, an oversight in the original 1965 legislation, this bill would allow pharmacists to obtain provider numbers to bill Medicare directly for their professional services.

Conclusion

The previous discussion outlined desirable elements of an ideal system that would compensate pharmacists for the services they routinely perform in the delivery of pharmaceutical care. Although significant gains have been made in recent years, pharmacists who wish to pursue compensation for their professional services must recognize that they are still entering poorly charted waters. Most government and private third-party payers still do not have well-defined policies for paying pharmacists for their professional services. This is not to say that payers have no interest in pharmacists' services. Rather, for the most part they simply do not understand what these services are or how they will benefit them and their beneficiaries. That is, they do not understand how these services do, in fact, add value to the bundle of health care goods and services for which they already pay. Overcoming this barrier and demonstrating to payers the value of pharmacists' services represents a priority—perhaps *the* priority—for pharmacy practice-related research in the years ahead.

Until generally accepted policies exist, payment for pharmacists' cognitive services will continue to be achieved one service, and one payer, at a time. But despite the absence of standard compensation policies, a growing number of pharmacists have been successful at getting paid for the non-distributive professional services they provide to patients. As a result of their collective experiences, an effective if still somewhat cumbersome system for getting paid for professional services has emerged.[49,50]

In his economic treatise, *Wealth of Nations*, Adam Smith commented on pharmacists and the value of their professional services:

> *Apothecaries' profit is become a bye-word, denoting something uncommonly extravagant. This great apparent profit, however, is frequently no more than the reasonable wages of labour. The skill of an apothecary is a much nicer and more delicate matter than that of any artificer whatever; and trust which is reposed in him is of much greater importance. He is the physician of the poor in all cases, and of the rich when the distress or danger is not very great. His reward, therefore, ought to be suitable to his skill and his trust, and it arises generally from the price at which he sells his drugs. But the whole drugs which the best employed apothecary, in a large market town, will sell in a year, may not perhaps cost him above thirty or forty pounds. Though he should sell them, therefore, for three or four hundred, or at a thousand per cent profit,*

this may frequently be no more than the reasonable wages of his labour charged, in the only way in which he can charge them, upon the price of his drugs. The greater part of the apparent profit is real wages disguised in the garb of profit.[51]

Although pharmacy practice has undergone dramatic changes in the 225 years since those words were written, the fundamental basis for compensating pharmacists has not. In general, the value of pharmacists' professional services, and certainly those related to dispensing prescriptions, is still interwoven with and obscured by the price of the products they sell. If pharmaceutical care is to evolve from a practice philosophy to a widely adopted and accepted practice reality, the future of compensation for pharmacists' cognitive services must break from this tradition.

For this to occur, standard compensation systems must evolve that encourage and reward pharmacists and pharmacy organizations to expend the time and effort required to provide this level of care. For the reasons described earlier, it is essential that payment for pharmacists' professional services be based on the value of the services themselves, and not on drug products that may or may not have been delivered in relation to the services.

The adoption and use of standard pharmacy services terminology and related electronic claims transmissions standards will help speed the evolution of new payment systems. Likewise, the growing body of pharmacy practice-based research will allow the pharmacy profession to better characterize and quantify the economic value of pharmacist care services and better articulate this value to patients and payers.

Although standard third-party compensation policies for professional pharmacy services are still evolving, pharmacists would be wise not to await the resolution of this process before embarking on the implementation of pharmaceutical care in their practices. Not only do patients need these services but, in something of a chicken-or-egg dilemma, the number of pharmacists who routinely perform them is likely to influence the speed at which new payment systems develop. An axiom of standards development in any industry is that use determines need. Thus, the more pharmacists who are routinely engaged in providing these services, the greater will be the recognized need for standard mechanisms to document and bill for them. So, while not a completely self-fulfilling prophecy, pharmacists are, through their collective practice behaviors, in a position to significantly influence their own destiny when it comes to securing compensation for pharmaceutical care.

References

1. Brodie, DC. Drug-use control: keystone to pharmaceutical service. *Drug Intell Clin Pharm.* 1967; 1:63–5.
2. Study Commission of Pharmacy. Pharmacists for the future. Ann Arbor: Health Administration Press; 1975.
3. Hepler CD, Strand LM. Opportunities and responsibilities in pharmaceutical care. *Am J Hosp Pharm.* 1990; 47:533–43.
4. APhA Board of Trustees. *Am Pharm.* 1991; NS31:29.
5. U.S. Department of Health and Human Services Office of the Inspector General. The clinical role of the community pharmacist; 1990.

6. Kotler P, Bloom PN. Marketing Professional Services. Englewood Cliffs: Prentice-Hall; 1984.

7. Kotler P. Marketing management: analysis, planning and control. Englewood Cliffs: Prentice-Hall; 1984.

8. Willett MS, Bertch KE, Rich DS et al. Prospectus on the economic value of clinical pharmacy services. *Pharmacother.* 1989; 9:45–56.

9. Hatoum HT, Catizone C, Hutchinson RA et al. An eleven-year review of the pharmacy literature: documentation of the value and acceptance of clinical pharmacy. *Drug Intell Clin Pharm.* 1986; 20:33–48.

10. Manasse HR. Medication use in an imperfect world: drug misadventuring as an issue of public policy, part l. *Am J Hosp Pharm.* 1989; 46:929–44.

11. Manasse HR. Medication use in an imperfect world: drug misadventuring as an issue of public policy, part 2. *Am J Hosp Pharm.* 1989; 46:1141–52.

12. APhA Academy of Pharmacy Practice and Management, Cognitive Services Working Group. Payment for cognitive services: the future of the profession. *Am Pharm.* 1989; NS29:34–8.

13. Kidder SW. Cost-benefit of pharmacist-conducted regiment reviews. *Consult Pharm.* 1987; Sept/Oct:394.

14. Rupp MT, DeYoung M, Schondelmeyer SW. Prescribing problems and pharmacists interventions in community practice. *Med Care.* 1992; 30:926–40.

15. Rupp MT. The value of community pharmacists' interventions to correct prescribing errors. *Ann Pharmacother.* 1992; 26:1580–4.

16. Rupp MT, McCallian DJ, Sheth KK. Developing and marketing a community pharmacy-based asthma management program. *JAPhA.* 1997; NS37:694–9.

17. Schafermeyer KW, Schondelmeyer SW, Thomas J. An assessment of chain pharmacies costs of dispensing a third party prescription. West Lafayette: Purdue University Pharmaceutical Economics Research Center; 1990.

18. Carroll NV. Costs of dispensing private-pay and third-party prescriptions in independent pharmacies. *J Res Pharm Econ.* 1991; 3:3–16.

19. Srnka QM. Implementing a self-care consulting practice. *Am Pharm.* 1993; NS33:61–71.

20. Rosenthal WM. Implementing bone mineral density testing in the community pharmacy. *JAPhA.* 2000; 40:737–45.

21. Marcrom RE, Horton RM, Shepherd MD. Create value-added services to meet patient needs. *Am Pharm.* 1992; NS32:48–59.

22. Campbell RK. Pharmaceutical services for patients with diabetes: developing a diabetes program for your pharmacy, module 2. *American Pharmacy.* 1986; NS26(suppl 2):1–11.

23. Bennett JA. Developing a successful home infusion practice. *Drug Topics.* 1993; 62–73.

24. Knowlton CH, Zarus SA, Voltis O. Implementing a pharmacy-based therapeutic drug monitoring service. *Am Pharm.* 1993; NS33:in press.

25. McCurdy M. Oral anticoagulation monitoring in a community pharmacy. *Am Pharm.* 1993; NS33:61–72.

26. Rosenthal WM. Establishing a pharmacy-based laboratory service. *JAPhA*. 2000; 40:146–56.

27. Canadian Pharmaceutical Association (CPhA). Alternative reimbursement schemes for pharmacy services: a discussion paper. Ottawa: CPhA; 1991.

28. Poston JW. Quebec Provincial Drug Benefit Program Update (personal communication). Canadian Pharmaceutical Association; 1992.

29. Gariepy Y. Quebec turnaround (letter). *Am Pharm*. 1993; NS33:5.

30. American Medical Association. Physicians' current procedural terminology. Chicago: American Medical Association; 2001.

31. Chalmers RK. Chair report of the AACP/ACPE conference on certificate programs. *Am J Pharm Edu*. 1990; 54:80–3.

32. Suveges LG, Blank JW. Development of a conceptual model for certificate programs in pharmacy. *Am J Pharm Ed.*1992; 56:109–13.

33. Ukens C. Signed, sealed. *Drug Topics*. January 3, 2000:15.

34. Bertin RJ. Credentialing in pharmacy. *J Manage Care Pharm*. 2000; 7:22–31.

35. National Committee for Quality Assurance. NCQA releases final disease management accreditation and certification standards. http://www.ncqa.org/Communications/News/dmfinalstds.htm (accessed 2001 Dec 18).

36. Raisch DW. Relationships among prescription payment methods and interactions between community pharmacists and prescribers. *Ann Pharmacother*. 1992; 26:902–6.

37. Hillman AL. Health maintenance organizations, financial incentives, and physicians' judgments. *Ann Intern Med*. 1990; 112:891–3.

38. Kao AC, Green DC, Zaslavsky AM, et al. "The Relationship Between Method of Physician Payment and Patient Trust." *JAMA*. 1998; 280:1708–14.

39. Yesalis CE, Lipton DP, Norwood GJ et al. Capitation payment for pharmacy services, part 1: impact on drug use and pharmacist dispensing behavior. *Med Care*. 1984; 22:737–45.

40. Yesalis CE, Norwood GJ, Helling DK et al. Capitation payment for pharmacy services, part 2. *Med Care*. 1984; 22:746–54.

41. Roe BB. The UCR boondoggle: a death knell for private practice? *N Engl J Med*. 1981; 305:41–5.

42. Glaser WA. Designing fee schedules by formulae, politics, and negotiations. *Am J Public Health*. 1990; 80:804–9.

43. Hsiao WC, Braun P, Kelly NL et al. A national study of resource-based relative value scales for physician services: final report. Boston: Harvard University; September 27, 1988.

44. Becker ER, Dunn D, Braun P et al. Refinement and expansion of the Harvard Resource-Based Relative Value Scale: the second phase. *Am J Public Health*. 1990; 80:799–803.

45. Marcus M, Koch AL, Schoen MH et al. A proposed new system for valuing dental procedures: the relative time-cost unit. *Med Care*. 1990; 28:943–51.

46. McMahon LF. A critique of the Harvard resource-based relative value scale. *Am J Public Health*. 1990; 80:793–8.

47. U.S. Congress Office of Technology Assessment. Quality of medical care: information for consumers. Washington DC: Government Printing Office. Publication OTA-H-386; 1988.

48. NCPDP Professional Pharmacy Services Work Group WG-10. Scope statement for Pharmacy Services Terminology task group TG-1 approved 2/7/94 at the Annual Meeting in Scottsdale, Arizona; 1994.

49. Rupp MT. Documentation and billing for pharmaceutical care services in Remington: The Science and Practice of Pharmacy, 20th ed. Baltimore, MD: Lippincott Williams & Wilkins; 2000.

50. Rupp MT. Pharmacist care claim form user's manual: a guide to pharmacist care documentation and compensation, 3rd ed. National Community Pharmacists Association; 2000.

51. Smith A. In: Campbell RH, Skinner AS, eds. Adam Smith: inquiry into the nature and causes of the wealth of nations. Indianapolis: Liberty Classic Press; 1981.

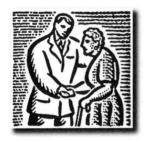

Chapter 14:
Competence for
Pharmaceutical Care

Susan M. Meyer, Ph.D.

What Does It Mean to Be Competent?

Contemporary Competence

Competence is the capability to perform a particular function. Demonstrating competence to practice pharmacy means one has command of the requisite knowledge base and possesses the skills, values, and attitudes necessary to provide pharmaceutical care. The desired outcomes of an educational program designed to prepare practitioners for the contemporary practice of pharmacy then, necessarily, include the knowledge base and those skills, values, and attitudes required of practitioners. Maintaining contemporary competence does not mean staying as capable to provide pharmaceutical care as one was at the time of graduation and first licensure, but rather staying as competent as current graduates year after year. It is incumbent on professionals to maintain contemporary competence.

Experience, Proficiency, and Efficiency

Pharmacy practitioners can be loosely organized into three interrelated categories on the basis of their relationship to the educational process: practice faculty, practitioner, and student. Across these categories, some competencies are shared and some are unique to a category depending on role expectations and functions related to the provision of pharmaceutical care.

Practice faculty, or educator–practitioners, are often specialists; that is they possess education and training beyond that of the generalist, often in focused areas of practice. Specialists gain efficiency and proficiency with experience, but may lose their breadth or generalist skills. Educator–practitioners are teachers and scholars who maintain a viable practice, usually in their specialty areas, as part of their academic responsibilities. The pharmacist who serves as a preceptor or practitioner–educator may share the same level of experience, efficiency, and proficiency as practice faculty. A key component to the practitioner–educator's role is the commitment to assisting with the preparation of future pharmacists. A pharmacist's competence to teach others about rendering pharmaceutical care is grounded in greater depth and breadth of competence.

Students are preparing to become practitioners; upon graduation they will be beginners who possess a specific, well-defined set of knowledge, attitudes, skills, and values. Students do not share experience, efficiency, or proficiency with practice faculty and pharmacists. New graduates enter a continuum of lifelong learning for maintaining contemporary competence and, ideally, increasing proficiency and specialized expertise.

Practitioners, while gaining experience, may fail to maintain contemporary competence. New graduates into the profession may possess greater knowledge or skill in certain areas than practitioners with considerably more experience. It is essential that these practitioners, whether practice faculty or pharmacists, grow in their ability to meet contemporary practice needs and demands.

What Competencies Are Required to Render Pharmaceutical Care?

Contemporary competence for pharmacists can be defined in different contexts and has been defined by multiple organizations. In the broadest sense, pharmacists must be competent as health care professionals. The Pew Health Professions Commission[1] published a report that recommended "twenty-one competencies for the twenty-first century" that will be required of all health care professionals, within the context of their particular professions.

Educational Outcomes for Professional Degree Programs in Pharmacy

The American Association of Colleges of Pharmacy (AACP) Commission to Implement Change in Pharmaceutical Education defined in its Background Paper II[2] two types of abilities necessary to perform pharmacy practice functions: general ability-based competencies and professional competencies. Further developing the concepts articulated by the AACP Commission to Implement Change in Pharmaceutical Education, the AACP Center for the Advancement of Pharmaceutical Education (CAPE) Advisory Panel on Educational Outcomes[3] delineated the general ability-based outcomes and professional practice-based outcomes. Following is a list of general abilities included in their report.

- *Thinking abilities* including logical and analytical thinking, problem solving, and decision-making. In order to function as a citizen and professional, the practitioner must
  - Identify, retrieve, understand, analyze, synthesize, and evaluate information needed to make informed, rational, and ethical decisions;
  - Solve problems within the context of scientific, social, cultural, legal, clinical and ethical issues; and
  - Display habits, attitudes, and values associated with mature clinical thinking.
- *Communication abilities* including writing, reading, speaking, listening, and using data, media, and computers. The practitioner must not only communicate effectively in speaking and writing, but also choose strategies and media that are appropriate to the purpose of the interaction and to the culture, language, and type of audience.

- *Values and ethics* guide professional behavior and, therefore, have a direct impact on rendering pharmaceutical care. The practitioner must possess personal values and demonstrate professional ethics in providing pharmaceutical care.

- *Social and contextual awareness* is the ability to place health care and professional issues within appropriate historical, cultural, social, economic, scientific, political, and philosophical frameworks. The practitioner must demonstrate sensitivity and tolerance in multicultural interactions and settings.

- *Social responsibility* is demonstrated through participation in efforts to help individuals and to improve society and the health care system. The practitioner must continue personal and professional growth, develop leadership abilities, and advocate improved professional approaches to meet the pharmacy-related needs of society and individual patients.

- *Social interaction* requires the practitioner to function effectively in interactions with individuals, within group situations, and within professional organizations and systems.

- *Self-learning* fosters the ability to adapt to and promote change. As a result, improvement and continued learning enhances the practitioner's ability to serve individual patients and the public.

The practice of pharmacy demands that practitioners draw upon professional competencies that enable them to perform the functions that practice comprises. These professional competencies are summarized below.

- *Provide pharmaceutical care.* Practitioners must be able to
  - gather, organize, and interpret data in order to make judgments and decisions that benefit individual patients and populations;
  - perform ongoing patient evaluation to identify drug-related problems;
  - monitor the safety and efficacy of therapeutic plans;
  - collaborate with physicians, other health care professionals, patients, and/or their caregivers to formulate a pharmaceutical care plan;
  - accurately prepare prescriptions; and
  - provide counseling to patients and/or caregivers relative to proper therapeutic self-management.

- *Manage the practice,* including pharmacy operations, medication distribution and control systems, personnel, fiscal, and physical resources.

- *Manage medication-use systems,* participating in the health care system's process for reporting and managing medication errors and adverse drug reactions, conducting drug use evaluations, and contributing to health outcomes research initiatives.

- *Promote public health.* Practitioners have a responsibility to provide patients with poison control and treatment information and promote public awareness of health and disease.

- *Provide drug information and education,* sharing knowledge with students, colleagues, other health professionals, and patients.

This rich mix of competencies that define a professional is essential for contemporary pharmacy practice. These competencies do not define the specific conceptual or technical knowledge necessary to create, maintain, or retrain the contemporary practitioner. The content varies depending on practice focus, evolving science, and current treatment practices and standards.

The American Council on Pharmaceutical Education (ACPE) is the national body responsible for the accreditation of professional degree programs in pharmacy. Through the monitoring and evaluation of degree programs relative to the Accreditation Standards and Guidelines for the Professional Program in Pharmacy Leading to the Doctor of Pharmacy Degree,[4] specifically standards 9, 10, and 11, the Council articulates an expectation of certain competencies for graduates of accredited programs.

Competencies by Practice Environment and Specialty Area

Practitioner organizations provide resources that articulate competencies for their members. For example, the American Pharmaceutical Association (APhA) provides on its Web site (www.aphanet.org) *Principles of Practice for Pharmaceutical Care* and the American Society of Health-System Pharmacists (ASHP) publishes *Best Practices,* guidelines specific to various practice environments (see http://www.ashp.org/bestpractices/guidelines.html).

How Do You Become and Stay Competent?

The Mission of Pharmaceutical Education, first proposed by the AACP Commission to Implement Change in Pharmaceutical Education in its Background Paper I,[5] states that educators are responsible for preparing students to enter into the practice of pharmacy and that the mission of pharmacy practice is to render pharmaceutical care. It is therefore concluded that to enter practice is to render pharmaceutical care.

Professional Education

An individual can become competent to render pharmaceutical care in several ways. For the novice, a professional education in an accredited pharmacy program provides the accepted pathway in the United States. It is beyond the scope of this chapter to provide a discussion on selection of a pharmacy program; the reader is referred to *Pharmacy School Admission Requirements,*[6] the student's section of the AACP Web site (www.aacp.org), and the catalogs and Web sites of individual colleges and schools of pharmacy for more information.

Postgraduate Professional Education and Training

Postgraduate professional education and training provides opportunities for pharmacists to maintain contemporary competence and develop new and expanded competencies through continuing education, certificate programs, nontraditional degree programs, residencies, and fellowships.

Continuing professional education and certificate programs are focused on the professional needs of individuals seeking knowledge and skills needed for new practice and educational roles. In the past, these programs have involved primarily journal articles and one-day seminars. Today, these traditional approaches to continuing professional education offer only one avenue for developing new knowledge and skills. Certificate programs are structured and systematic postgraduate educational and training experiences for pharmacists that are generally smaller in magnitude and shorter in duration than degree programs, but are more extensive in expected outcomes, time, and effort required for completion than traditional continuing-education formats.

Degree programs, specifically programs leading to the doctor of pharmacy (Pharm.D.) degree, are another mechanism by which practitioners acquire contemporary competencies. Nontraditional degree programs, which are accessible and flexible, hold promise for practitioners to pursue contemporary knowledge and skills that build on their experience. Nontraditional programs provide the opportunity for pharmacists to pursue the didactic portion of their education via a variety of methods (e.g., regional live courses, weekend/evening courses, print-based home study, video-based home study, and Web-based courses). Several programs also award academic credit for satisfactory performance on challenge examinations and for demonstrated prior learning. Select nontraditional programs also provide alternate options for the completion of the experiential components of the curriculum.

Pharmacy practice residencies are organized, postgraduate experiences in defined areas of practice. Residencies exist primarily to train pharmacists in professional practice and management activities. Residencies provide experience in integrating pharmacy services with the comprehensive needs of individual practice settings and advance practice skills and knowledge. A residency is typically 12 months in duration. Pharmacy practice residencies offer major benefits to the profession and society—as a mechanism to prepare practitioners to meet patients' needs; as an efficient way to explore and develop new roles; as a way to test innovation; and for the development of practitioners and educators. Most residency programs are currently institution-based, although several exist in long-term care and community pharmacy practices. ASHP, a pioneer in the accreditation of pharmacy practice residency programs, currently recognizes two types of programs: residencies in pharmacy practice (with emphasis on pharmaceutical care) and specialized pharmacy residency training.

Traditional approaches to continuing education will continue to play an important role in assisting practitioners in keeping up with developments in areas where they are already competent. This is in contrast to the development of new competencies such as those offered through curricular approaches to continuing education, such as certificate programs. Maintaining disciplinary competence is important, especially for those practitioners who have focused on one particular practice area and developed a specialized competence. Often, this specialized competence is maintained and further developed by participating in scholarly research. Experienced faculty may develop, maintain, or fine-tune disciplinary competence through participation in a sabbatical (paid leave from normal employment responsibilities) to participate in a concentrated study or research in a particular area. New faculty or those intending to become faculty who wish to develop a particular disciplinary and research competence may complete a fellowship, often two years in length. Practice faculty, like other pharmacists, maintain and evolve their competence, both in their discipline and in practice, through interaction and scholarly discussion with colleagues and students.

In addition to their responsibility to maintain competence as practitioners, practice faculty also have a responsibility to maintain their competence as educators. Teaching competence may be developed and maintained through a variety of mechanisms. Many colleges and schools are located on university campuses with instructional development centers. These centers often offer faculty development programs and college teaching workshops on instructional design and development, particular instructional strategies, assessment methods, student advising, and curriculum development. As institutional and curricular changes occur to meet the challenge of educating future practitioners, so too must the educational processes used change. These changes necessitate faculty development and maintenance of teaching competence in the context of new educational paradigms.

Assessment of Competence

Because competence is more than a knowledge base, assessment of contemporary competence must be valid and reliable and must require the individual to do more than recall memorized facts. Assessment may be performed for a variety of purposes

- To influence and serve as a motivation for personal improvement by diagnosing areas of weakness. Assessments for this purpose should be conducted frequently to facilitate continuous learning improvement.

- To determine the degree of competence exhibited by a practitioner or student to facilitate appropriate placement in an educational program. If a student or practitioner is able to demonstrate certain competencies, then he or she might be placed in a more advanced educational program than the one in which those competencies are addressed and developed.

- To measure the degree of learner achievement at the end of an instructional process, such as a final exam for assigning a course grade.

- To measure competence to practice, such as a licensing exam or a relicensure process.

How Is Professional Competence Recognized?

A mobile, complex society supported by a technological economy is, by nature, dependent on formal recognition of competence to identify qualified individuals. This is necessary to protect against incompetence and fraudulent professional behavior and to encourage learning and continuing competence. These are important professional reasons for practitioners to have their competence to practice recognized publicly.

In the United States, licensure by government agency, credentialing by educational institutions, and certification by voluntary and professional associations serve these social needs.[7] Formal credentials fall into three categories.

- *Documents of certification, licensure, or registration* are issued by agencies of government to persons who meet specific requirements. In pharmacy, the most common example is the license to practice pharmacy granted by a state board of pharmacy. Such a license provides evidence that the state has granted a person permission to engage in a specified activity; practice by the uncredentialled is prohibited.

- *Diplomas attesting to degree or certificate status conferred by educational institutions or providers for successful completion of an organized program of study or for equiva-*

lent educational achievement may, in some cases, be a requirement for governmental or professional credentialing. The doctor of pharmacy degree in pharmacy is such an example. Additionally, practitioner organizations such as ACCP and ASHP award fellow status to member practitioners who have distinguished themselves and who meet specified criteria for such recognition.

- *Documents of certification or registration awarded by a professional organization* attest that the holder meets certain requisites or professional standards. This credential represents an advisory opinion by the issuing agency that the holder is qualified to engage in specified practices. Professional certification may duplicate, complement, or supplement credentials offered by government agencies or institutions of higher learning. Examples in pharmacy include

  - Board of Pharmaceutical Specialties certification recognizes competence in several specialized areas of pharmacy practice, including nuclear pharmacy, nutrition support pharmacy, oncology, pharmacotherapy, and psychiatric pharmacy.
  - Commission for Certification in Geriatric Pharmacy certifies practitioners in geriatric pharmacy.
  - National Institute for Standards in Pharmacist Credentialing (NISPC) was established in 1998 by APhA, the National Association of Chain Drug Stores, the National Community Pharmacists Association, and the National Association of Boards of Pharmacy to create a consolidated, nationally recognized credential for pharmacists seeking certification in a variety of disease states. NISPC currently offers disease-state certification in asthma, anticoagulation, and diabetes.

The credentialing processes for all three categories are essentially the same. Each process involves three parties: the authority issuing the credential; the person to whom the credential is issued; and the persons, groups, or agencies benefiting from or using the judgments of the credentialing authority. Each process also involves the same three steps—definition of the competencies (knowledge, attitudes, skills, behaviors, and values) to be recognized, assessment of each individual to determine whether he or she meets the requisites, and the issuance of a document to attest the individual's possession of the requisites. A fourth step, periodic recredentialing, may be required. The credential is not a guarantee that the holder will perform satisfactorily or well in every situation. It indicates that those who are credentialled have the capability to deliver adequate services with substantially more consistency than those who do not hold the credential. In other words, credentialing cannot be expected to provide absolute protection to society, but it has social utility because it increases the likelihood that satisfactory services will be delivered.

An important distinction between the terms "certification" and "certificate" must be made. Certification is the process of credentialing individuals for possession of defined competencies. As such, certification attests to the achievement of a specified outcome. Examples from pharmacy include certification in specialty pharmacy practices as recognized by the Board of Pharmaceutical Specialties and disease-specific management as recognized by NISPC. Certificates, on the other hand, document completion of programs that provide the opportunity to acquire new knowledge and skills. A residency certificate is awarded by hospital pharmacy departments that provide ASHP-accredited residency programs and a certificate of Home Health Care is awarded by NCPA for completion of its course in this subject area. Within the profession of pharmacy, confusion over the distinction between these two types of credentialing and inappropriate use of the terms remains.

To the practitioner, public recognition of competence through credentialing confers pride in accomplishment and the knowledge that the mastery of requisite knowledge and skills is in the public interest. Further, credentialing is substantially interlinked with economic and social rewards in society. The overall social good of the credential, however, is to minimize risks to the public health, safety, and welfare by identifying those qualified to practice pharmacy. The competencies associated with rendering pharmaceutical care do indeed respond to this social need. Practitioners can document their competence and be publicly recognized as competent for practice via any or all of the mechanisms described above.

In most health professions, including pharmacy, there is no requirement for the demonstration of contemporary competence beyond the initial demonstration of competence required for licensure. Explicitly, health professions in general have avoided implementing a process of relicensure. There are public pressures, however, to develop national systems for demonstration of contemporary competence at regular intervals throughout a practitioner's career.[8] While regulation of health care practitioners and voluntary certification programs are important to the protection of patient and public safety, processes beyond initial licensure that have evolved have been described as insufficient at the very least. Pharmacy has evolved a culture of credentialing beyond licensure that lacks cohesiveness, common definitions, and standards.

Recognizing the variability among credentialing approaches in pharmacy, eleven of the pharmacy organizations in the United States created the Council on Credentialing in Pharmacy (CCP) in 1999. The CCP's stated mission is to "provide leadership, standards, public information and coordination for the profession's voluntary credentialing programs."[9] Envisioned is a professional culture in which "credentialing programs in pharmacy that meet established standards of quality will contribute to significant improvement in the pharmaceutical care of patients and the overall public health." Whether or not a standardized system of voluntary credentialing and/or relicensure evolves in pharmacy remains to be seen.

Summary

All pharmacy practitioners must be capable of rendering pharmaceutical care and competence for practice must be demonstrated and documented regularly by pharmacists. This statement represents both a societal and professional mandate. Contemporary competence for practice is dynamic and requires individual efforts aimed at life-long learning and assessment of competence. Public and professional recognition of such contemporary competence to render pharmaceutical care serve as both safeguards and motivations for self-improvement.

References

1. Pew Health Professions Commission. Recreating health professional practice for a new century: the fourth report of the Pew Health Professions Commission. San Francisco, CA: Pew Health Professions Commission; 1998.

2. American Association of Colleges of Pharmacy. Background paper II: entry-level, curricular outcomes, curricular content, and educational process. *Am J Pharm Educ.* 1993; 57:377–85.

3. American Association of Colleges of Pharmacy Center for the Advancement of Pharmaceutical Education. Educational outcomes. Alexandria, VA: AACP; 1998.

4. American Council on Pharmaceutical Education. Accreditation standards and guidelines for the professional program in pharmacy leading to the doctor of pharmacy degree. Chicago, IL: ACPE; 1997.

5. American Association of Colleges of Pharmacy. Background paper I: what is the mission of pharmaceutical education? *Am J Pharm Educ.* 1993; 57:374–6.

6. American Association of Colleges of Pharmacy. Pharmacy school admission requirements. Alexandria, VA: AACP; 2001.

7. Miller JW, Mills O. Credentialling educational accomplishment. Washington, DC: American Council on Education; 1978.

8. Pew Health Professions Commission. Strengthening consumer protection: priorities for health care workforce regulation: Pew Health Professions Commission Taskforce on Health Care Workforce Regulation. San Francisco, CA: Pew Health Professions Commission; 1998.

9. Council on Credentialing in Pharmacy. Credentialing in pharmacy. Washington, DC: Council on Credentialing in Pharmacy; 2000.

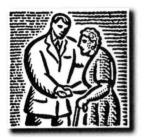

Chapter 15:
Pharmaceutical Care and Evidence-Based Pharmacotherapy

Calvin H. Knowlton, R.Ph., M.Div., Ph.D.

This chapter attempts to describe the current context for the ongoing innovation diffusion of pharmaceutical care, and how the concept of predictive pharmacotherapy outcomes systems (PPOS™) could propel the diffusion. PPOS provides an extra "data point" for prescribers to consider when selecting medication. In addition to historical opinion-based prescriptive decisions that are supported by data points, such as (1) a review of the static literature; (2) expert, personal, clinical experience; and (3) the effects from pharmaceutical manufacturer's marketing strategies, PPOS uses technology to harvest real-time information about the predictive results of using certain medications in similar situations. The key to successful utility, however, rests upon the ongoing comprehensive pharmacist assessment and monitoring of pharmacotherapy.

Resonance of Past and Present

Consider the following assertions:

- We have fallen far short of ensuring safe and appropriate drug therapy in society.[1]
- Most of the problems arising from drug mismanagement result from the fact that pharmacy practice is often poorly integrated into the overall health care delivery system.[1]
- Pharmacy practice must restore what has been missing for years: a clear emphasis on the patient's welfare.[2]
- In addition to clinical knowledge and basic skill, there must be an appropriate philosophy of practice and organizational structure within which to practice.[2]
- Pharmacists need both to cultivate a healthy skepticism toward the products they dispense and to seek a broader mission.[3]
- One of the reasons why the changes in the health care system have been so painful for contemporary health professionals is that the changes have undermined their sense of autonomy and independence.[4]
- As resources devoted to health services become more scarce, a redistribution of authority and accountability for the cost and quality of care will take place.[4]

- The first technological revolution of the twentieth century could be considered to be atomic technology; the second is undoubtedly computer technology; and the third is certainly biotechnology. How will that influence pharmacy's future?[5]
- Pharmacists will have a greater role in counseling, in monitoring patient compliance, and in the effectiveness of medication.[5]
- I know of no time outside of war when business has stood with government on the social goal of reducing health care costs.[6]
- HMOs are vulnerable because their one cost advantage over traditional fee-for-service care—the use of fewer hospital days—is eroding.[7]
- There is a need to create higher expectations among patients and payers about pharmaceutical services that patients should receive. There is a need to actively demonstrate and communicate pharmacy's value in health care. There is a need for pharmacists to develop standards for pharmaceutical care.[8]

These statements were extracted from the handouts and consensus views of the participants at the Pharmacy in the 21st Century Planning Conference, held in Williamsburg, Virginia, on October 11–14, 1989. They could be statements from today.

From my perspective, that 1989 conference marked the beginning of the pharmaceutical care movement. Participants identified the barriers to moving the profession from compounding and counting to caring. These obstacles were clustered into roughly the following domains—four domains over which we had some control and three domains over which we had input but not control.

Pharmaceutical Care Barriers within Our Control

- Academic—competency for practicing pharmaceutical care
- Regulatory—permission for practicing pharmaceutical care
- Structural—facility and space in which to practice pharmaceutical care
- Systems—processes and time to practice pharmaceutical care

Pharmaceutical Care Barriers Generally outside of Our Control

- Contextual—societal expectations to demand pharmaceutical care
- Financial—compensation to incent the practice of pharmaceutical care
- Technological—information access to integrate pharmaceutical care

From 1989 until now, the profession has done a remarkable job creating and executing scores of national, regional, and individual plans spawning the steady, but stealth-like, metamorphosis to pharmaceutical care. Happenstance or serendipity has not driven this reprofessionalization. Thoughtfully crafting and implementing a shared vision was needed to proceed rationally. And it did.

Changing the professional mission of pharmacy from a pill focus to a patient focus could not be accomplished haphazardly. Organized leadership with a keen sense of harmonious focus on achieving the goal—in spite of an expected ongoing onslaught of future role ambiguity and existing role protectionism—was requisite. And we have had it in pharmacy. Let the doubting Toms look at the results, from 1989's dream to today:

- Our schools and colleges of pharmacy, led by their national association, now teach and mentor patient-focused pharmacy practice. They less and less ignore or relegate community pharmacy to the "pathetic track" of practice options.

- Boards of pharmacy, led by their national association, have re-energized each of us with empowerment for collaborative practice in many new ways. They have listened to our pleas and are on the right track, with momentum. They, like those of us in practice, haven't arrived, but they clearly overcame the structurally focused inertia that had been typified by the anachronistic counting of beakers and spatulas.

- Grass-root community practitioners, led by numerous national and state associations, have remodeled pharmacies, both chain and independent, to accommodate new space wherein the consultative aspects of pharmaceutical care can be performed. Our grass-root pharmaceutical care entrepreneurs found accessible dollars were available to germinate pharmaceutical care if they initially cloaked it under the rubric of disease management.

- Collaboration across all segments of the profession—a harmony of various pharmaceutical care obstetricians—(this collaboration) has guided the birth of an array of policies, procedures, and certifications to help the initial standardization of the nascent provision of pharmaceutical care.

The profession has done it. The vision is no longer a dream. The pilgrimage has begun. Academics and association leadership have laid the tracks to the pharmaceutical care destination. Practitioners continue to get on board. The first trains have left the station. More are leaving every day.

Yet, we are not able to reach our destination in isolation. We are part of an environment, a cultural system that requires us to press harder, to integrate better, if we are to succeed. And we will succeed. Our challenge is to confront these cultural externalities—over which we have input, but not control—with the same resolve we have used to begin changing the infrastructure of the profession. The good news is that these externalities are in flux—and their unrest is clearly in our favor. There couldn't be a better context for ongoing change. To use a golf metaphor, the ball is teed up.

The Positive Context for Ongoing Change[a]

The glass is more than half full. The three contextual borders of demographic, financial, and technological bode well for accelerated change to pharmaceutical care.

Demographic: *"Will you still need me, will you still feed me, when I'm 64?"*[b]

First, consider demographics. By 2025, the proportion of all Americans who are elderly will be the same as the proportion in Florida today—America, by 2025, in effect will become a nation of Floridians. Also, by 2025, the number of Americans over age 85 will grow from 3 million to 20 million. The percentage of the U.S. population over 65—now 12%—will double.

Absent some elder-specific pandemic, such as "hoof in the south" disease—a potential massive mortal fungal malady spread to snow birds secondary to the warmth and moisture of southern winter sun—these are foreboding facts. The population is aging.

The stress and strain on the health care system to care for these high-demand, highly informed, baby-boomers will be stretched to the breaking point. In 1995 dollars, persons between 24 and 44 each spent an average of $1,000 per year on health care. Persons aged 80–84 spent more than $12,000 per year on health care. Do the numbers: Twelve times the spending on health care in a population that will be six times its current size.

As boomers age, their need for health care will grow almost logarithmically. Couple that with their assertive skepticism, which replaces the "passivity and respect" of the previous generation of health care users such as my parents, and demand for services will eclipse supply. The escalating incidence of drug-related problems, without comprehensive, accessible pharmaceutical care, is honestly unimaginable.

The reality is that the demographics are in our favor. Medication management is more important every year.

Financial: *"After a few years of success in controlling the costs of health care, the U.S. once again faces the challenge of what, if anything, to do about skyrocketing health care expenditures."*[9]

After demographics, consider the major payer, Medicare. In 1996, for the first time since the program's inception in the 1960's, Part A tax receipts were insufficient to cover the expenses incurred by its 36 million recipients. In general, 1996 was a boom time, and yet the money was short. What will happen over the next 20 years when the recipient pool increases from 36 million persons to 80 million persons?

When you add to that the rapid developments in medical technology and pharmaceuticals, especially biopharmaceutics and pharmacogenomics, it is not a stretch to believe that projections for health care indicating an increase from just under the current 15% of the Gross Domestic Product (GDP), will easily exceed the projected 25% of GDP in 2030.

The reality is that our financial experiment with managed care rationing is not working. Health care is not akin to gas rationing in the 1970's. The current managed care backlash is more than palpable.

The same is true with pharmacy spending. In 1990, patients paid for 65% of all prescriptions. Today, patients pay for just over 10% of all prescriptions. It is a dysfunctional market—create demand in the user and/or the prescriber, yet both are insulated from the medication cost. Then, set up a third-party payer that will try to contain costs by (a) imposing dispensing fee controls and (b) stifling access by interjecting self-anointed formularies. Ironically, formularies based upon rebate extraction from the manufacturers, who just reset the insulated price points higher to cover the rebate costs. With all this economic awkwardness, pharmacy spending is, and will be, very high.

Just like with managed care, the reality is that our experiment with pharmacy benefit management is not working. Fourteen to twenty-two percent annual increases in drug spending are not considered, by most, to be reflective of medication management. The chilling effect of the ongoing pharmacy expenditure escalation is on our side. Pharmaceutical care is about outcomes, including the cost-effectiveness of the medication portion of the care plan. Pharmaceutical care makes a difference in total costs, while enhancing quality—which we, and many others, are nicely demonstrating, documenting, and publishing.

Although rising cost may provide a necessary ingredient to demand some systemwide change, pharmacy costs alone are not sufficient to compel a societal demand for pharmaceutical care.

However, the reality is that the unrelenting upward financial pressures on the health care system and on the pharmacy line item are in our favor.

Technological: *First comes outcome; then comes income.*

The utmost element catalyzing our ongoing change to pharmaceutical care is technological.

The technological revolution is also on our side. It is all about the integration of pertinent pharmacotherapy-related data. Datapenia for us is coming to an end—as it must to fully engage pharmaceutical care. Outcomes are vapor-speak without data. Health care is largely a transaction industry, based on the transfer of information. Between the Internet and wireless communication, it will be a matter of very short order when real-time pharmacotherapy and other health data are universally accessible across the globe. Information technology will enable outcome-based best practices, globally, to be continually score-carded and revised.

Pharmaceutical care is a collaborative medication management practice that will easily tap into the Internet. The systematic provision of pharmaceutical care, in the digital culture, will remove mindless algorithms and formularies that assume everyone is equal. New medications, based upon pharmacogenomics, will permit individualized dosing. Applied pharmaceutical care will be executed using real-time, evidence-based digital grounding as its touchstone.

Virtual health care webs will give rise to global centers of excellence focused on specific diseases or maladies, along with enabling the creation of local and regional communities that will amass medical intellectual capital to be applied locally to clinical problems.

Pharmacists will enter specifics about a patient's health history plus numerous other variables including DNA-based profiling and will get back a predictive medication portion of the care plan—truly Rosabeth Kanter's view of mass customization.[10–12]

Mass customization, in the chronic care sector of predictive pharmaceutical care, has to do with having an in-depth knowledge about individual patients and widespread digital knowledge about possible courses of treatment, along with their correlated, projected outcome.

The reality is that Internet and wireless digital technologies will serve to propagate the diffusion of an additional pharmaceutical care strategy termed Predictive Pharmacotherapy Outcomes—where prescribing options will be aligned with outcomes. Outcomes will be aligned with income. Be clear that predictive digital evidence systems will replace current opinion-based prescribing, which currently masquerades as fact.

There are three distinct technological components necessary to evolve a PPOS—complete demographics, historical and current pharmacotherapy, and pertinent endpoints and outcomes.

Complete demographics means *ICD-9* diagnoses, traditional medication history, normative personal descriptors, such as age, and pharmacotherapy meaningful DNA profiling (e.g., related to drug-metabolism liver enzymes).

Pharmacotherapy electronic records, in a PPOS environment, need to include both profiled and dispensed medications. Each prescription must be *ICD-9* linked to a precise indication for that patient—not the FDA-approved indication. All medications must be tracked for reasons for discontinuation—that is, why has the regimen been changed from drug A to drug B.

Clinical endpoints, that are clustered with and determined by the diagnoses, are routinely monitored and entered by the patient. What should be monitored is determined by the literature and expert opinion. For instance, in a chronic pain patient, appropriate endpoints (0–10 scale) might include worse pain level in the last 24 hours, bowels, anxiety, tiredness, dyspnea, and nausea and vomiting. Clinical outcomes are related to Quality of Life metrics. These might include such domains as general activity, mood, walking ability, sleep, enjoyment of life, and appetite.

Triangulation of these three components—demographic, pharmacotherapy, and endpoints/outcomes—is the first technological step in building an expert system that one can probe, real-time, to provide meaningful predictive pharmacotherapy insight for the prescribing process.

In a different light, technician-driven robotic dispensing from regional central fill operations will be used much more to displace most of local prescription processing—much as the wholesalers are starting to do now. Control over dispensing, rather than being controlled by dispensing, is the welcomed relief foreshadowed by new automated dispensing models that are quickly diffusing across the globe.

The reality is that technology is on the side of advancing pharmaceutical care both in terms of adoptive customization of global best practice (i.e., predictive pharmacotherapy outcomes) and in terms of loosening the shackles of manual dispensing.

The Prejudices Against Readiness for Change

There are three forms of prejudice against readiness for change that will influence our predictive pharmaceutical care metamorphosis efforts in the near term. They may be classified as professional, system, and cultural.

Professional Prejudice: *"The important thing about the Change Wheel is that it has to keep turning. All of the spokes are necessary to build momentum and keep change rolling forward."*[10]

The diffusion of pharmaceutical care innovation is a professional remaking, within a broader social context. It threatens the authority of other roles. It is an alteration in the structure and function of a social system, which does not realize the need for change.

Opinion leaders and change agents within the pharmacy profession have made great strides, focused within our profession, to implant the concept. While new ideas are adopted and rejected, this one has converted many early adopters.[13]

The key for our future success is widespread communication (outside of pharmacy) of information regarding the value associated with the outcomes of pharmaceutical care. Again, however, we must have definitive outcomes, not wistful vapor outcomes.

Pharmaceutical care can flourish in an interdisciplinary environment, where areas of discrete cognition and expertise are honored. Although the pharmaceutical professional literature now strongly reflects increased attention to pharmaceutical care, the health care professions—that collection of individually rewarded and motivated workers we call a team—profoundly lack a sense of our contribution. This is our fault, not theirs. Again, definitive outcomes speak with resolve to those outside of pharmacy.

I still believe that we should move, as others have before us in nursing and optometry, toward independent prescriptive authority—but, this time using a different strategy. Until, and if, the U.S. health care system changes, collaborative practice is the exception. Ours is a system of disjointed individualism. Systems are constructed for silo-based economic rewards. Decision-making follows from autocratic protection of the silos. The exception may be best exemplified by the Medicare Hospice Benefit that mandates an interdisciplinary, collaborative approach.

In the current individualistic professional environment of zero-sum, new responsibilities for pharmacists mean taking responsibilities (and control and financial capital) from others. Although persuasion can be powerful—especially in light of a fairly well-publicized medication-use process systems failure—fear of losing revenue, power, and prestige to pharmacists is more persuasive.

System Prejudice: *"The current health care delivery system, composed of isolated providers and controlled by managed care organizations whose systems resemble a chewing-gum-and-duct-tape arrangement, is simply inadequate to care for the coming needs of the population."*[12]

The uphill battle we fight to legitimize pharmaceutical care confronts public policy, legislative, regulatory, custom, and reimbursement challenges—in short, the current health care system. The most direct way to evaluate or penetrate the system is to follow the dollars within the system.

One of the foremost barriers to professionwide assimilation of pharmaceutical care continues to be the compensation arrangement of the system. While this is nothing new to pharmacy, it has taken on a different face.

The first wave of compensation challenges came to community pharmacy when the prescription processing fees were eroded by the pharmacy benefits managers (PBMs). The second wave is harder to grapple with because it has to do with paying for substitute services within a managed care system. The argument goes like this: (1) I am paying the physician for ensuring optimal medication therapy; (2) I understand that the literature shows a problem with optimal medication therapy; (3) We need to get the physician, whom I'm already paying, to fix it; and (4) We have no substitute resources to pay pharmacists to take over this role.

The pharmaceutical value proposition needs a boost. As the economy slides and health care costs continue to increase, one might think that the notion of reducing total costs with pharmaceutical care might make inroads. Do not think that this logic will prevail. It is not a rational health care system. While profound medication-use systems problems and poor outcomes continue to be identified,[14] we still do not have pharmaceutical care outcomes data sufficient to broadly influence system reform. We have more work to do.

Cultural Prejudice: *"Mass Customization combines in-depth knowledge about individual patients and widespread knowledge about possible courses of treatment [and outcomes]."*[15]

Lastly, consumer engagement will be a powerful mechanism to overcome the disconnect with the managed care health care system. Society needs pharmaceutical care. They just don't know it yet.

The data keeps pouring in regarding how challenged our health care processes have become relating to medications. Morbidity and mortality from non-optimized medication management is rising and it will continue to escalate, as our aging grows closer.

What can we do to elicit a societal urgency toward a crescendo to the Tipping Point for pharmaceutical care? How can we get momentum for pharmaceutical care in our favor? It will take consumer education, advocacy, and activism. It will also take lobbying for passage of favorable policy. However, it will take more than legislative dictates encouraging compensation for the diffusion of pharmaceutical care.

We need to assert a new value proposition for society—a value proposition that compels the wide dissemination of pharmaceutical care that is based upon technology-empowered predictive outcomes of pharmacotherapy. We need to leap-frog other health care providers with a new application. With the new application in place, the system will re-align and pharmaceutical care will "tip." The new value proposition for pharmaceutical care is predictive pharmacotherapy outcomes.

Predictive Pharmacotherapy Outcomes

Dr. Richard Penna posits that the nexus of pharmaceutical care is embodied in the question from the pharmacist to the patient: "How are you doing?"[16]

The rejoinder to this question is what does the pharmacist currently do with this information, and what can be done with it? Herein lies the new value proposition.

The time is ripe for pharmaceutical care. The time is ripe only if we choose to use the new technologies to broadly integrate information that heretofore is neither systematically collected nor used for expert-type decision-making regarding pharmacotherapy. PPOS is a viable strategy for pharmaceutical care.

The infrastructure necessary for sustainable improvement to occur in the care for persons taking medication, is taking form. Someone will be in control of the pertinent information that predicts outcomes. As such relates to pharmacotherapy, pharmacists ought to be in here.

Consider the implications. Consider who might be the nexus for this data. It's too much for the PBMs. It's too episodic for physicians. Pharmacists have ongoing contact with patients, like no other segment in health care. We ought to systematically collect, integrate, and harvest the aggregated data. It certainly could be pharmacy groups that congeal and data-integrate around centers of excellence that perform the same disease management services. It could be state or national associations. Consider how pharmacy groups might be the nexus. The alternative logical group, as the resultant individualization from pharmacogenomics takes root, is the pharmaceutical manufacturers.[17]

There is much opportunity for pharmacists to use the new Web and wireless technology to populate and mine this database. There is much opportunity for us to have authentic prescriptive authority based upon a rich repository of outcomes evidence. Consider who else might perform this integration, if we do not.

The "How are you doing" query that initiates the pharmaceutical care encounter becomes the platform for harvesting pertinent information that pharmacists can use to empower the patient to make decisions—decisions made from options we provide and that are based upon the evidence of predictive outcomes. These are informed outcomes based on evidence.

We need to continue our relentless press for change in the professional, cultural, and system elements that facilitate and impede the pharmaceutical care diffusion process. The stage is set for the "gold standard" of evidence-based, predictive pharmaceutical care to emerge. There is much to do to make it happen. The profession needs to take a second wind and get on with it.

References

1. Pharmacy in the 1990s: A challenge to the profession in California. Proceedings of the pharmacy in the 21st century conference, October 11–14,1989; Williamsburg, VA.

2. Hepler CD, Strand LM. Opportunities and responsibilities in pharmaceutical care. Proceedings of the pharmacy in the 21st century conference, October 11–14,1989; Williamsburg, VA.

3. Fried JF. The future of the health professions: implications of changing patterns of mortality and morbidity. Proceedings of the pharmacy in the 21st century conference, October 11–14,1989; Williamsburg, VA.

4. Goldsmith J. American health care delivery in transition. Proceedings of the pharmacy in the 21st century conference, October 11–14,1989; Williamsburg, VA.

5. Montague MJ. The impact of biotechnology on the practice of pharmacy in the year 2000. Proceedings of the pharmacy in the 21st century conference, October 11–14,1989; Williamsburg, VA.

6. Hughes EF. The challenges facing American medicine: the search for a new equilibrium and its implications for physician executives. Proceedings of the pharmacy in the 21st century conference, October 11–14,1989; Williamsburg, VA.

7. Schwartz WB. A serious threat to HMO's health. Proceedings of the pharmacy in the 21st century conference, October 11–14,1989; Williamsburg, VA.

8. Highest ranking consensor session statements. Proceedings of the pharmacy in the 21st century conference, October 11–14,1989; Williamsburg, VA.

9. Blumenthal D. Controlling health care expenditures. *N Engl J Med.* 2001; 344:766–9, Mar 8, 2001. Health Policy 2001.

10. Kanter RM. E-volve: succeeding in the digital culture of tomorrow. HBS Press; 2001.

11. Gilmore JH, Pine BJ. The four faces of mass customization, in markets of one. HBR Press; 2000.

12. Friend DB. Healthcare.com: Rx for reform. Boca Raton: St. Lucie Press; 2002:50–1.

13. Rogers E. Diffusion of innovations, 3rd ed. Free Press; 1983.

14. Institute of Medicine. To err is human: building a safer health care system. Kohn LT, Corrigan JM, Donaldson MS, eds. Washington, DC: National Academy Press; 2000.

15. Ibid, 10.

16. Knowlton CH, Penna RP. Pharmaceutical care. New York, NY: Chapman & Hall; 1996.

17. Kline R. The upcoming challenge of pharmacogenetics. *Health Affairs.* April 2001.

Footnotes

[a]Much of this section is derived from the thinking of David B. Friend, Healthcare.com: Rx for reform. Boca Raton; St. Lucie Press; 2000.
[b]Lennon/McCartney. Sony/ATV Songs LLC; 1967.

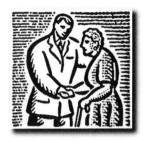

Chapter 16: Impact of Pharmaceutical Care on Managed Care

Peter M. Penna, Pharm.D.
Diane Giaquinta, Pharm.D.

Introduction

Managed care began its existence in this country during the westward expansion as railroad, mining, and lumber companies came to understand that they would have to provide health care to the workers and their families, especially for those in remote outposts, if they wanted to retain these employees. These companies hired physicians and others to provide service, thereby creating the concept of provider-funded health care. In the early part of the twentieth century, several pioneering physicians and communities expanded this concept by purchasing and building clinics and hospitals and selling memberships. These new organizations included the Western Clinic in Tacoma, Washington, the Grange in Elk City, Oklahoma, and the Ross-Loos Clinic in Los Angeles.

In the 1930's, the Kaiser company won the contract to build the Grand Coulee dam in Washington, as well as a water system in southern California. For these projects, health care was provided for the employees and their families, again as a tactic to draw and retain qualified workers. When Kaiser became a major ship builder during World War II, the company continued and formalized the concept of providing health care and formed the Kaiser Foundation Health Plan. During this time, other prepaid health care organizations were formed, including the Blue Cross and Blue Shield plans, the Group Health Association in Washington D.C., Maxicare, and Group Health Cooperative of Puget Sound in Seattle. In 1954, the first Independent Practice Association (IPA) was formed in the San Joaquin Valley of California to compete with Kaiser and to provide services to other health plans.

The federal Health Maintenance Organization (HMO) Act was passed in 1973, spurring the entry of for-profit insurance companies and other organizations into the health care business. Examples include Aetna, United Health Care, CIGNA, PacifiCare, etc. These organizations sponsored prepaid pharmacy benefits and introduced basic pharmacy management programs, such as contract networks and drug utilization review (DUR). In the 1980's the concept of separate pharmacy benefit management (PBM) companies was established to provide full management services to insurance companies, employers, and HMOs on a carved out basis. Today, there are a number of different types of organizations under the managed care umbrella, including HMOs, IPAs, preferred provider organizations (PPOs), integrated delivery systems, point-of-service (POS) programs, PBMs, etc. They all have in common some aspects of prepaid health care or incorporate accepted business practices to the provision of services.

Managed care enrollment has been growing steadily, although there has been significant controversy associated with it, including concerns about quality of care, withholding of services, freedom of choice, financial pressures, etc. It is now the dominant system for providing health care in this country; but it has been struggling, as it tries to create more member friendly programs with less restrictions, open networks, less prior authorization, etc.

Pharmacy in Managed Care

In the early years of managed care, pharmacy was not a covered benefit. The conventional wisdom was that drugs could not be provided in a way that met member expectations while still maintaining financial viability. In the early 1950's, Group Health Cooperative of Puget Sound decided to offer a drug benefit, and structured it on a traditional hospital formulary system. Only those drugs on the formulary would be provided, and they must be obtained at pharmacies owned and operated by Group Health. Selected nonprescription drugs were also included on the formulary and provided as a covered benefit. The experience showed that the benefit could be provided in a cost-efficient manner such that member and provider expectations were largely met. After publicizing the program results, other similar plans soon developed their own pharmacy benefits. In those early days, most plans provided a drug benefit with "first dollar" coverage. No co-payment was required.

Today, pharmacy is an integral part of managed care programs, but brings with it a number of issues, problems, and opportunities. The following is a partial list:

- Depending on the specific organization, drugs are now the second or third largest component of medical spending, eclipsing primary care costs and, in some cases, hospitalizations.

- The rate of increase has been above 10% for most organizations for the past five years and longer.

- All too often, the value that a given pharmaceutical brings to a managed care organization's (MCO) population of patients is ill defined, creating problems for a pharmaceutical company trying to justify its pricing.

- There is a growing impression among some employers that drugs offer the greatest return-on-investment for an MCO in terms of positive outcomes for its members. Others remain skeptical and require proof before they will accept this concept.

- There are growing concerns by MCO members (and their payer employers) that managed care is not doing enough to prevent drug misadventures. There is evidence that more money is spent on the problems resulting from drug therapy than on the drugs themselves.

- The increasing complexity of new drugs, especially those still in the development stages from biotechnology research, is challenging the capabilities of the Pharmacy and Therapeutics (P&T) staff support function.

- Regulatory agencies, payers, members, and legislative bodies are questioning and challenging the drug formulary decision-making process.
- Members want everything covered at no added cost.
- There is often disagreement between MCOs and their pharmacy providers over compensation for pharmaceutical care services, the need for these services, and the quality with which they are provided.
- There is an impression within the public that health plans are more concerned about the drug product and its financial implications than they are about the quality of care.

As a result of the above and other conflicting priorities, managed care pharmacy is often caught in the dilemma of having to manage short-term costs at the expense of short- and long-term quality initiatives. Nevertheless, this segment of pharmacy practice has built an enviable toolbox that has been and can be used to improve quality and maximize positive outcomes, as well as manage costs—often through the provision of pharmaceutical care services.

Managed Pharmacy Tools

There are a number of activities that managed pharmacy programs do to manage their members' drug therapy and to improve outcomes. The following lists the most commonly used tools:

- pharmacy network management;
- mail service programs;
- pharmacy benefit design;
- generic drug incentives;
- formularies and associated P & T processes;
- exception and prior authorization programs;
- point-of-sale-edits;
- contracting with pharmaceutical manufacturers;
- DUR and drug utilization evaluation programs;
- physician profiling and academic detailing;
- population management (patient profiling, identifying patients at highest risk, case management);
- quality management/improvement programs including NCQA and HEDIS measurements;
- disease management and care management programs;
- data management, integration, and mining;
- outcomes research and management; and
- compliance and adherence and persistency programs.

Many of these activities are operational processes that have little to do with pharmaceutical care (e.g., network management, benefit design, mail service, preferred generics programs, and contracting with manufacturers). The remaining activities do have some type of application to pharmaceutical care. It is important to understand that some of these are meant for the entire population while others are designed to impact specific or individual patients. Activities that have the greatest ties to pharmaceutical care are

1. *Formularies and associated P&T committee development processes.* The application of sound principles of formulary development and decision-making coupled with the use of the P&T committee to develop appropriate drug-use policies can serve as a major support of pharmaceutical care in MCOs. P&T committees, whose members are experts in evidence-based decision-making, can form the basis for rational use of the best pharmaceuticals and can assist in the development of programs that help ensure optimal outcomes from the use of drugs. Managed care pharmacists play vital roles in this process. First, qualified clinical pharmacists serve as staff support for the committee. In this function, they develop drug monographs for committee deliberation on the basis of their analyses of the literature and other data. They also identify problems and opportunities with drug therapy for their health plan members and design approaches for P&T consideration. They help construct step therapy and other protocols and guidelines for rational drug treatment for selected diseases and conditions. Finally, pharmacists also serve as members of P&T committees, bringing their unique perspectives to the deliberations.

2. *Exception and prior authorization programs.* Restrictive formularies should make available the best drugs to meet the needs of the majority of the health plan's members. Of necessity, not all drugs are available, but ethical formulary design considerations require that allowances be made for those few patients for whom only a nonformulary agent will work or will provide the best outcome. This can be accomplished by an exception program in which a health plan pharmacist (or physician) can authorize coverage of a nonformulary drug. Similarly, prior authorization programs can be used to facilitate coverage of selected pharmaceuticals when certain criteria are met by the patient. Such criteria are usually determined by the staff support pharmacist through the P&T committee and help identify those patients who will be the best candidates for a particular drug. For example, most MCOs use prior authorization for human growth hormone. Typical criteria might require documented primary or secondary growth hormone deficiency and that the patient be under 15 years old. There would be another set of criteria for patients suffering from AIDS-related cachexia.

Most pharmacists would probably agree that growth hormone should not be used by someone who wants to "bulk up," or by children whose parents want them to grow beyond their natural (and normal) size so that, for example, they might be a better high school football player. Preventing inappropriate drug use in cases like these are good, although unusual, examples of pharmaceutical care. In many health plans, the prior authorization process can be automated if a step therapy protocol exists where a therapeutically rational sequence of drug use can be defined. The development of the step therapy protocol is usually the responsibility of the pharmacy department (with input from appropriate medical specialists), which is a good example of pharmaceutical care applied to a population of patients or members.

3. *Point-of-sale edits.* The vast majority of managed care prescriptions are filled using an electronic claims processing system. Not only is the claim adjudicated (checked for eligibility, formulary status, co-payment calculation), but a concurrent DUR is also conducted. This includes scans for drug interactions, duplicate therapy, allergies, over or under utilization, and other alerts. This particular feature forms one of the main "disconnects" between managed care pharmacy and their network providers. It is commonplace for this concurrent DUR program to identify potential drug interactions and other problems related to the patient's therapy. Typically, the pharmacist serving the patient when this occurs does not receive any extra reimbursement for efforts to deal with the identified interaction. At the same time, there are so many DUR alerts that the pharmacist is inundated, resulting in well-publicized situations where significant problems, such as drug interactions, are overlooked.

4. *DUR programs.* This term typically encompasses retrospective, concurrent, and prospective review processes. The basic objective is to define how a drug is being used, then determine how it can be used more effectively in order to enhance outcomes. Using data from the health plan's prescription claims system, it is relatively easy to categorize drug prescribing and use by physician, drug, dosing and dosage form, patient and patient characteristic (age, sex, location), concomitant drug therapy, location filled, refill history, etc. Careful development and application of such information can be used to improve quality and manage costs. The process might begin when the P&T staff support pharmacists note new reports of adverse drug reactions in the literature for a particular very popular drug. In preparation for a discussion at a P&T committee meeting about this problem, they would not only define what is scientifically known about the drug-related problem but also develop some data on who is taking the drug, who is prescribing it (by individuals and specialties), and any other information that will help the P&T committee define the problem and develop tactics to address it. In a situation like this, warning letters (or calls) might be sent to physicians along with a list of the patients under their care who are at risk. In severe cases, patients might be contacted directly by a health plan pharmacist. Managed care pharmacists have a unique opportunity to apply the principles of pharmaceutical care by appropriate use of DUR programs.

5. *Physician profiling.* Physician profiling and the production of "report cards" are valuable activities for managed care pharmacists practicing pharmaceutical care. It is relatively easy for a health plan to analyze its database to identify problem prescribing and take corrective action. Such profiling could be done to target a specific type of concern, such as those physicians who have problems with polypharmacy, dosing errors, under-prescribing, etc. For example, if the health plan can generate a list of their members who have had a recent myocardial infarction (MI), it would be very easy to determine if their physicians routinely prescribe a beta-blocker. Physicians who don't can then be contacted to remind them of generally accepted medical guidelines and standards. If done correctly, patient care and outcomes will improve.

Profiling can also take the form of a report card where a physician is compared to his or her peers (by specialty, location, patient population). Although report cards typically focus on the financial implications of prescribing (e.g., prescribing rates for specific drug classes, generic utilization, formulary compliance, overall drug pmpm), they can also address clinical quality issues, such as the aforementioned use of beta-blockers post MI. One of the best ways of using the results of profiling is academic detailing. Under this practice, a health plan pharmacist will visit selected physicians to provide information, much like a pharmaceutical manufacturer's representative might do. Although academic detailing might not be considered pharmaceutical care in the traditional sense, it can help ensure that patients are getting better outcomes.

6. *Population management (patient profiling and case management).* Similarly, the pharmacy's claims database can be used to identify patients who might benefit from some type of intervention by the health plan's pharmacists. Examples include identification of members who are at risk for adverse reactions due to overutilization, underutilization, and noncompliance. The pharmacists then need to determine how best to address these types of problems, given the public's sensitivity for the confidentiality of patient-specific data. The plan may choose to send a letter from one of its pharmacists or even a medical director, work through that patient's physician or network pharmacy, or have one of its pharmacists contact the patient directly.

One of the major uses of patient profiling is to identify members at risk, which is one of the key components of disease management programs. For example, if the plan is embarking on an asthma management program, and if it has a list of its asthmatic members, it is very easy to identify patients who are not on an inhaled corticosteroid and those who are not compliant with their therapy, as well as those who may be taking contraindicated drugs. These individuals can be targeted for the plan's asthma management program, which should have pharmacist involvement.

7. *Disease management programs.* As a continuation of the above, disease management programs can be a fruitful environment for pharmaceutical care. The AMCP in its "Concepts in Managed Care Pharmacy" series, defines disease state management as "a continuous, coordinated, evolutionary process that seeks to manage and improve the health status of a carefully defined patient population over the entire course of the disease. This care process encompasses the entire spectrum of health care including disease prevention efforts as well as patient management after the disease has developed." Chronic conditions, such as asthma, diabetes, AIDS, and depression are the usual diseases for such offerings. Usually, there is a well defined and accepted treatment guideline or algorithm that forms the basis of the program. These are the result when professional experts are able to reach consensus on the best approach for a population of patients who are diagnosed with a specific disease. Then, the health plan's information sources are used to identify patients who might benefit from enrollment in the program, followed by monitoring to ensure that outcomes are improving. The health plan's pharmacists need to be integral team members in these efforts, if they are to be

successful. Pharmacists need to take responsibility for providing their unique perspectives on the use of drugs in the target population, focusing on obtaining the best outcomes for all enrolled individuals. The principles of pharmaceutical care are very applicable in disease management programs, and indeed, should be considered mandatory if the program is to be successful.

8. *Data integration.* Much of what has been stated above is based on the fact that managed care pharmacy has created the richest, most accurate, and up-to-date database in all of health care. The prescription files have served as a model for other health care disciplines that want to create or upgrade their information systems. Although the pharmacy database can provide very useful information for the application of pharmaceutical care, it becomes logarithmically more powerful when integrated with other medical databases so that a much more complete picture of individual patients and their health care providers can be created. One of the major tools for managing health care is the capability to gather data and convert it into information so that health outcomes can be improved. An integrated database would have information from hospitalizations, emergency room visits, physician office visits, laboratory tests, and other ancillary services, as well as pharmacy. Tied to this would be the member eligibility and the provider databases. Using information "mined" from this resource, a health plan can do a much better job determining which patients to put into disease management programs, as well as measure the results of these efforts. For example, in the asthma program cited above, a better definition of patients at highest risk can be obtained if emergency room visits and hospitalizations for asthma are factored in. Unfortunately, integrated databases are all too often still in the planning stage, but offer the hope of a greater capacity to improve care and outcomes. Since pharmacy was the leader in creating automated databases, it has a legitimate claim to inclusion in any integration programs. Such participation is key if pharmacists are to use this information for pharmaceutical care.

9. *Outcomes research.* As mentioned at the beginning of this chapter, managed care pharmacy is under intense pressure because of escalating expenditures for pharmaceuticals. Many of its customers expect that it will solve this problem. Although drug spending is escalating, it is believed that drugs are the most cost-effective form of treatment. If this is true, then consideration should be given to promoting the appropriate use of pharmaceuticals rather than trying to decrease drug use. The problem, of course, is that there is limited proof of this concept for most drugs. Nevertheless, those health plans that have sophisticated or integrated databases can determine when the use of a specific drug does lead to better results than its competitors. Since the goal of pharmaceutical care is improved outcomes, those plans with the capability to mine their databases can have a significant impact. The problem is that even when a plan does have an integrated database, there may be limited resources (i.e., information technology personnel) to conduct the mining operations needed to answer outcomes questions

10. *Compliance/persistency programs.* Although managed care has other tools available to promote pharmaceutical care, the last tool we will mention in this chap-

ter deals with programs that enhance member compliance and adherence to their medications. It is well known that compliance and adherence is a major problem, especially for those members who have an asymptomatic chronic condition like hypertension or a lipid disorder. Using its database, a managed care pharmacist can readily determine which members are not taking their chronic medications as prescribed. Although there may be legitimate reasons why a given patient has stopped taking a prescription, such a list of apparent noncompliers can be used as a starting point to address the problem. Unfortunately, growing restrictions on patient confidentiality have limited the ability to directly contact noncompliant patients. Each patient is an individual, and that requires a customized approach to enhance compliance while respecting patient confidentiality. Clearly, this can be a very fruitful area for pharmaceutical care to focus on to determine optimal methods to reach these patients.

In summary, managed care has some powerful tools that can be used to facilitate the provision of pharmaceutical care to its members. It does have a major challenge in this regard however, in that there are often conflicting agendas from the MCO for their pharmacy department, especially with pharmaceutical expenditures at an all time high. There is the expectation that they must first manage costs, making it difficult to focus on programs that improve the quality of the care provided to the plan's members.

The Format for Formulary Submissions

As mentioned earlier, there have been increasing concerns about the formulary decision-making processes used by managed care. Specifically, questions have been raised about the quality and wisdom of many decisions (i.e., the capabilities of P&T committee members to use the principles of evidence-based decision-making). Generally, a decision is made based on the safety and efficacy of a drug, and if these are judged equivalent to competing products, then drug cost is used as a tiebreaker. There is growing recognition that effectiveness, rather than just efficacy, should be used to compare competing products and to make a decision regarding formulary acceptance. In addition, a movement has begun that tries to incorporate into the equation the value that a pharmaceutical brings to the health plan and its members. In other words, the ultimate outcomes that a health plan can expect from using one drug versus another should be determined. This concept was first developed in Australia, in the early 1990s, and then adopted widely by other countries including the United Kingdom, France, Canada, New Zealand, and others. In this country, it was pioneered in 1996 at Regence BlueShield in Seattle. After the concept was successfully demonstrated there, the AMCP formed a task force to formalize these principles and published the *Format for Formulary Submissions*. While some may argue that the *Format* is not a true application of the principles of pharmaceutical care, others believe that using expected outcomes in the P&T process helps create an environment where pharmaceutical care can flourish. As such, many view the *Format* as a major step forward in helping health plans ensure that their members have access to the drugs that are most likely to give the best results. Clearly, the adoption of the *Format* process will be major support to health plans wishing to provide pharmaceutical care to its members.

AMCP's Framework for Effective Drug Therapy Management

In 1999, the AMCP embarked on a project to define pharmacy's role within managed care and published another report, "Pharmacy's Framework for Drug Therapy Management in the 21st Century." When the task force was assembled to carry out this charge, one of the first things it did was to identify the different types of customers using managed care pharmacy and to ask them about their expectations from their pharmacy programs. As a result, opinions were obtained from MCO members, employers, academicians, governmental officials, nurses and physicians, health plan administrators, and pharmaceutical manufacturers. The expectations that these various customers identified could be grouped into several common themes. They expect pharmaceutical services and products that are

- safe (including prevention and/or resolution of problems);
- effective;
- accessible;
- coordinated among the various providers;
- responsive (with information and education for appropriate drug use);
- affordable; and
- thoughtful, caring, and respectful.

It is significant that these are very similar to the expectations identified in the Institute of Medicine's report on quality health care in America. It listed the expectations that drugs and drug therapy be safe, effective, efficient, timely, patient centered, and equitable. It's also interesting to note that all of the expectations identified by the AMCP task force can be addressed, to at least some extent, by application of pharmaceutical care. At the same time, it's discouraging to discover that such expectations have been left unfilled. Customers told the task force that there were disconnects throughout the drug-use process, poor communication between physicians and pharmacists, and little means to continuously measure and address problems of compliance and outcomes. These can be specific threats to those patients with multiple diseases, who are seeing several physicians, and who use the services of more than one pharmacy. As stated in AMCP's document, "Effective drug therapy management is necessarily oriented to a continuous, longitudinal care management plan rather than episodic encounters with patients seeking one or more prescription drugs." A piecemeal approach is clearly substandard.

As the "Framework" taskforce studied the problem of how to satisfy the customer expectations identified above, it developed approaches and solutions that seemed to aggregate themselves in seven distinct categories or domains. Each of these domains includes very specific tasks, activities, and responsibilities to help achieve satisfaction of the requirement of a specific domain. It's significant that the vast majority of these activities would be considered components of pharmaceutical care. The seven domains are as follows:

1. Employ fundamental skills to support effective drug therapy management.
2. Offer health promotion and disease prevention programs.

3. Select appropriate drug therapy after screening and patient assessment.

4. Provide health information and drug therapy that are effective, accurate, and convenient.

5. Monitor adherence to drug therapy, prevent adverse events, and adjust drug therapy.

6. Provide and manage drug benefits through appropriate drug-use policy and benefit design.

7. Use and develop evidence from studies and research to ensure drug therapy management contributes to population health.

It is important to note that the "Framework" is not just for pharmacists but for anyone or any institution which participates in managing drug therapy to ensure the best outcomes.

Application of Pharmaceutical Care in Managed Care

Managed care pharmacists have some unique opportunities to apply the principles of managed care for their members. Most have a variety of tools that can help to ensure that their members achieve desired results. At the same time, there are very real limitations in terms of time, staff resources, and other priorities. As MCOs develop areas for their different units to address, pharmacy can use the results of the customer surveys referenced in the "Framework" discussion above to convince senior management of the need to focus on providing safe, effective, results-oriented drug therapy programs for their members. Meeting the needs of customers is a basic tenet of any business. The fact that managed care's customers are asking that their pharmacy programs address issues such as safety, efficacy, coordination of care, and accessibility is a very powerful inducement for the MCO to adopt the principles espoused in pharmaceutical care.

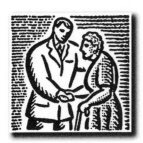

Chapter 17: Informatics: The Integration of Technology into Pharmaceutical Care

Bill G. Felkey, M.S.

Brent I. Fox, Pharm.D.

"Medical informatics is the rapidly developing scientific field that deals with the storage, retrieval, and optimal use of biomedical information, data, and knowledge for problem solving and decision making."

Blois, M.S., and E.H. Shortliffe. The computer meets medicine: Emergence of a discipline. *Medical Informatics: Computer Applications in Health Care;* 1990:20.

". . . The understanding, skills, and tools that enable the sharing and use of information to deliver healthcare and promote health."

British Medical Informatics Society— http://www.bmis.org/

Introduction

At a time when pharmacists are venturing further into new areas of direct patient care and increased interaction with other members of the health care team, they are also facing pressures from the health care system that threaten their ability to provide the very services they have worked for years to develop. The information age in which we live has brought about changes in the depth and breadth of our knowledge of medicine, especially that information pertaining directly to medications and their use. The ability to remain up-to-date with this information for applying the best practice approaches to patient care is something that health care professionals must develop. Increased prescription volumes, shrinking revenue margins, and a national shortage of pharmacists have created an environment that, on one hand demands an efficient dispensing process and, on the other hand stretches pharmacists to give each patient individual attention to ensure appropriate medication therapy.

At the same time, pharmacists have the opportunity to play a more proactive role in patient care. Pressures in health care have put a strain on the entire health care system such that pharmacists are being given the opportunity to assume roles that they may not have played in the past. As we accept these new roles, we must be ready and equipped to provide contributions that not only improve patient outcomes but also demonstrate our value.

The ability to place patient-specific information at the point of care in real-time is essential to the provision of pharmaceutical care. Informatics will play a key supporting role in the provision of pharmaceutical care. This chapter discusses that role.

Technology Taxonomy Supporting the Process of Pharmaceutical Care

Technology usually either replaces a task that humans perform or extends human capabilities to be more efficient and effective in their performance. We must then answer the question, "While I'm doing pharmaceutical care, what is my computer supposed to be doing?"

Key to the provision of pharmaceutical care is the establishment of a therapeutic alliance between the patient and the pharmacist.[1] The role of technology in pharmaceutical care usually begins after this relationship has been firmly established. This technology can potentially be overutilized and dehumanize the provision of pharmaceutical care. Some pharmacists are so enthralled with their computer that they figuratively hug it instead of the patient. Other pharmacists are computer illiterate and resist the appropriate use of technology out of fear that they will never quite master the appropriate integration of computers into their practice. The most beneficial use of technology increases pharmacist efficiency and produces an environment that supports the establishment of the therapeutic alliance.

Documentation is a critical component of the pharmaceutical care process. The axiom is, "If you didn't document it, you didn't do it." Every pharmacy system, whether it is a dispensing system, or an application to support the provision of pharmaceutical care, is essentially a database. A well designed pharmacy system not only allows essential documentation, it promotes it. Some applications assist pharmacists throughout the appraisal process to identify drug-related problems. Once a drug-related problem(s) is identified, the system prompts the pharmacist for action until an intervention has been made. Once an intervention has been made, the system directs that an evaluation of the intervention be performed. Following the evaluation of the outcomes of the intervention, the system prompts for an appropriate monitoring interval and follow-up activity. This system thereby drives an appropriate care process and forces documentation as a byproduct of the transactions performed with its database.

The process of patient appraisal is an obvious focus for implementation of technology. Several chain pharmacies, health systems, and physician offices are beginning to use Web pages for patients to fill out the necessary information to begin a drug profile or medical record. This can be accomplished through a Web browser and be verified by the pharmacist during a medication history interview, providing that the patient and the pharmacist agree to the appropriate consents and releases. Prior claims data can be incorporated to supplement the patient's self-reported data.

Following the steps of information gathering, the identification and classification of problems requiring interventions from the pharmacist can be supported by information technology. The purpose of information is to support clinical decision-making. Thus, the application of evidence-based practice guidelines, drug utilization review (DUR) flags, and access to tertiary literature resources during decision-making is important for the profession.

With over two million articles being published in biomedical literature every year, it is difficult to imagine the scope of effort it would take to "keep up" with this ocean of new information. Detecting potential drug-related problems, therefore, requires both a thought process on the part of the pharmacist and DUR support provided through the computer system. What are the medication problems that can be addressed by a pharmacist? The profession has been using the following problems in **Table 17.1** as a rubric for pharmacist intervention addressing potential medication problems[2]:

Table 17.1. The Seven Major Drug-Related Problems

1. Additional drug therapy needed
2. Unnecessary drug therapy
3. Wrong drug
4. Dosage too low
5. Adverse drug reaction
6. Dosage too high
7. Compliance

When we examined what support existed to assist pharmacists in the identification of potential medication problems, we found that there were 15 DUR modules available from First Databank (**Table 17.2**). These modules can be used in pharmacists' dispensing systems as a flagging function to assist in the identification of potential drug-related problems.

Technology supports the evaluation of outcomes by connecting pharmacists with patients and outcome monitoring devices remotely, or by allowing the measurement of outcome data within the walls of the pharmacy. A range of technology including electronic blood pressure devices, blood glucose devices, asthma and cholesterol monitoring devices, and compliance tools exist to facilitate outcomes measurement. This technology should perform within clinically useful limits without significant false positive or negative rates. Clinical practice guidelines ensure that care management is supported by evidence-based, empirically derived literature, when available.

Computers supply a logistical resource for organizing the provision of care. Monitoring schedules can be entered into a calendar tracking program and daily "to do" lists can be created by a practice system that gives attention to the priorities implicit in the patient population being served. Thus, the organization of care currently being provided, as well as reminders for long-term follow-up care, is supported.

The Environment and Infrastructure

The average pharmacist experienced a 32% increase in his or her prescription workload in the years between 1993 and 2000.[3] This increase occurred concurrently with the decision

Table 17.2. First DataBank's DUR Modules. Claims Based on First DataBank Information—www.firstdatabank.com

A Representative Listing of DUR Capabilities for Integration into Pharmacy Practice

Drug–Drug Interaction Module

Drug–Food Interaction Module

Drug Interactions Database

Min–Max Dosing

Drug Image Database

Drug Imprint Database

Drug Name Identifiers
    Master Parameters Database

Dosage Range Check

Drug Allergy Module

Patient Education Module

Intravenous Module

Counseling Messages Module

Duration of Therapy Module

Prioritized Label Warnings

Prescriber Order Entry Module

These modules make up the National Drug Data File (NDDF) from First DataBank. The NDDF contains data including ingredients, strength, dosage form, route, and detailed descriptive fields on every FDA-approved drug in the U.S. It is the largest drug knowledge base in the world.

of the profession to provide pharmaceutical care as its mission. Technology companies have had a difficult time implementing management systems that are focused on supporting pharmaceutical care. Instead, some pharmacists have even turned off their DUR support on their dispensing systems because they don't want to be "slowed down" by computer-generated interruptions.

In the same time period described above, patients have seen the cost of their prescriptions more than double. With the widespread use of the Internet, many of these patients have become health information seekers (as this is the most prevalent use of the Internet by consumers). They have also adopted a consumerist attitude, determining that they will use the power of the Internet to obtain the answers to their questions and to obtain the best prices for the drug products they consume. Some pharmacists have expressed understandable concern that consumer access to this resource is a threat to the profession. In practice, patients are quickly overwhelmed by the information on their computer screens, and they need the caring assistance of a pharmacist to help them prioritize and customize the information.

Workloads and limitations on pharmacists' abilities to delegate responsibilities have been at least partially responsible for large investments in automation. Outpatient initiatives include in-store automation or robotic pill counters. A recent movement involves the use of central fulfillment dispensing pharmacy, as well as central processing for prescription problems that can outsource, thereby, taking work out of the store. Another initiative involves the integration of ready-to-label products (unit-of-use packaging) to speed up the dispensing process while implementing barcodes to increase safety.

The Point of Care

One of the most exciting opportunities for adopting and diffusing technology into the everyday practice of pharmacy is being described as a point-of-care initiative. Although many pharmacies have access to the Internet through a workstation in the pharmacy, it is often the case that this workstation is remote and, therefore, not usable in direct patient care matters. Placing a computer workstation at the point of care allows the practitioner to have the information available when it's needed and where it's needed.

A point-of-care device could consist of a palmtop, personal digital assistant (PDA), subnotebook, notebook computer, or a desktop computer. Ideally, these devices would contain core reference materials in medical, pharmacy, and patient education topics. These resources can either be contained offline on the internal storage capacity of the device or could be accessed through intranet or Internet sources. At the time of publication, there were over 700 medical and pharmacy resources that fit on a palmtop device. Many of these resources are updated on a daily or monthly basis so that pharmacists have access to the latest information for clinical decision support.

The addition of a wireless infrastructure for portable devices makes it possible for computer technology to be ubiquitous in health care. These devices bring with them a promise of greater flexibility in providing care. They also must be equipped with software that can ensure the privacy of confidential information.

Other important assets to a pharmacist include numerous patient education resources and an emerging support for prescriber order entry systems. Significant advances in natural speech recognition software have progressed to the point that it can aid in the documentation of care rendered to patients. The majority of patients learn best by visual means, and yet, they often leave pharmacies with a minimal leaflet of printed information and very little verbal explanation. Multimedia resources exist for supplementing the counseling provided by a pharmacist and can be used to show people not only what to do with their medication but how to do it.

Prescriber order entry of prescriptions into a computerized environment is being touted as the best first step to address the problem of medication errors due to illegible prescriptions.[4] A typical order entry application requires that prescribers select a patient name from a screen that was preloaded by a receptionist; then they enter an indication, after which a screening module assesses formulary considerations and any potential drug-related problems. A list of potential medications is then presented to the prescriber for selection. Selecting a desirable therapy from a list of those possible concludes the order entry process and transmits the prescription to the pharmacy by a variety of telecommunication channels ranging from hardcopy printouts to direct entry into the pharmacy management system.[5] Additionally, interesting possibilities exist in these systems for the marketing of advanced pharmaceutical care services.

Information Systems and the Profession of Pharmacy

Pharmacy is a knowledge-driven profession. Because it is difficult to imagine any scenario of the future of health care that is not supported by technology, every pharmacist should have a working knowledge of informatics. Informatics deals with the acquisition, organization, and dissemination of information. As a career path, health care technology and informatics will remain a strong choice, using the knowledge base of both a pharmacist and an information scientist.

Although computers seem complicated, they can be understood if one recognizes that each computer consists of five components. These components are standard across the continuum of computers, whether we are talking about the earliest vacuum tube, room-size computer, or future computers with flexible displays not yet conceived by the average computer user. All computers have some method of input that allows humans to give commands to a computer. Keyboards, mice, touch screens, and speech recognition are all examples of *inputs*. The opposite of input is output. Computers typically produce *outputs* on display monitors, printers, and speakers. Third, all computers have memory that enables the computer to do work on its system. *Memory* is temporary in nature, and the more memory the computer possesses, the more that can be accomplished. In order to keep a record of work done, the computer must have a *storage* device. Hard drives, floppy diskettes, zip drives, and writable CD-ROM devices are classified as storage in a computer. The brain of the computer is its *processor*. Within a family of processors, such as a Pentium, one will find a variety of clock speeds with the higher number clock speed representing the faster processor.

Beyond the basic hardware of computers, there are different operating systems that are employed by various computer systems. Operating systems translate the commands given by users into actions. One of the information goals in health care is the integration of information systems. A barrier to this integration is the variety of operating systems that are employed in today's computers. Each operating system is analogous to a language. Multiple operating systems result in multiple languages and an increased risk of information loss or delay.

The vision of the Internet has been described as every computer talking to every other computer in the world. Health care information systems projects should attempt to involve the Internet in their design. The developers of pharmacy systems are beginning to examine the use of the Internet for application service providers (ASP) that would allow processing to take place over the Internet and thus decrease the necessary power of local computers in health care facilities.

Computers that work to support the provision of pharmaceutical care do so at many layers of complexity. The simplest level of data processing is called transaction processing. Performing an intake on a prescription involves several transactions. At the end of the process, paying for the prescription is a transaction. The next level of data processing is called management information systems. Administrators for an organization need to know trends in the transactions to be able to predict the success of the organization. Management information systems can also be used to determine staffing needs and other business needs. The next highest level of data processing involves decision support where the computer provides information prospectively while transactions are occurring. DUR modules are good examples of decision support systems. The highest level of data processing involves the use of artificial intelligence and/or expert systems. These systems use applied mathematics and inference engines to assist people in decision-making.[6]

The Internet

There are over 20,000 valuable health care Web sites and nearly one billion individual Web pages that are focused on health or health-related issues.[7] To understand the functional features of the Internet, we find it useful to consider the three Cs of the Internet: content, communication, and commerce.

There is no longer a question about how rich the Internet is as a content resource. Since 1999, the Internet has housed more information than exists in the entire history of print for mankind.[8] The main issue about Internet content is the concern of the quality of the information obtained. Although certain tools actually filter out inaccurate, biased, or outdated resources, it is the pharmacist's responsibility to ascertain the source reliability and credibility of any Internet content used in patient care or patient education activities. The pharmacist must further assess the usefulness of a set of data to the totality of the patient.

The Internet has given rise to new levels of connectivity and even the capability of using its massive communication resources to open channels with patients that were never possible before. Communication tools ranging from e-mail, voice over Internet telephony, and videoconferencing continue to make the world smaller. The opportunity for patients to collaborate with professionals concerning their own health care is very exciting. Patients may access their own medical records and even be asked to take active roles in their self-care management because of the communication channels provided by the Internet.

The attribute of the Internet for supporting commerce has made the global commodization of goods and services a reality. People are investing in the stock market without knowing where their brokerage firm resides. Specialty Web sites identify the best prices on the planet for a given item and supplement the buyer's knowledge by listing independent comparisons, business ratings, shipping costs, availability, and pertinent contact information on hundreds of thousands of products. However, no system is completely without bias or infinitely accurate; the pharmacist must actively continue to critically interpret these activities for patients.

Access to the Internet continues to be a barrier for some, but over 30% of Americans have broadband (high speed) access to the Internet from home, work, or school.[9] An even higher percentage of American homes have regular dial-up access. The ability to have full-time high bandwidth connectivity is possible now in many pharmacies. As the richness of resources available to pharmacies increases, it will become commonplace in all pharmacies to use this infrastructure.

Intranets and Extranets

While the Internet represents the infrastructure that is connecting every computer on the planet, the implementation of intranets and extranets is facilitating more secure and efficient access to necessary resources and support. Intranets require user identification and various levels of passwords and encryption for entry on a Web site. Extranets, like intranets, require access authorization, but usually connect organizations to their business partners for support in their rendering of care. It is mandatory to protect the confidentiality of patients in this process by removing patient identifiable information from any transaction shared between the health care provider and business stakeholder.

Informatics Skills

Pharmacists possess a unique knowledge base that allows them to identify, resolve, and prevent drug-related problems. Like any knowledge base, it is subject to decay unless it is kept up-to-date. Pharmacists must learn effective information skills to continually nurture their abilities to use their knowledge base in the provision of pharmaceutical care. Application of the skills will ensure pharmacists have a greater role in telehealth in general, and telepharmacy in particular. Telehealth has been defined as "the use of electronic information and telecommunications technologies to support long-distance clinical health care, patient and professional health-related education, and public health and health administration."[10] The qualities that make information valid and reliable include those listed in **Table 17.3**.

Table 17.3. Characteristics of Useful Information

Accurate	Information that is error free
Complete	Information containing all important facts
Economical	Production of the information is feasible
Flexible	Information can be used for a number of purposes
Reliable	Information can be depended upon
Relevant	Information is important to the decision-maker
Simple	Information is not overly complex
Timely	Information is delivered when it's needed
Verifiable	Information can be checked for correctness
Accessible	Information can be obtained easily, in the right format, and in a timely manner
Secure	Information access is limited to authorized users

We believe that pharmacists can be key information purveyors in a collaborative, multidisciplinary team of practitioners. Pharmacists are uniquely positioned to participate in obtaining positive outcomes and in the management of pharmacotherapy. Using tools such as telephony and through the connectivity offered by prescriber order entry, pharmacists should be able to resolve drug-related problems in near real-time modes of delivery. One critical factor in determining how the profession will progress rests in its ability to access the emerging electronic medical records. Pharmacists need access to patient diagnostic information and lab results. They need to be able to write to the records so that other practitioners, and ultimately the patient, can benefit from the pharmacist's care.

Informatics Opportunities

In order to play a key role in the management of information in health care, pharmacists will need to acquire research skills to enable them to access the best information resources. Some of their access to information resources will take them to pharmacist portals that contain only the most beneficial products to support their practice. Other sites will supply them with the resources to effectively communicate with patients to help them know what to do, how to do it, and assist them in becoming motivated to be adherent with their therapies.

The incorporation of information technology can often begin with the development of a Web site. The realization of the mission of the pharmacy can be undercut if the site promises resources to patients that cannot be delivered. A successful Web site has internal mechanisms in place to deal with an e-business approach to health care. Having connectivity with business partners and other stakeholders associated with the pharmacy tends to be a precursor to successful transactions with patients.

A new opportunity emerging for pharmacists involves telecommuting. It has been shown that as much as a 30% increase in productivity can be achieved by telecommuters when compared with the work done in the actual workplace.[10] Telecommuting requires an activity-based job description and careful screening to determine the suitability of the pharmacist for this type of work. Some people thrive on the social aspects of the traditional workplace, and care must be taken to ensure the telecommuter feels he or she is still a part of the organization.

Keyword: Integration

Due, in part, to the complexity of health care organizations, there is a huge need for integration to be considered when implementing technology support. At one point in time, large mainframe computers dominated the health care landscape. Then, as the information needs of clinical departments became more pronounced, specialized departmental solutions were acquired. The pendulum has now swung back to the need for a repository that requires an integrated environment to be successful.

There is a general lack of standards that impedes progress. There are many regulatory issues that remain unresolved. Legislation, such as the Health Information Portability and Accountability Act, will have an enormous impact on health care as it seeks to ensure patient privacy in medical records and add security in the handling of patient identifiable information, yet allow information records to become more portable. Additionally, legislation requires increased access to medical records by individual patients.

Conclusion

Pharmacy is a profession whose primary purpose is to use information to make patient care decisions that lead to positive health outcomes. This chapter has presented the need in pharmacy for systems and processes that move information more efficiently and effectively. The tools of informatics equip the profession to meet both current and future challenges while increasing the level of pharmaceutical care provided. Although daunting, these challenges represent a real opportunity for the profession to increase its role as a direct provider of care. As steps are taken to virtual integration of information storage and retrieval, boundary lines will blur, facilitating communication among providers of care. The profession of pharmacy will be better positioned for these changes with a working knowledge and understanding of informatics.

References

1. Berger BA. Building an effective therapeutic alliance. *Am J Hosp Pharm.* 1993; 50:2399–403.
2. Cipolle RJ, Strand LM, Morley PC. Pharmaceutical care practice, 1st ed. New York: McGraw Hill; 1998:78–111.
3. The pharmacist workforce: a study of the supply and demand for pharmacists. Washington, DC: Bureau of Health Professions, Health Resources and Services Administration, U.S. Department of Health and Human Services. http://bhpr.hrsa.gov/healthworkforce/pharmacist.html (accessed 2001 September 25).
4. Institute for Safe Medication Practices. A call to action: eliminate handwritten prescriptions within 3 years! Electronic prescribing can reduce medication errors. http://www.ismp.org (accessed 2001 March 14).
5. Electronic prescribing and the pharmacy. NACDS Chain Pharmacist Practice Memo. 2000; 4(10):1–3.
6. Carr HC, Snyder CA. The management of telecommunications: business solutions to business problems, 1st ed. Boston, MA: Irwin/McGraw-Hill:1997:22–6.
7. Pastore M. The mess known as online healthcare. Markets: Healthcare [periodical online].http://cyberatlas.internet.com/markets/healthcare/article/0,,10101_379231,00.html (accessed 2000 November 23).
8. Gates B. Keynote address. Telecom '99. Redmond, WA. 1999 October.
9. Pastore M. One-third of online Americans surfing at high speeds [periodical online]. http://cyberatlas.internet.com/markets/broadband/article/0,,10099_790641,00.html (accessed 2001 September 26).
10. Office for the Advancement of Telehealth. http://telehealth.hrsa.gov/welcome.htm (accessed 2001 September 26).
11. Stair RM, Reynolds GW. Principles of information systems, 5th ed. Boston, MA: Course Technology; 2001:7.
12. Felkey BG, Fox BI. Telehealth for Pharmacy Care. In: Pharmacotherapy Self-Assessment Program, 4th ed, book 2. Kansas City, MO: American College of Clinical Pharmacy; 2001:117–41.

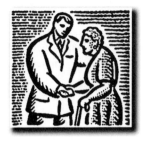

Chapter 18: Performance Improvement

Stephanie A. Zarus, Pharm.D.

"The responsibility for achieving and ensuring consistent quality belongs in the hands of those who perform the activities."[1]

W. Edwards Deming

The value of pharmaceutical care is determined by the perceived benefits and quality of the goods and services offered in relation to its direct and indirect costs. To show continued value, baseline performance markers must be defined and outcomes must be tracked and evaluated on the basis of these markers. This strategy supports ongoing performance improvement. It is not possible to know when something has improved unless there is a basis of measure for comparison.

This chapter will present the concepts and methods of performance benchmarking to enable ongoing improvement in pharmacy-related functions. The goal is to equip the reader with the tools to target an organizational process for performance improvement and to outline the steps by which one engages in process definition, redesign, assessment benchmarking, measurement, and outcome documentation. Before describing the systems approach, this chapter will review the human components of performance improvement. This includes knowledge and skill development, as well as supportive measures to change attitudes and practice behaviors.

Understanding the Human Component of Performance Improvement

Whether one speaks of pharmaceutical care or other services, it is important to first understand the background regarding human performance expectations. Generally, people expect to perform a process in a specific way and to receive routinely a particular outcome. This process is subject to personal interpretation. The pharmaceutical care challenge is to set pharmacy-based outcome expectations and improve the systems to enable routine achievement of expected outcomes.

Consumers expect to get diagnosed correctly and to return home with an appropriate prescription, which has been filled accurately. Society has set this expectation. Before the climate of open disclosure of health care processes, consumers rarely gave thought to the processes involved in the health care system and certainly had little knowledge or expectation of pharmaceutical care. Likewise, pharmacists had always expected nurses and prescribers to communicate clearly the prescription orders needed for dispensing. Clinical collaboration and care planning remain on the fringe of pharmacy practice.

In the current climate, pharmacy technicians expect that they will support the pharmacist regarding medication preparation and packaging, but not necessarily health outcome monitoring. This list of expectations goes on throughout the health care system. Each person in the system performs processes within their knowledge boundaries, expecting others to do the same as they strive toward some resultant pre-defined health-related event. Pharmaceutical care positions pharmacists to improve upon past performance and reset societal expectations regarding the pharmacist's role in achieving positive health outcomes.

There are three human factors that establish performance expectation. These factors can also be barriers to change.[2]

1. *Social: customs and culture.* The way people feel and behave is determined by their social customs and culture. Each person has his or her own definition of how to act in a given environment. To establish a performance standard regarding how one behaves, a profession or an organization must set basic social standards. For example, what defines professionalism in pharmacy practice? Is it how pharmacy staff are dressed? Is it how staff address customers and vendors? Is it how data is documented or how a product appears upon dispensing? Or is it how well the prescription will meet an indicated goal for the consumer?

   A corporate culture that is defined and known by all employees can be maintained as a normal, routine practice. However, if there is no clear definition of social culture or responsibility in an organization, then any given performance is based on personal judgment and not subject to collective standards.

   A corporation that publicly announces its passion for achieving positive health outcomes through medication management has taken the first step toward establishing the corporate culture performance marker.

2. *Technical: knowledge of standard of practice.* What a person does relates to knowledge of what has been expected of him or her (or others) in the past and the technical standards of the position. We can all agree on the components of a completed, labeled prescription. Pharmacy staff members know the components of a prescription. What may not be formally established is a routine workflow for the integration of each position that allows for efficient dispensing with near zero order variance (nearly complete accuracy on every dispensing).

   A standard of practice, a routine stepwise approach regarding dispensing workflow and the integration of what each person and system does along the process chain, is required to establish a foundation for performance expectations. Workflow documentation and understanding forms the technical benchmark upon which performance is measured.

3. *Managerial: policy deployment and goal setting.* Finally, there are managerial factors that establish performance expectations. A person may behave in a manner

acceptable to recipients and may be technically proficient in meeting a position's skill set, but that same individual may fail to meet expectations by ignoring policies or missing targeted goals. The establishment and deployment of policies along with specific goal setting allows for individuals to perform routinely in an expected manner. The documentation of standard operating procedures, corporate policies, and tactical plans form the managerial benchmark upon which performance is measured.

When things do not go as expected, the current health care climate allows for individuals to bypass the root cause of the unmet expectation (defining the social, technical or managerial factor at play) and to become defensive, or to formulate accusations. In a similar vein, when something outside of the routine is asked of health care providers in the system, many formulate barriers to meeting expectations and are reticent to move beyond those barriers.

The challenge is to understand the factors that establish performance expectation— to use this knowledge to identify barriers to performance improvement and to design, implement, and monitor a performance improvement plan. The goal is to reset performance expectations by changing the social (how one acts), technical (what one does), and managerial (how one does it) components of the workplace.

Ultimately, understanding the human component to performance improvement is to understand the interplay between what one knows, the skills one has, the attitude one displays, and the resultant behavior. Where the goal is provision of pharmaceutical care, the corporate mission is to develop staff who know pharmaceutical care, have the skills necessary to provide pharmaceutical care, possess the attitude necessary to deliver pharmaceutical care, and engage in behavior necessary to successfully provide pharmaceutical care. A complete performance improvement (PI) program actively manages these human components, along with the complementary system components.

Understanding the Systems Components of Performance Improvement

Performance improvement is a discipline that allows for a system or process to be identified, targeted, and enhanced with a measurable change in outcome because of the enhancement. Performance improvement embraces team-driven problem solving using goal-oriented system redesign with a customer focus and measurable outcomes.

In *The Road Less Traveled*, Peck writes that life is difficult and that we should recognize that each day is made up of a series of events—some expected, some surprises.[3] The basis of a sound performance improvement program allows for everyone in the system to accept the notion that growth comes from knowing what has happened and plan to improve upon the knowledge of that occurrence.

Target an Organizational Process for Redesign

To target a process for improvement, there should be measurable data that forms a benchmark for the current system and a goal for where the organization wants the system to be.[4] It is important that there is a clear understanding of how the process currently works and what the performance goal will achieve. A performance goal may be to enhance any process area (e.g., productivity, cost, quality) or outcome. It is important to evaluate how an improved performance goal in one area may negatively impact another performance marker elsewhere in the system. It would certainly be less than prudent to implement a new prescription processing procedure that promised reduced processing time if the new procedure resulted in doubling the cost of dispensing with no further gain elsewhere in the system. Performance improvement focuses on organizational excellence. It provides a framework to systematically evaluate trends, target systems or processes, redesign the target, and keep an ongoing measure of the outcome.

Performance Improvement Initiatives through Quality Assurance

A performance improvement program will typically have a quality assurance (QA) system designed to track reported events (variance from the expected). A QA tracking system can establish a target for performance improvement. For example, over the course of a month it appears that you have been hearing people complaining about errors in the prescription labeling from your pharmacy. Recording each event reported allows you to know the exact number of prescription labeling variances, when they occurred, and by whom. It allows you to define the scope of the problem, systematically analyze the cause of the events, and target a performance improvement plan.

Root Cause Analysis: Problem Definition

The process of searching and identifying the true cause of a problem is called a root-cause analysis. A QA focused PI plan begins with documentation of the current performance level and the expected performance level. Then an analysis of what caused the variance in performance is initiated. An analysis of the events preceding the occurrence is documented. This process is called a root cause analysis. The root cause analysis establishes specific factors responsible for the variance.

In the case of the reported variances in labeling, one would review the source of the variance. Was the labeling on the source prescriptions prepared according to policy? Was the print acceptable? Did the labeling match the prescription request for accuracy?

Problem Resolution

Once the problem is defined and the causes well documented, a resolution plan can be initiated. In the labeling example, a review of prescriptions dispensed during the time frame in question reveals a printer driver failure that resulted in the dropping of the letter "e" from the labeling process. In this case, a performance improvement plan would include the following steps:

1. Process for checking label printer and warning for system malfunction
2. Process for reviewing labels for accuracy
3. Process for identifying and correcting affected labels and ensuring patient understanding of prescription labeling

Monitoring Plan

Often a solution to a problem can create downstream variances in goods or service. For this reason, a PI plan includes a method for monitoring the effects of the changes that are implemented.

Following the labeling example, one finds that the warning system designed to alert staff of a printer malfunction randomly causes an alarm to sound. Annoyed by the alarm, staff turn off the warning function, thereby eliminating the warning system component of the PI plan. Printer-related errors now go undetected.

An effective performance improvement plan would include involving staff in monitoring each component of the plan with documentation of the outcome. Corrective action would have been taken before staff abandoned the plan.

Pharmacy staff has an important role in reporting and tracking quality-related events. This retrospective approach to monitoring service levels helps to target areas for performance improvement. In addition, the pharmacist and staff have the responsibility to participate in ongoing performance improvement programs.

Performance Improvement Initiatives Aligned with Corporate Mission

The pharmacy mission statement should include a framework to incorporate that the highest quality services are provided to achieve positive health outcomes with responsible deployment of resources. The mission statement, and related measurable goals, provide a foundation for ongoing performance improvement. The performance-related goals establish the measurable benchmarks for the value of the pharmaceutical care provided.

Setting Benchmarks and Measuring Outcomes of Performance Improvement

Incorporating the Demming model into pharmaceutical care can provide a guide for setting and measuring PI outcome goals. This goes beyond the latent recognition of PI needs from QA systems and creates a prospective identification of PI opportunities.

Again, effective performance improvement first requires that an organization has established expectations or benchmarks in core areas. There are many ways to systematically look over a pharmacy practice and compartmentalize it into workable core areas. A common way is to split the practice into departments (finance, marketing, human resources) or workflow functions (profiling, compounding, preparation, packaging, billing) to create a framework for benchmarking.[4]

Once the specific target areas are determined, management establishes performance improvement goals, such as reduce frequency of negative outcomes, improve efficiency of resources, eliminate redundancies, reduce mistakes, increase productivity, and increase satisfaction.[1]

With these factors in mind, it becomes necessary to define what endpoints go into meeting the expected outcomes of the performance improvement goal. For example, to reduce the frequency of negative outcomes in the pharmacy, one would need to define a negative outcome. In traditional pharmacy practice, this could be defined as a dispensing error. In pharmaceutical care, this could be defined as inappropriate adjuvant therapy. Whatever the endpoint selected, the concept is to track the number of reported variances in relation to the total exposures (e.g., all prescriptions dispensed by the pharmacy). Another (process) endpoint could be to track the number of times staff are observed not adhering to dispensing practice workflow guidelines.

A standard spreadsheet program can be used to help monitor performance based on changes made to social, technical and managerial factors. A sample spreadsheet is included in **Figure 18.1.**

Setting PI-Based Pharmaceutical Care Goals

Pharmaceutical care performance-based goals go beyond the process of dispensing and focus on related health outcomes. Again, the same principles apply.

1. Define the performance goal and the measurement indicators.

2. Define the process for achieving the goal.

3. Redesign current performance standards to achieve the new goal. Implement the process redesign and pay attention to social, technical, and managerial components of the redesign.

4. Measure the performance indicators on a regular basis.

5. Document the outcome of the performance improvement plan.

6. Adjust the plan as necessary with continued monitoring and reporting.

Outcome	Reduce Frequency of Negative Events Occurring in the Pharmacy Dispensing Area			Month 1		Month 2	Month 3	Comments
	Endpoints	Dispensing Errors	Adherence to PI Plan					
Baseline measure	Date	X reported errors/total dispensed	X observed occurrences/time measured					
Social change: Quiet Zone								
Technical Change: Automated counting Machines; Bar coding								
Managerial Workflow policy and procedure for filling and checking								

Figure 18.1. Performance Monitoring Tool.

To set PI-based pharmaceutical care goals, consider markers that are easily measurable. In setting the goals, the pharmacy sets the value measures. For example the pharmacy with a PI goal to "be responsible for positive medication-related outcomes" would have a system for measuring pertinent medication-related outcomes in order to know that the goal was met.

A more focused measurable goal may be that 90% of patients receiving morphine for pain control are counseled about constipation. To enable this performance measure to be met, the following elements of a PI plan would be in place:

1. A policy and procedure for achieving the performance measure

2. Staff training regarding the performance measure

3. A system for documenting and reporting the performance measure

4. A system for monitoring the performance level

On a predetermined interval (monthly, quarterly, etc.) an assigned person or team monitors the performance improvement based pharmaceutical care goals. Performance monitoring includes a review of achievement of goals (a report of the recorded indicators) with modification of goals and establishment of new markers where necessary. Remediation for persons or systems that interfere with goal attainment is provided.

Outside Influences Guiding Performance Improvement in Pharmaceutical Care

The Joint Commission for the Accreditation of Healthcare Organizations defines nine dimensions of care for pharmacy.[5] The nine JCAHO dimensions for quality care are (1) efficacy of a treatment in relation to a condition, (2) appropriateness of a medication to meet a patient's need, (3) availability of the treatment, (4) effectiveness with which the services is provided, (5) timeliness with which the services is provided, (6) safety for the person to whom services are provided, (7) efficiency in care, (8) continuity in care, and (9) respect and caring.

These dimensions can be considered when defining pharmaceutical care performance improvement initiatives. Since the pharmaceutical care staff and systems are responsible for achieving positive medication-related outcomes, a variation of the JCAHO dimensions may be called for. Consider developing benchmarks that define the pharmacy staff responsible to

- ensure access to medication that is accurate and timely,
- ensure competence in the provision of pharmaceutical care,
- provide support of patient needs as the primary function,
- use resources efficiently, and
- respect and care for patients, clients, and each other.

Each of these performance measures may have a clinical, financial, marketing, and human relations component. These components come together in the development of performance benchmarks. Once the performance improvement program is underway, there are three primary components to successful maintenance: (1) communicate and document the issue, plan, and resolution to all parties involved; (2) monitor resolutions and report positive and negative outcomes; and (3) rework resolutions until positive outcomes result.

From experimentation and re-evaluation, migration toward improvement is found. A sound program requires the openness to report variances and a system to track, report, and evaluate them. Performance improvement provides documentation tactics to continually fine-tune people and systems toward desired outcomes.

References

1. Walton M. The Deming management method. New York, NY: Perigree Books; 1986.

2. Dobyns L, Crawford-Mason C. Quality or else: the revolution in world business. Boston, MA: Houghton Mifflin Company; 1991.

3. Peck S. The road less traveled. New York, NY: Simon Schuster; 1978.

4. Harrington JH, Harrington JS. High performance benchmarking: 20 steps to success. New York, NY: McGraw-Hill; 1996.

5. Joint Commission on Accreditation of Healthcare Organizations: A guide to performance improvement for pharmacies. Oakbrook Terrace, IL: Joint Commission; 1995.

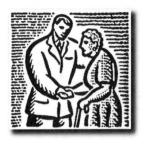

Chapter 19: Ethics and Pharmaceutical Care

Robert A. Buerki, R.Ph., Ph.D.
Louis D. Vottero, R.Ph., M.S.

Throughout the development of American medical services, pharmacy—like all professions—has continually struggled to define its relationship with the American society. At the center of this negotiating process has been the fundamental concern for balancing professional autonomy with the public's demand for accountability. Society grants discretionary power and privilege to pharmacists premised on their willingness and ability to contribute to social well-being and to conduct their affairs in a manner consistent with broader social values. As the American pharmacy profession continues to refine and articulate the practice philosophy of pharmaceutical care, it continues also to emphasize its pursuit toward a wider range of practice activities that carry with them a greater degree of professional autonomy. Pharmacists who respond to this level of professional practice and embrace the unique caring aspects of this new practice philosophy will be challenged to demonstrate group and individual ethical behavior far beyond the present expectations of society.

Pharmacy as a Moral Community

Like other professionals, members of the pharmacy profession are bound together by a common course of training, traditional values, and communal aspirations all of which lead to an agreed upon professional purpose. It is reasonable, even in a pluralistic society such as ours, to view all professions as moral communities whose members "are distinguished as individuals and as a group by widely shared goals, beliefs about the values of these goals . . . about the appropriate means for achieving them, and about the kinds of relations which in general should prevail among themselves, and in many cases between themselves and others."[1]

This view of professionals as moral agents was more simply stated by Pellegrino and Thomasma[2] who examined the fundamentals of the professional client relationship and summarized that "any act which applies knowledge to persons involves values and consequently falls into the moral realm." Likewise, pharmacy educators have long envisioned the moral nature of professional pharmacy using exhortations of virtue such as "the character and personality of pharmacists are of primary importance" (in 1927) and concluding (in 1950) that "the outstanding factor determining the future of the profession of pharmacy is fundamentally moral in nature."[3,4] In his analysis of pharmacy's societal purpose, pharmacy educator Donald C. Brodie[5] stresses a pattern of professional behavior that demonstrates a "commitment to the common good." More recently, the American Association of Colleges of Pharmacy's Commission to Implement Change in Pharmaceutical Education embraced pharmaceutical care with its "emotional commitment to the welfare of patients as individuals who require and deserve pharmacists' compassion, concern, and trust" as a new philosophy of pharmacy practice.[6]

Professional autonomy, correctly understood, is not a right of the profession but is a socially granted privilege. Its proper use has become a moral duty of the profession. This moral dimension helps to shape the relationship between the profession as a group, its members, and the individuals who receive professional services. Although the ultimate responsibility for action rests with individual practitioners, promoting ethical conduct is not the sole responsibility of the individual since this ignores the importance of social structure in shaping individual consciences and behavior. For professions, the focusing and articulation of appropriate behavioral norms to individual practitioners are the cornerstones of the trust between individual professionals and their clients. Society places its trust not only in individual pharmacists but also in the profession of pharmacy, relying upon that profession to guarantee that its members fulfill their agency obligations.[7]

Importance of a Professional Ethic

Self-regulation and self-discipline are generally viewed by the public as essential requisites for a profession, especially when a professional assumes duties that are linked to the personal health of the individual, involving life-and-death decisions in a literal sense. Furthermore, despite the increasing sophistication among segments of the American public, few individuals are able to judge the quality of the professional services they receive. As a result, a professional ethic is one of several generally accepted criteria that serve to distinguish a profession from other occupations or business endeavors.

Professionals are given certain legal prerogatives by society, such as a license to practice and a quasimonopoly to operate in a certain professional arena. In return for these prerogatives, a profession accepts responsibility to maintain a standard of conduct beyond conformity to law or technical skill. This standard of conduct, this common concern for collective self-discipline, this control of a profession from within, is known as professional ethics.

Professional ethics may be defined as rules of conduct or standards by which a particular group regulates its actions and sets standards for its members. Ethics control a particular group in society, not society at large; control of this group is from the group itself.

The system of ethics is closely related to and overlaps with two other systems designed to control society: laws and morals. Laws are regulations established by a government to apply to and control all people within a certain political subdivision, not a particular group in society. Control of the people is external to any group within society. By contrast, morals are generally accepted customs of right living and conduct, and an individual's practice in relation to these customs. Morals control individuals within society by means of internal, personal controls. These distinctions are summarized in **Table 19.1**.

Table 19.1. Comparison among Systems of Ethics, Law, and Morals

System	Application	Control Source	Form
Ethics	Specific group	Within the group	Codes of ethics
Law	Political subdivision	Outside the group	Legislation
Morals	Individuals	Religious beliefs, conscience	Religious writings

Of the three systems, law would seem to have the greatest payoff to society because sanctions for noncompliance include not only fines but imprisonment. Nevertheless, the system of law does not cover all areas of professional endeavor or all potential risks a professional encounters. Thus, no matter how broadly laws and regulations are written or how detailed they might seem, there are still areas that must be covered by a system of voluntary self-discipline, the system of ethics.

Society also expects a profession, through its collective members, to generate its own statement of acceptable and unacceptable behavior, usually in the form of a code of ethics—a detailed, explicit operational blueprint of norms of professional conduct, a recital of desirable and undesirable actions having an impact on the character of a profession and its functional reliability. The behavior pattern established in a code of ethics is generally enforced through a peer-review mechanism associated with a professional academy, organization, or association. One measure of professionalization is the extent to which such a peer-review mechanism actually works to control a profession.

Codes of Professional Ethics[a]

Codes of professional ethics are visible and explicit enunciations of professional norms, embodying the collective conscience of the profession, and serve as testimony to the group's recognition of its moral dimension. Since the middle of the nineteenth century, organized professional pharmacy in America has promulgated codes that reflect the collective values and aspirations of practitioners committed to raising the overall standards of pharmacy. More recently, dedicated practitioners acting through the Joint Commission of Pharmacy Practice expressed their intent to review and restate a code of ethics for the profession of pharmacy. The American Pharmaceutical Association (APhA), a member of the Joint Commission, was asked to carry out the intent which produced the current Code of Ethics for Pharmacists.[8]

Three types of professional codes may be identified in the literature: aspirational, educational, and regulatory.[7] Codes of ethics that are primarily aspirational focus upon practice ideals to which member practitioners should strive, thereby placing a strong emphasis on human achievement. An educational code will have fuller statements of principles, perhaps with commentary or interpretations that are useful in dealing with problems encountered in professional practice. A regulatory type of code is framed upon sets of detailed rules intended to govern professional conduct, and serves as a basis for resolving grievances. In reality, any single code of professional ethics may combine all three of these types. Up to the present time, the typical code of ethics developed for American pharmacy has combined a regulatory-educational tone, with only an occasional aspirational expression.

Structure can also affect the utility of a code of ethics. If a code is too long, it becomes unwieldy and unusable; if a code of ethics is too short, it may be too abstract or idealized to be useful and may avoid dealing with sensitive areas. The ideal code of ethics usually consists of a concise, generalized code supplemented by a manual of interpretations or case histories. Both medicine and law use this latter approach, an approach that has yet to be attempted in pharmacy.

The 1994 Code of Ethics for Pharmacists represents a strong shift away from traditional regulatory statements toward statements that are more aspirational and educational. Although codes of ethics may have any number of functions, the primary function of any code should be to promote ethical behavior and to serve as a deterrent to unethical behavior. There is no question that this function is the underlying reason for the propagation of nearly all codes.

At times, other functions are necessary for the fullest expression of a profession's ethical responsibilities. For example, it is possible that a code, through its summary statements of principles and direction-setting, may be used as an enabling document offering guidance to practitioners. The recently adopted Code of Ethics for Pharmacists, in describing the patient–pharmacist relationship as a covenant, may prompt pharmacists toward avenues of action that would otherwise be difficult to discern. Codes might be used as a foundation for public evaluation, or even to strengthen or hasten professional socialization. Some codes are designed to enhance a profession's reputation and trust and may preserve or entrench professional biases. Codes might be used to create a support system for the practice of the profession or to serve as the basis for adjudication procedures for resolving difficult cases.

The Developing Ethic of American Pharmacy

As America emerged as an increasingly complex society, pharmacy practitioners sought a new professional structure combining the strengths of the English laissez-faire system with the multinational potpourri of the American experience.[9] This structure first emerged with the founding of the Philadelphia College of Pharmacy in 1821 in response to perceived threats of pharmacists being labeled as neglectful or indifferent, and eventually leading to its 1848 Code of Ethics, which attempted to advance "professional conduct and probity."[10,11] The 1852 APhA Code of Ethics, modeled after the Philadelphia example, asked those who honored it to "protect themselves and the public from the effect of an undue competition, and the temptation to gain at the expense of quality," thereby establishing guidelines for professional practice that were clearly beyond the realities of pharmacy practice of that time.[12]

For nearly seven decades this Code of Ethics for American pharmacy remained intact, obscure, and generally ignored by practitioners and educators alike. In 1921, APhA President Charles LaWall wrote a new and comprehensive code for the Association that was adopted the following year.[13] This new Code, and its subsequent revisions, continued to reflect societal concerns as organized pharmacy attempted to define an ever-expanding standard of professional practice. New educational requirements for pharmacy students and various drug laws passed on the federal and state level, especially the 1906 Pure Food and Drugs and the 1914 Harrison Narcotic Act, presented serious challenges to practicing pharmacists. Rapidly expanding enrollments in American schools and colleges of pharmacy by students of questionable motivation in the years following the enactment of national prohibition prompted a detailed reference to the "dispensing and sale of narcotic drugs and alcoholic liquors" in the 1922 APhA Code.[13] By the same token, the 1952 revision reflected the emergence of brand-name pharmaceuticals and subsequent state-based antisubstitution legislation as it urged pharmacists to recognize the "significance and legal aspects of brand names and trade-marked products."[14]

By the mid-1960's, it became apparent that a reactive approach to developing an ethical code had resulted in increasingly detailed standards of practice. This fact, coupled with the new five-year degree in pharmacy and a greatly revised consensus on the merits of generic drug products, prompted APhA to convene a conference on ethics to reconsider its Code. The Code that eventually emerged from these discussions was streamlined and focused upon the protection of the public rather than upon proscriptive guidelines for pharmacy practitioners. For example, the new Code placed a positive duty upon the pharmacist to "render to each patient the full measure of his ability," removing the traditional restriction to "not discuss the therapeutic effects or composition of a prescription with a patient."[15] In 1975, the Code was amended to remove any restriction on the advertising of professional services. The offending statement was replaced with a principle stating that communications by the pharmacist should be truthful, signifying the appearance of the first clearly stated moral principle in an American pharmacy code of ethics. The 1981 version of the APhA Code of Ethics incorporated society's increased sensitivity to cultural attitudes and removed all masculine pronouns.

In some sense, the 1981 APhA Code of Ethics was outdated when it was approved by the association membership. By this time, the clinical practice of pharmacy had assumed national significance and support for the six-year degree in pharmacy had swept the profession. In addition, major developments in medical ethics during the 1970's and 1980's had developed highly respected centers of research for professional bioethics, all of which moved the practicing pharmacist closer to questions about complex ethical dilemmas, such as patient autonomy and self-determination.

More recently, the introduction of pharmaceutical care as a standard for professional pharmacy practice provides still another reason to reexamine the moral and ethical implications implicit within American pharmacy. Pharmaceutical care in its fullest sense redefines the pharmacist–patient relationship and expands the boundary of pharmacy practice into levels that clearly involve value-based professional care decisions that are beyond enhanced therapeutic outcomes and the more traditional pharmacy practice values of compassion, faithfulness, and fairness. Indeed, if an ethic of care is implicit in the pharmaceutical care philosophy, then additional virtues such as kindness, sensitivity, attentiveness, tact, patience, reliability, responsiveness, and human relating will need to emerge as foundational values of ethical pharmacy practice.[16,b]

Newer Principles in a Pharmacy Ethic

Framers of the earliest codes of professional practice presumed that their codes would reflect their patients' best interests. Primarily based upon the ancient Hippocratic principle of doing good and avoiding evil, these codes essentially reflect paternalistic attitudes that pose challenges to patient autonomy and question professional veracity. For example, the basic principle that underlies the Hippocratic oath enjoins physicians to work for the benefit of the sick according to their "ability and judgment" without necessarily including patients in the decision-making process surrounding their therapy.

This somewhat exclusive focus for a pharmacy ethic has been examined and challenged as self-serving. In 1985, pharmacist–ethicist Robert M. Veatch[17] brought this concern to the attention of a symposium of pharmacists during a national meeting and challenged them to "respond to the critical questions of the day," especially as they moved "beyond the traditional conception of our profession." Veatch argued persuasively that several additional ethical principles beyond beneficence—"doing good" in Hippocratic terms—must be considered in developing an ethic for the current practice of pharmacy. Such principles include autonomy, veracity, and justice.

The principle of autonomy is considered paramount in formulating a contemporary code of professional conduct. The autonomous person has the right to decide what—if any—medical treatment he or she will accept. The ethical value associated with this principle may be expressed through the patient's right to informed consent, the knowledge base upon which a patient may rationally choose or refuse treatment. Given the sophistication of our current medical system and its complex modern pharmaceuticals, many practitioners unintentionally violate this right by assuming their patients would not understand the technical details underlying their treatment plan. Other practitioners assume that their patients are not interested in such details. Still other practitioners are guided by the traditional paternalistic view that they know what is in the best interest of their patients, with or without their consent.

The principle of veracity—or truth-telling—was first reflected in the 1981 APhA Code of Ethics, which encouraged the pharmacist to "strive to provide information to patients regarding professional services truthfully, accurately, and fully." Curiously, the Code endorsed truth-telling only as it applied to a pharmacist's professional services, but in Veatch's words, it was the closest that the Code came to "acknowledging moral obligations that potentially may have harmful consequences."[17] In contrast, the 1994 Code of Ethics for Pharmacists frankly states that "a pharmacist acts with honesty and integrity in professional relationships," explaining that pharmacists have "a duty to tell the truth and to act with conviction of conscience."[18]

Within the professional arena, pharmacists are often torn between conflicting values: Full disclosure of all possible harmful side effects of a potent prescription medication may seriously interfere with a patient's compliance with the drug regimen or result in refusal to even take the medicine. Certainly, pharmacists are obliged to warn their patients of potentially life-threatening side effects, but may use professional judgment and discretion in discussing side effects that may not be clinically significant. By the same token, the use of placebo therapy, as ordinarily defined, relies upon the violation of this principle for its successful effect.

The principle of justice, as applied to the practice of medicine and pharmacy, is primarily associated with the allocation of goods and services. The questions associated with allocating access to a kidney dialysis machine provides an intellectual challenge to students of professional ethics, but the allocation of professional services to an ever-increasing aged population provides a less dramatic, but equally pressing need for applying the principle of justice. Drug compliance among the marginally indigent population often depends upon pharmacists extending credit or making other special arrangements for providing expensive maintenance drugs. The principle applies to the pharmacist's relationships with patients at all levels of the socioeconomic scale, ranging from the wealthy to those receiving public assistance. To selectively deny professional services to Medicaid recipients or other "undesirable" patients on the basis of their inability to pay violates the principle of justice in its fullest sense.

Each of these principles is independent and of equal importance in establishing the basis for more concrete ethical rules and guidelines. In many cases, however, two or more of these principles may apply to a single complex moral dilemma. Thus, in attempting to solve such a dilemma, the practitioner should recognize that each principle may not be totally binding in and of itself and must be tempered by reason and personal judgment. Many practitioners, inured by years of study in the objective world of pharmaceutical sciences, find it difficult to resolve these dilemmas because of unfamiliarity with the principles of professional ethics, as well as their uneasiness with the subjective nature of ethical decision-making. For this reason, many pharmacists find it useful to employ a formal process of conflict resolution to assist them in balancing the conflicts among ethical principles.

Veatch proposed four possible strategies: (a) rank-ordering the principles according to one's perceived priorities (which may prove impossible in practice); (b) balancing the competing principles according to one's personal beliefs (which he finds "discomfortingly vague"); (c) collapsing the principles into one larger all-encompassing principle (which may result in the loss of specificity); and (d) balancing beneficence and nonmaleficence (the so-called "consequentialist" principles) against autonomy, veracity, and justice (the so-called "non-consequentialist" principles), using the former to break any resulting ties.[17] Nevertheless, many pharmacists ultimately behave in a manner reflecting the values and attitudes that are associated with the professionalization process.

The 1994 Code of Ethics for Pharmacists

The 1994 Code of Ethics for Pharmacists adopted by the members of APhA and the American Society of Health-System Pharmacists is strikingly different from all code statements previously adopted by pharmacists. Earlier codes were very practice specific, and often narrowly focused merely on practice events encountered by pharmacists with patients, physicians, other health care professionals, or fellow pharmacists. Although common to many other professional codes, this approach tends to narrow the scope of ethical concern. The 1994 Code of Ethics for Pharmacists, with its preamble and eight principles, avoids this detailed approach and instead uses general recommendations and general norms as the framework.[c]

Preamble

Pharmacists are health professionals who assist individuals in making the best use of medications. This Code, prepared and supported by pharmacists, is intended to state publicly the principles that form the fundamental basis of the roles and responsibilities of pharmacists. These principles, based on moral obligations and virtues, are established to guide pharmacists in relationships with patients, health professionals, and society.

The three sentences that compose this straightforward expression of purpose establish a solid foundation for the ensuing eight statements of ethical principles. The first statement is a simple, clear declaration of the role that pharmacists play in medication use, namely to "assist individuals in making the best use of medications." This obviously refers not just to the patient but all individuals who are linked by the medication-use system, including physicians, nurses, administrators, pharmaceutical manufacturers, insurance executives, hospital administrators, government officials, and all others who formulate drug-use policy. Such a sweeping statement of role responsibility positions pharmacists as critical to all drug therapy situations. The second and third sentences recognize publicly that the Code was prepared by pharmacists and that its principles are "based on moral obligations and virtues." This declaration of a moral foundation for a professional code of ethics is unique among American health professions and sets the aspirational tone that is carried forward throughout the Code.

Principle I. A pharmacist respects the covenantal relationship between the patient and pharmacist.

This bold beginning principle sets the stage for the rest of the Code by defining the relationship that exists between a patient and a pharmacist: no earlier code makes this kind of clear defining statement. By establishing the patient–pharmacist relationship as a covenant, the Code serves notice that pharmacists respond to this relationship by observing certain moral obligations; that pharmacy practice is not merely transactional.

The concept of a covenant relies upon giving and receiving the gift of trust. In return for this gift, pharmacists promise to help individuals achieve optimum benefit from their medications, to be committed to their welfare, and to maintain their trust. Some may question the use of the term covenant in defining the pharmacist–patient relationship, suggesting the term is overinflated or too religious to use in a secular society. A few may prefer to define the relationship more as a social contract. Others may question the idea of the gift of trust, believing instead that it is an earned professional practice outcome. Nevertheless, since the nature of the pharmacist–patient relationship forms the bedrock of professional practice, its nature and the resulting moral obligations deserve sincere reflection by every pharmacist.

Principle II. A pharmacist promotes the good of every patient in a caring, compassionate, and confidential manner.

This principle recognizes the well-being of the patient as a primary practice imperative and places this concern at the center of professional pharmacy practice. To carry this out, a pharmacist must consider both the needs defined by science and the needs stated by the patient. Furthermore, the principle expects pharmacists to honor the dignity of the patient and accomplish all practice tasks with a caring attitude and a compassionate spirit. Finally, the Code exhorts pharmacists to focus on serving the patient in a private and confidential manner. Unlike the previous APhA Code of Ethics where patient confidentiality was dependent on serving the patient's best interest, this principle removes this dependency and makes confidentiality more absolute.

Principle III. A pharmacist respects the autonomy and dignity of each patient.

Respect for patient autonomy, especially the right of self-determination, may very well be the defining moral value for medical practice in this new century. Principle III emphasizes this particular ethical value and pledges that pharmacists will respect patient autonomy and in doing so promote the right of self-determination. Since the passage of the 1990 Omnibus Budget Reconciliation Act, pharmacists and other health care professionals have been challenged by federal and state law to provide their patients with the kind of information that is needed to make the difficult decisions that affect their health. This principle not only reinforces this attitude but also promotes individual self-worth through encouraging patients to participate in making choices about their health that coincide with their own values or beliefs. Indeed, meaningful communication with patients about their intended therapy is a core component of the pharmaceutical care practice philosophy and shared decision-making stands as one of its important intended goals.

Principle IV. A pharmacist acts with honesty and integrity in professional relationships.

The virtues of honesty and integrity have long been associated with professional pharmacy practice. The pharmacist not only must tell the truth and act with conviction of conscience but also must avoid discriminatory practices and behavior or work conditions that impair professional judgment. Furthermore, actions that compromise dedication to autonomy and self-determination, such as placebo therapy or other forms of beneficent deception, will test the spirit of the most ethical pharmacist.

Principle V. A pharmacist maintains professional competence.

In the presence of a patient who is in need of pharmaceutical services, a pharmacist makes an implicit public "profession" that he or she has special skills and knowledge that will contribute to the patient's best interest. This declaration of a special competence and its use in the interest of others is the central act of a profession, carrying with it all the obligations that make the declaration authentic.[19] Thus, a pharmacist has a duty to possess and maintain competent knowledge and abilities, especially as new medications, devices, and technologies become available and as health information advances.

Principle VI. A pharmacist respects the values and abilities of colleagues and other health professionals.

This principle recognizes the complexities of contemporary medical practice and emphasizes the need for pharmacists to willingly accept the limits of their knowledge and practice competencies. In these cases, pharmacists ask for the consultation of colleagues or other health professionals or refer the patient to the most appropriate service. Furthermore, this principle directs pharmacists to be aware and acknowledge that colleagues and other health professionals may differ in the beliefs and values they apply to the care of the patient and in doing so observe their moral accountability as individuals.

Principle VII. A pharmacist serves individual, community, and societal needs.

The primary obligation of a pharmacist is to individual patients; however, this does not diminish the need for pharmacists to extend beyond the individual to the community and to society. Increasing public concerns for human health and welfare, resource use, technology, justice, and the place of humans in nature are forcing all health professionals to consider these more global issues. Pharmacists will recognize their basic obligation to participate in public policy decisions that affect priorities of health care reform and contribute to developing a perspective on global health problems.

Principle VIII. A pharmacist seeks justice in the distribution of health resources.

The final principle is a simple statement of the principle of justice or equity within the practice domain of health resources. Any medical code needs an expression of justice or equity, and pharmacy, like most health professions, has ignored this dimension since previous codes focused nearly exclusively on providing benefits to individuals. Questions now confronting pharmacists make it impossible to escape this issue any longer, especially at the level of policy. Who should decide if everyone has the right to prescriptions under a national drug plan? By including this principle of justice, the Code exhorts pharmacists to be fair and equitable when health resources are allocated, balancing the needs of patients and society.

Conclusion

Pharmacists practicing in the American health care system of the twenty-first century are encountering serious ethical challenges within their professional practices that might include issues such as terminal sedation, confidentiality, and alternative medicine. Novice and experienced pharmacists alike face choices and responsibilities in the process of making value-laden, ethical decisions. Pharmacists who embrace a professional practice that builds upon moral principles and virtues will find expanded opportunities for ethical decision-making as they strive to meet the challenges of pharmaceutical care.

References

1. Gamenisch PF. Grounding professional ethics in a pluralistic society. New York: Haven Publications; 1983.
2. Pellegrino ED, Thomasma DC. A philosophical basis of medical practice: toward a philosophy and ethic of the healing professions. New York and Oxford: Oxford University Press; 1981.
3. Charters WW, Lemon AB, Monell LM. Basic material for a pharmaceutical curriculum. New York: McGraw-Hill Book Company, Inc.; 1927.
4. Elliott EC. The general report of the pharmaceutical survey, 1946–49. Washington, DC: American Council on Education; 1950.

5. Brodie DC. Pharmacy's societal purpose. *Am J Hosp Pharm.* 1981; 38:1893–6.
6. Commission to Implement Change in Pharmaceutical Education. Background paper II: entry level, curricular outcomes, curricular content and educational process. In: Penna RP, ed. The papers of the Commission to Implement Change in Pharmaceutical Education. Alexandria, VA: American Association of Colleges of Pharmacy; 1994:10–34.
7. Frankel MS. Professional codes: why, how, and with what impact? *J Bus Ethics.* 1989; 8(2/3):109–15.
8. Code of ethics adopted, bylaws amended. *Pharm Today.* 1994; 33:1, 12.
9. Buerki RA, Vottero LD. Ethics. In: Wertheimer AI, Smith MC, eds. Pharmacy practice: social and behavioral aspects. 3rd ed. Baltimore: Williams & Wilkins; 1989.
10. England JW, ed. The first century of the Philadelphia College of Pharmacy, 1821–1921. Philadelphia: Philadelphia College of Pharmacy and Science; 1922.
11. Smith DB, Ellis C, Troth SF. A code of ethics adopted by the Philadelphia College of Pharmacy. *Am J Pharm.* 1848; 20:148–51.
12. Code of ethics of the American Pharmaceutical Association. Proc Natl Pharm Conv, Phila, Oct 6, 1852. Philadelphia: Merrihew and Thompson, Printers; 1852.
13. Code of ethics of the American Pharmaceutical Association (adopted August 17, 1922). *J Am Pharm Assoc.* 1922; 11:728–9.
14. Code of ethics of the American Pharmaceutical Association. *J Am Pharm Assoc Pract Pharm Ed.* 1952; 13:721–3.
15. APhA code of ethics. *J Am Pharm Assoc.* 1969; NS9:552.
16. Sharpe VA. Justice and care: the implications of the Kohlberg-Gilligan debate for medical ethics. *Theor Med.* 1992; 13:295–318.
17. Veatch RM. Ethical principles in pharmacy practice. In: Buerki, RA, ed. The challenge of ethics in pharmacy practice, no. 8, new series. Madison, WI: American Institute of the History of Pharmacy; 1985.
18. Code of Ethics Review Committee. Proposed: code of ethics for pharmacists. *Am Pharm.* 1994; NS34:79.
19. Pellegrino ED. Toward a reconstruction of medical morality: the primacy of the act of profession and the fact of illness. *J Med Philos.* 1979; 4:32–56.

Footnotes

[a]For a fuller treatment of this topic, see Vottero LD. The 1994 code of ethics for pharmacists and pharmaceutical care. In: Haddad AM, Buerki RA, eds. Ethical dimensions of pharmaceutical care. New York and London: Pharmaceutical Products Press; 1996:153–69.

[b]The best single source for comparing the various versions of the Code of Ethics of the American Pharmaceutical Association is Buerki RA, Vottero LD. Ethical Responsibility in Pharmacy Practice. Madison WI: American Institute of the History of Pharmacy; 1996:149–62.

[c]American Pharmaceutical Association. Code of Ethics for Pharmacists, from a placard issued by the Association.

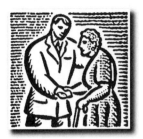

Chapter 20: The Diffusion of Pharmaceutical Care: A European Perspective

Marion Schaefer, Ph.D.
Frank Verheyen, Ph.D.

Pharmaceutical care has become a worldwide movement with its main roots in the United States where its ability to grow and come to full bloom was influenced mainly by the social and political climate in the second half of the last century.

Following the Thalidomid disaster in the early 1960's, there was an increased awareness of the potential harmful effects of drugs. Consequently, clinical pharmacology emerged as an independent scientific subject focusing on the risk–benefit relation of drugs. Later in the 1980's, this patient-focused methodology was supported by the growth of pharmacoepidemiology—the examination of drug-use experience in population groups. Soon it became obvious that the chemical and biological properties of a substance are only partly responsible for adverse drug reactions. It was equally important to avoid undesired events due to medication errors or "wrong" behavior by the patient. This broader focus also promoted clinical research and refined the design of clinical trials.

Meanwhile the cost of health care, too, had also become an issue. The medical sciences found new approaches to diagnose and treat diseases and new and more expensive drugs were introduced into the market. Avoiding the undesired effects of drug use was no longer the issue of a more rational drug therapy but was complemented by the demand to use drugs as effectively as possible. In order to ensure rational and outcome-oriented drug use in this sense, more specific care programs were needed.

This setting offered an opportunity for Hepler and Strand to publish their noteworthy definition of pharmaceutical care in 1990. The term traveled fast around the world accompanied more slowly by a deeper understanding of the concept, its methods, and philosophy. Probably the most important event on this journey was the International Congress of the International Pharmaceutical Federation in Tokyo in 1993 where the Section of Community Pharmacists offered the first one-day workshop on pharmaceutical care. This workshop, with participants from all over the world, was written about in professional journals in many countries, marking an important step into a future with pharmaceutical care, especially in Europe.

It would be unjust, however, to ignore European attempts to control and improve drug use in their respective countries at that time. Supported by the World Health Organization (WHO), the change from a drug product focus to a more patient-oriented perspective had led to more patient counseling activities and communication among health care professionals. At the same time, drug utilization studies were performed to detect and explain differences in drug use in European countries. To undertake investigations in this area, instruments like the defined daily dose and the Anatomical-Therapeutical-Chemical Classification were developed and applied. The strengthening of the theoretical background of patient care, however, had limited impact on the general practice.

The steps of the diffusion of the concept of pharmaceutical care in Europe can be understood from the following timetable:

Steps of the Diffusion of Pharmaceutical Care in Europe

1991 - Sweden released a document on good pharmacy practice.

The European Council organizes a seminar recommending changes in curricula to meet the needs of a more patient-oriented care.

1993 - The annual Congress of the International Pharmaceutical Association (FIP) in Tokyo released the "Guide to Good Pharmacy Practice" and offered workshops on pharmaceutical care.

1994 - Foundation of the Pharmaceutical Care Network Europe during the FIP Congress in Lisbon.

1995 - The European Council organizes a seminar titled "The pharmacist and the challenge by new social trends."

1996 - The European Association of Faculties of Pharmacy (EAFP) established a task force to implement pharmaceutical care into the curriculum.

1999 - First International Working Conference on Pharmaceutical Care in Hillerod, Denmark.

2001 - Second International Working Conference on Pharmaceutical Care of the Pharmaceutical Care Network Europe (PCNE) in Hillerod, Denmark.

This development of patient-oriented pharmaceutical care on the European level is reflected in most European countries, although in a different timeframe.

Steps of the Development of Pharmaceutical Care in Different European Countries

Austria

1998 - Pharmaceutical care of asthma patients initated by the Austrian Chamber of Pharmacists.

Belgium

1991 - The Katholieke Universiteit Leuven starts teaching pharmacy practice methodology, communication sciences, and drug information from a patient's perspective.

Denmark

1992 - Inclusion of pharmaceutical care service into the Danish professional standard.

1994 - The asthma project is started, providing for the first time a comprehensive pharmaceutical care service that included the documentation of added value.

1995 - Development of a model for pharmaceutical care at the counter and a non-disease-specific consultation model for the elderly.

2000 - Introduction of a fee-for-service by the Pharmaceutical Association for providing pharmaceutical care to diabetes and asthma patients.

Finland

2000 - Start of a four-year project to improve patient counselling in community pharmacies (Tippa-Project).

Germany

1993 - The Association of German Pharmacists (ABDA) released a statement demanding the improvement of individual drug therapy by pharmaceutical care.

1994 - The Foundation of Pharmaceutical Care is established to promote pharmaceutical care research and the practice.

1995 - First study on Pharmaceutical Care for the Elderly in Berlin initated by the Insititute of Pharmacy at Humboldt University.

Iceland

1994 - First country to put the concept of pharmaceutical care into legislation through the Pharmaceutical Act No 93/1994.

Ireland

1996 - The Health Authorities conclude the "Community Pharmacy Contractor agreement for the Provision of Services under the Health Act, 1970" with the community pharmacists who supply medicines to patients in the State schemes.

Norway

2001 - The Norwegian Association of Pharmacists develops two pharmaceutical care programs on behalf of the new pharmacy chains in Norway, Apokjeden AS.

Poland

2001 - The Faculty of Pharmacy at the Medical University of Gdansk in cooperation with the Polish Pharmaceutical Society and Pharmaceutical Chamber of Gdansk organized a nationwide conference on pharmaceutical care.

Portugal

1999 - The Portuguese Pharmaceutical Society and the National Association of Pharmacies declare the implementation and evaluation of Disease State Management / Pharmaceutical Care Programmes in Portuguese pharmacies as being one of the four top priorities in their political/professional agenda.

Slovenia

1997 - A Chair of Social Pharmacy is established at the Faculty of Pharmacy, University of Ljubljana in order to focus on pharmaceutical care and pharmacy practice.

2000 - Implementation of a postgraduate program for community pharmacists focusing on pharmaceutical care and developing new service programs and models for pharmacy practice.

Spain

1995 - Fifth Congress on Pharmaceutical Sciences dedicated to pharmaceutical care.

2000 - Establishment of a Spanish Network for Primary Care.

Sweden

1991 - Annual theme campaigns, or disease management programs, containing elements of pharmaceutical care begin.

2001 - The documentation of drug-related problems of patients with prescriptions becomes mandatory in all Swedish pharmacies.

Switzerland

2000 - Pharmaceutical care is introduced into the new curriculum for pharmacists. At Basel University a Pharmaceutical Care Research Group is established.

2001 - The Federal Social Insurance Office introduced a new service-oriented remuneration for community pharmacies.

The Netherlands

1991 - Adaptation of the concept of pharmaceutical care for The Netherlands simultaneously amending the university curriculum.

1994 - Research into the effects of pharmaceutical care started at the University of Groningen.

1997 - Pharmaceutical care standards and protocols are released by the Royal Dutch Association for the Advancement of Pharmacy (KNMP).

2000 - KNMP and the Minister of Health agree that pharmacists are care providers.

United Kingdom

2000 - The Department of Health publishes the document, "Pharmacy in the future—implementing the NHS plan."

In Scotland, the Scottish Government established a Pharmaceutical Care Model Schemes Development Team.

In Northern Ireland, pharmacists are paid by the government for managing the medicines of patients with cardiovascular disease under a national scheme.

Pharmaceutical Care Projects and Studies in Europe

In 1998 van Mil identified 35 research or implementation projects on pharmaceutical care throughout Europe. Since then the number of studies has increased (e.g., in Germany there were 8 projects in 1998 and 17 in 2001). The wide variety of projects encompasses case controlled studies, implementation studies, feasibility studies, and practice research projects. Two of the studies on pharmaceutical care, for asthma patients as well as for elderly patients, included several European countries in the original design.

Pharmaceutical Care for the Elderly

This study was the first large-scale, multicentre study to investigate the effects of pharmaceutical care provision by community pharmacists to elderly patients in Europe. It was based on the Dutch OMA study developed by van Mill and Tromp and was supported by the BIOMED program of the European Union. Participating countries included Denmark, Germany, Ireland, The Netherlands, Northern Ireland, Portugal, and Sweden. The study focused on improving health care for elderly patients. To achieve this goal, a care model was developed to detect and solve drug-related problems to optimize drug therapy and to minimize drug-related problems. Patient education on drug use and information regarding drug therapy and health behavior was intended to improve self-monitoring and compliance. By introducing the provision of pharmaceutical care, health-related quality of life in elderly patients should improve.

The data of 1290 intervention group patients and 1164 control group patients could be pooled for further statistical analysis. A general decline in health-related quality of life was observed; however, significant improvements were achieved in patients involved in the pharmaceutical care program in some countries. Intervention patients also reported better control of their medical conditions. Cost savings associated with pharmaceutical care provision were observed in most countries. The new comprehensive service was well accepted by intervention patients, and patient satisfaction with the service improved during the study. The pharmacists involved in providing pharmaceutical care had a positive opinion on the new approach, as did the majority of general practitioners surveyed.

Therapeutic Outcomes Monitoring for Asthma Patients

This project focused on therapeutic outcome monitoring for asthma patients in Belgium, France, Iceland, Malta, Northern Ireland, the Netherlands, Denmark, and Germany. It aimed to demonstrate the effectiveness of community pharmacy-based interventions on lung function, health-related quality of life, and self-management in asthma patients. Furthermore, patients were educated regarding knowledge about asthma and drug therapy.

In Germany, 26 intervention and 22 control community pharmacies provided pharmaceutical care services to 161 and 81 patients, respectively. It could be demonstrated that pharmaceutical care led to improved inhalation technique. Asthma specific quality of life (physical symptoms, psychological distress, functional status) and the mental health summary score of the SF-36 improved significantly in the intervention group. At 12 months, the intervention group showed significant improvement with regard to self-efficacy and knowledge. The self-perceived asthma severity in the patients in the intervention group decreased and the evening peak-flow improved.

Other Indication-Oriented Studies

Pharmaceutical care studies in different indications are needed to give evidence for the beneficial effects of this expanded function. Such studies require thorough preparation with regard to the definition of relevant outcome parameters and a sound design to test the given hypotheses. Different European countries are currently investigating the effect of pharmaceutical care on patients with angina pectoris, congestive heart failure, hypertension, diabetes, neurodermatitis, osteoporosis, elevated lipid level, and arthritis.

Another variation tries to apply pharmaceutical care to self-care concepts or to focus on special risk groups like children or pregnant women. Contrary to indication-oriented studies, this approach is less suitable to produce outcome data but very valuable with regard to special information needs of these groups.

When the first investigations were initiated in Europe, it soon became obvious that there was a lack of validated instruments to be used for the evaluation of the care process as well as the measurement of outcomes. Differences in the organization of health care in the participating countries also led to an interesting and fruitful discussion as it was expected that they would have an impact on study outcomes. These were the main two reasons, which subsequently led to the founding of PCNE in 1994.

Pharmaceutical Care Network Europe

PCNE started as an informal group of researchers active in the field of pharmaceutical care. The purpose of PCNE was and is to integrate pharmaceutical care through projects carried out in one or more countries simultaneously. So far, researchers from 17 European countries are active in PCNE. The work of PCNE encompasses all steps of project development: studies on a national or international basis are developed, implemented, and evaluated. Comparative studies between several countries are planned and designed on a sound scientific and methodological basis considering the feasibility and practicality of practice research.

PCNE tries to establish a network around its projects and offers the opportunity for the researchers from those European countries who are involved in projects and share their experiences. Therefore, two working conferences were organized. The first international working conference on "Outcome Measurements in Pharmaceutical Care" in 1999 focused on the development of the following instruments to appropriately reflect outcomes and processes related to pharmaceutical care:

- Patient satisfaction questionnaire,

- Attitudes towards medicines questionnaire,

- Assessment of behavior and coping strategies,

- Assessment of the use of medical resources and economic impact, and

- Assessment of drug-related problems from patients' perspectives.

The second international working conference on "Quality Issues in Pharmaceutical Care Research" in 2001 tried to contribute to the further development of pharmaceutical care research and to provide a multifaceted view on pharmaceutical care research by means of lectures focusing on pharmacoepidemiology, health economics, organizational theories, and patients' satisfaction. Workshops tackled methodological and scientific issues: the intervention process, drug use indicators, health status instruments, assessment of changes in drug use, and design of pharmaceutical care studies.

Because of the activities in the field of pharmaceutical care, PCNE was granted observer status to the EuroPharm Forum. This cooperation becomes even more important since only support by professional organizations can be expected to ensure the broader implementation of pharmaceutical care. In that respect, collaboration between EuroPharm Forum and PCNE comprises several aspects: EuroPharm Forum serves, for instance, as a platform for implementation of the projects developed or supported by PCNE. Furthermore, PCNE and EuroPharm Forum discuss and share experiences.

EuroPharm Forum

EuroPharm Forum was formed in 1992 by national pharmaceutical associations to improve health care in Europe. The activities of the Forum are aimed at the development of pharmacy practice, thus establishing a strong link to pharmaceutical care.

The main projects initiated or supported by EuroPharm Forum are as follows:

- Ask about Your Medicines

   This project is a Europe-wide campaign to encourage the public to seek information to help them to derive maximum therapeutic benefit from a course of medication.

- Asthma Services

   This project provides technical support for pharmacists in dealing with asthma patients in everyday practice at the pharmacy. A task force was established in

1996. The main focus of the Pharmacy-based Asthma services protocol and guidelines (now available as an official WHO document) is to provide a systematic and structured approach to pharmacy-based asthma services, including documentation of services, patient outcomes, and implementation strategies.

- CINDI—Hypertension Management

  This project, a multidisciplinary approach, aims to achieve an optimal hypertension control through more active involvement of pharmacists in the prevention, detection, and management of hypertension.

- Diabetes Care

  This project, operative since 1993, aims at improving the quality of diabetes care by integrating pharmacists in a national diabetes program.

- Pharmacists and HIV/AIDS

  This project provides strategies and guidelines for the activities of pharmacists in combatting HIV/AIDS. They include prevention, improved safe sexual behavior, risk reduction, and improved treatment by the provision of pharmaceutical care to patients.

- Smoking Cessation

  This project seeks to involve pharmacists in smoking cessation programs in the communities. The publication Smoke-free Europe 12, entitled "pharmacists and action on tobacco," details various types of smoking cessation activities that can be implemented at the national level, including the Pharmacists' Charter on action against smoking.

Lessons Learned from the Pharmaceutical Care Projects and Studies

As described above, pharmaceutical care research pursues two different strategies: (1) to develop, test, and extend the concept to new areas or indications of treatment and care with the goal of providing general evidence for a positive cost–benefit relation of the provided service and (2) to implement pharmaceutical care as a service provided by each pharmacy following more or less standardized guidelines of care with the goal of improving the practice of care in pharmacies. Consequently, the experiences gained in various projects and studies encompass different aspects like the impact of pharmaceutical care on health outcomes, methodological issues, and the optimal study design.

Barriers of Pharmaceutical Care in Every Day Practice

General experience gained from projects and studies so far indicate that it takes a special effort to maintain the motivation of participating pharmacists over more than six months and that continuous further education during the study is required. Furthermore, it was observed that the motivation of pharmacists and patients declined when they served as a control group. The case-control design, which is well known for clinical trials, is only partly suitable for pharmaceutical care studies as it proved to be difficult not to provide care when it is obviously needed. This also includes an ethical component, which led to a recommendation by the European Union to prefer other study designs.

Outcomes of pharmaceutical care studies often show trends rather than significant differences. This refers especially to the health-related quality of life, which declines with increasing age. Furthermore, patients who are recruited for pharmaceutical care studies often show a lower status of health compared with the so-called norm population. If services like pharmaceutical care can elevate the quality of life in single domains, the effect is often leveled when one looks at the spectrum of all domains. The relief of acute symptoms, like with asthma or dyspepsia, led to more significant differences in the pre- and post-evaluations or between case and control groups than is found with care programs for the chronically ill of higher age.

Conducting a feasibility study is one further key to the success of a pharmaceutical care project. It is also important to be precise and selective regarding the study focus and to decide whether it is necessary to have a control group to demonstrate the impact of the intervention.

The participation in a pharmaceutical care study or the attempt to implement the concept as a general practice requires both time and personnel resources. Furthermore, it may often become necessary to alter the workflow and to specify responsibilities. Therefore it makes sense to connect the implementation of pharmaceutical care with the process of quality assurance in the pharmacy.

Quality Assurance Concept

Pharmaceutical care can be implemented successfully in daily practice only if the organization of the workflow is adequate and personal responsibilities are sufficiently described. Therefore it was suggested, especially in Germany, to use quality assurance programs to support the implementation of pharmaceutical care in pharmacies. Suitable structure and process measures are closely related to outcome measures of pharmaceutical care and are sometimes even used as surrogate parameters. Vice versa, pharmaceutical care studies do not only demonstrate outcomes in terms of health status in patients but can also be used to organize structural and process components to ensure the quality- and patient-oriented provision of pharmaceutical care.

Meanwhile, a considerable number of pharmacies have been accredited. The description of processes, however, comprises hardly those which are relevant for pharmaceutical care. This situation should be changed when the provision of pharmaceutical care is accepted by those who have to pay the costs for this service. Implementing quality assurance programs in the pharmacy also contributes to the competition between pharmacists.

Computer-Based Programs for the Documentation of Pharmaceutical Care

As the lack of time, especially for documentation purposes, was mentioned frequently by practitioners as an impediment to the provision of pharmaceutical care, it soon became obvious that software programs had to be developed to support the provision and documentation of pharmaceutical care.

By using the medication profile, drug-related problems can be detected easier. Possible solutions must then be discussed with the patient and the physician. Furthermore, the documentation of the interventions helps the pharmacist determine whether the proposed solution can be successfully realized by the patient. The software programs serve as an individual care and counseling tool for pharmacist and patient. Appropriate software will facilitate the telecooperation between different health care professions, which for the time being is only partly developed within the medical profession.

Aggregate data reflecting the individual care process can be used later for epidemiological research, which will provide feedback information to optimize the care process. Thus pharmacists provide an added value for the benefit of the individual patient as well as science.

Programs for Further Education and Quality Management

The provision of pharmaceutical care depends greatly on well-trained pharmacists and quality management systems implemented in pharmacy. Therefore, a three-step approach seems essential to facilitate the implementation of pharmaceutical care.

1. Pharmaceutical care studies are accompanied by training modules and suitable methods of knowledge transfer required to conduct the study. Vice versa, experience about interventions and their impact generated through studies, can be used to improve the care process.

2. Professional bodies organize workshops on pharmaceutical care or sponsor nationwide conferences where experiences can be shared.

3. Materials are developed and published based on comprehensive training, usually with reference to special groups of indications.

Ideally, the training for pharmacists is based on a practice-oriented approach and integrated into continuing education programs and the implementation of quality management systems.

In 1998 The European Association of Faculties of Pharmacy (EAFP) declared the stimulation of best practice in its faculties as one of their objectives and set up a task force for implementing pharmaceutical care into the curriculum. Dick Tromp, from the University of Groningen, chaired the task force and presented the final report in May 1999. The task force decided not to agree on a unique definition of pharmaceutical care because of differences in the philosophy and the understanding of the main elements in European countries. The group gave detailed recommendations for introducing elements of pharmaceutical care into the curriculum of pharmacy students differentiating between the introductory and main modules. Teaching methods like problems-based learning were also mentioned. The task force hoped that the report would convince academic and administrative colleagues to support the implementation of pharmaceutical care in their institutions.

Reaction of Other Health Care Players

The attempts to implement pharmaceutical care caused ambivalent reactions among other health care professionals. In particular, cooperation with physicians seemed crucial for the successful implementation of pharmaceutical care. However, in most European countries, pharmacists face difficulties when trying to communicate with physicians. Most physicians were neutral or not interested in getting involved in pharmaceutical care usually because of misgivings regarding professional competence and competitive behavior. Some of them rejected the provision of pharmaceutical care and only a few physicians were very positive about the contribution of pharmacists providing pharmaceutical care services. Acceptance increased, however, over time when health care professionals were involved in well-organized pharmaceutical care studies.

Consumer groups are slowly organizing themselves in European countries and are striving for more political influence in health care issues. Hence, they show clear interest in the provision of pharmaceutical care and seek pharmacist support in getting consumer objectives incorporated in health policy programs.

The sickness funds (health care insurers), state authorities, and the ministries who should be interested in the outcomes of pharmaceutical care are still hesitant in most European countries. The reason for this reluctance is that most health systems usually focus on the physician when trying to optimize drug therapy. Furthermore, it is feared that pharmacists will seek additional reimbursement when providing pharmaceutical care. However, countries have different attitudes concerning this issue.

Outlook

There is a general agreement among pharmacists in Europe that pharmaceutical care is the right way into the future for both the profession and patients. Implementing the concept as a standard of practice requires substantial changes in the organization of health care, which will take time to be realized. The support by professional organizations and health policy to achieve this goal in due time varies among European countries. It can be expected, however, that new approaches like the introduction of accredited disease management programs may also promote the implementation of pharmaceutical care. The public discussion on the risk–benefit ratio of drugs, like the issue of Lipobay/Cerivastatine, may speed up the process.

In general, there are different prerequisites for the implementation of pharmaceutical care, which should be considered (**Figure 20.1**).

In 1999 the European Commission commissioned a project on the "Development of quality assured and quality assuring patient-oriented health promotion in primary health care—general practitioners and pharmacists." This report compiled

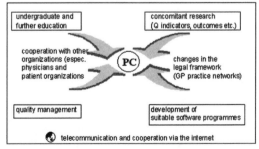

Figure 20.1. Steps to a Comprehensive Implementation of Pharmaceutical Care.

and assessed projects carried out in the respective European countries focusing on patient-oriented health promotion. The perspective of several European countries has been invited to facilitate the European-wide exchange of experiences in the field of health promotion. This process should lead to a more comprehensive knowledge about the contents of good and best practice, which might serve as role models for the national implementation of pharmaceutical care.

The future integration of the concept of pharmaceutical care into the complex field of health promotion might in the future lead to a better recognition by health care authorities as well as professionals.

Conclusions

The development of prudent policies to control health care costs in an aging society in all industrialized countries is required to overcome inefficiencies in the delivery of health care services. Reducing costs, however, should be possible while maintaining or even improving the quality of health care. For appropriate prescribing by physicians, dispensing and counseling by pharmacists, and drug use by patients, the concept of pharmaceutical care offers an opportunity to achieve these conflicting goals.

While the philosophy and aim of pharmaceutical care is increasingly accepted by pharmacists and at least tolerated by physicians, the practice of pharmaceutical care in the daily routine leaves much to be desired. This is mainly due to political decisions about the remuneration of pharmaceutical care, which are still pending in most European countries. So far, only the Netherlands and Switzerland have introduced a fee-for-service instead of linking the income of pharmacists to the turnover of their pharmacy. Although a fee-for-service formula may represent an improvement in achieving social objectives, it may not necessarily motivate pharmacists to provide pharmaceutical care on a more comprehensive basis. Further, patients have to get used to receiving comprehensive professional service at their pharmacy. Some are concerned about protecting the confidentiality of data on medical care as well as whether pharmaceutical care will be accompanied by sufficient explanation to maximize benefits associated with drug therapy.

The development of computer programs which facilitate the provison of care, and especially documentation of the process, will certainly promote the implementation of pharmaceutical care. Indeed, it is one of the main prerequisites. The breakthrough to a general practice of pharmaceutical care will come only when the system of remuneration in pharmacies is adapted in a way that is based on pharmaceutical care contributions rather than one designed to impede them.

This process will require more time in European countries and rely on the staying power of those who act as leaders in the field. Meanwhile, graduate and postgraduate education must be strengthened in a way that enables pharmacists to build up a sufficient knowledge base and meet the requirements of the pharmaceutical care model.

Pharmaceutical care is a concept that offers a benefit for all: patients, society, health insurance companies, physicians, and pharmacists with regard to the effectiveness of health care and drug safety in particular. To prove this result in due time, and to communicate the beneficial effects of pharmaceutical care, stands as one of the most important tasks for pharmacists not only in Europe but worldwide.

Bibliography

1. McElnay JC et al. Improving the well-being of elderly patients via community pharmacy-based provision of pharmaceutical care. A multicentre study in seven European countries. *Drugs&Aging.* 2001; 18:63–7.

2. Schaefer M. Paradigmenwandel in der pharmazie mit pharmaceutical care. *Pharm. Ztg.* 1994; 28, 3093–102.

3. Schaefer M, Belgardt Ch. Pharmaceutical care: bundesweite umfrage liefert daten und fakten. *Pharm. Ztg.* 1996; 50, 4758–64.

4. Schaefer M. Pharmaceutical care und datenmanagement. *Pharm. Ztg.* 1997; 41, 3519–26.

5. Schulz M, Verheyen F, Mühlig S et al. Pharmaceutical care services for asthma patients. A controlled intervention study. *J Clin Pharmacol.* 2001; 41, 668–76.

6. Bell HM McElnay J, Hughes CM et al. Provision of pharmaceutical care by community pharmacists in Northern Ireland. *Am J Health-Syst Pharm.* 1998; 55:2009–13.

7. Bell HM, McElnay J, Hughes CM. Pharmaceutical care provision by community pharmacists in the United Kingdom: a comparison of two regions. ACCP/ESCP International Congress on Clinical Pharmacy. Orlando, Florida; 1999:336.

8. Herborg H. The pharmaceutical care concept—personal views with a focus on development projects in Denmark. *Int Pharm J.* 1995; 148–9.

9. van Mil JWF et al. Development of pharmaceutical care in The Netherlands: pharmacy's contemporary focus on the patient. *J Am Pharm Assoc.* 1999; 39:395–401.

10. van Mil JWF, de Jong-van den Berg LTW, Tromp TFJ. Pharmaceutical care in the community pharmacy in the Netherlands. Pharmacy in the Netherlands (special issue); 1998:36–9.

11. Braun R, Schaefer M. Software für die pharmazeutische betreuung. *Pharm Ztg.* 1998; 143: 3458–64.

12. Verheyen F, Mühlbauer K, Schulz M. Pharmazeutische betreuung in Deutschland. *Pharm Ztg.* 1997; 142:3662–6.

13. van Mil JWF. Pharmaceutical care the future of pharmacy. Theory, research, and practice. Dissertation. Rijksuniversiteit Groningen; 2000.

14. van Mil JWF, Tromp TFJ. The Pharmaceutical Care Network Europe (PCNE). *Int Pharm J.* 1997; 11:10–1.

15. Müller-Jaeger A, Schaefer M. A trial of community pharmacists. Pharmaceutical care program to improve drug therapy and health-related quality of life for elderly patients: introduction and preliminary results from the OMA project in Germany. ACCP/ESCP International Congress on Clinical Pharmacy. Orlando, Florida; 1999:387.

16. van Mil JWF, Tromp TFJ, de Jong-van den Berg LTW. OMA pharmaceutical care in the elderly. Second International Symposium on the Role of the Pharmacist in Health Promotion and Disease Prevention. Malta; 1996:32.

17. Winterstein A, Jopp R, Schaefer M. OMA-Studie in Westfalen-Lippe. Ältere multimorbide patienten werden in apotheken gut betreut. *Pharm Ztg.* 2001; 146:833–41.

18. Winterstein A, Jopp R, Schaefer M. OMA-Studie. Gesundheitsbezogene lebensqualität als wichtiges zielkriterium. *Pharm Ztg.* 2001; 146:936–42.
19. Winterstein A, Jopp R, Schaefer M. OMA-Studie. Patienten profitieren von der pharmazeutischen betreuung. *Pharm Ztg.* 2001; 146:1024–33.
20. Herborg et al. Quality improvement of drug therapy for asthma patients in Denmark I. Analysis of patient outcomes. *J Am Pharm Assoc.* (in press).
21. Herborg et al. Quality improvement of drug therapy for asthma patients in Denmark II. Use of anti-asthmatic medication. *J Am Pharm Assoc.* (in press).
22. Schulz M et al. Pharmaceutical care services for asthma patients. *Eur J Clin Pharmacol* 1999; 55:A15.
23. van Mil JWF ed. Proceedings of the 1st PCNE International Working Conference on Outcomes Measurements in Pharmaceutical Care. HillerØd, Denmark; January 26–29, 1999.
24. Schulte van Werde M, Schaefer M. Pharmazeutische Betreuung und QMS. *Dtsch Apoth Ztg.* 1999; 139:2803–7.

Appendix 20.1. Useful Web Sites

www.pcne.org

www.who.dk/ch/pha/europha.htm

www.unvie.ac.at/phc

Appendix 20.2. Centers of Pharmaceutical Care in Europe

BELGIUM

Marleen Haems

KAVA

Consciencestraat 41

2018 Antwerpen

DENMARK

Hanne Herborg

Pharmakon

Danish College of Pharmacy Practice

42 Milnersvej

3400 Hillerød

Ellen Westh Sørensen
Royal Danish School of Pharmacy
Universitetsparken 2
2100 Copenhagen

FINLAND

Sirpa Peura
The Association of Finnish Pharmacies
Pieni Roobertinkatu 14 c
00120 Helsinki

GERMANY

Prof. Dr. Marion Schaefer
Humboldt Universität
Institut für Pharmazie
Goethestrasse 54
13086 Berlin

Dr. Martin Schulz
Center for Drug Information and Pharmacy Practice
ABDA
Carl-Mannich-Strasse 26
65760 Eschborn

GREAT BRITAIN

Prof. James McElnay
The School of Pharmacy
The Queen's University of Belfast
97 Lisburn Road
Belfast BT 7BL

Prof. Peter R. Noyce
School of Pharmacy and Pharmaceutical Sciences
University of Manchester
Oxford Road
Manchester M13 9PL

IRELAND

Dr. Martin Henman
School of Pharmacy
Trinity College
Dept. of Pharmacology
Dublin 2

THE NETHERLANDS

Prof. Dr. Th.F.J. Tromp / Foppe van Mil
Quality Institute for Pharmaceutical Care
Leylstraat 80
8265 BE Kampen

PORTUGAL

Prof. Dr. Maria Margarida Caramona
Faculdade de Farmacia
Laboratorio de Farmacologia
University of Coimbra, Largo de D. Diniz
3000 Coimbra

SLOVENIA

Mitja Kos
Chair of Social Pharmacy
Faculty of Pharmacy
University of Ljubljana
1000
Ljubljana

SWEDEN

Tommy Westerlund
Apoteket Björnen
Box 1052
SE-251 10 Helsingborg

Dr. Cecilia Bernsten
Socialstyrelsen
Ralambsvagen
310630 Stockholm

SWITZERLAND

Dr. Kurt Hersberger
Pharmazentrum
Universität Basel
Klingelbergstr.
504056 Basel

Dr. Olivier Bugnon
Swiss Pharmaceutical Association
Stationsstr. 12
3097 Bern-Liebefeld

Index

CL

362.
178
2
PHA